MINOR INJURIES

A Clinical Guide for Nurses

This book is offered with love to Lynda, Jude and Rebecca

For Churchill Livingstone:

Senior Commissioning Editor: Ninette Premdas
Project Development Manager: Mairi McCubbin
Project Manager: Joannah Duncan
Designer: Judith Wright
Specially commissioned illustrations: Ethan Danielson

Ideas for specially commissioned illustrations: Dennis Purcell

MINOR INJURIES

A Clinical Guide for Nurses

Dennis Purcell MA RN

Nurse Practitioner, Minor Injuries Clinic, Western General Hospital, Lothian University Hospitals NHS Trust, Edinburgh

Foreword by

Mark Cooper BN RGN

Clinical Educator, Accident & Emergency, Glasgow Royal Infirmary and PhD student, Nursing & Midwifery School, University of Glasgow

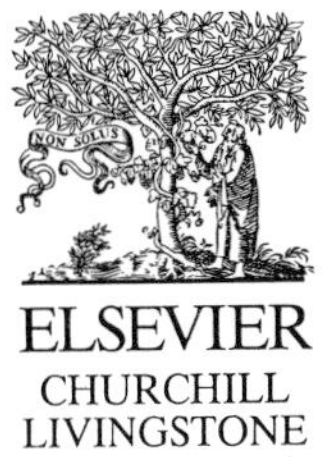

ELSEVIER
CHURCHILL
LIVINGSTONE

EDINBURGH LONDON NEW YORK OXFORD PHILADELPHIA ST LOUIS SYDNEY TORONTO 2003

CHURCHILL LIVINGSTONE
An imprint of Elsevier Limited

First published 2003
Reprinted 2004 (twice), 2005, 2006

ISBN 0 443 06277 3

British Library Cataloguing in Publication Data
A catalogue record for this book is available from the British Library

Library of Congress Cataloguing in Publication Data
A catalogue record for this book is available from the Library of Congress

Notice
Medical knowledge is constantly changing. Standard safety precautions must be followed, but as new research and clinical experience broaden our knowledge, changes in treatment and drug therapy may become necessary or appropriate. Readers are advised to check the most current product information provided by the manufacturer of each drug to be administered to verify the recommended dose, the method and duration of administration, and contraindications. It is the responsibility of the practitioner, relying on experience and knowledge of the patient, to determine dosages and the best treatment for each individual patient. Neither the publisher nor the editors assume any liability for any injury and/or damage to persons or property arising from this publication.

The Publisher

The publisher's policy is to use **paper manufactured from sustainable forests**

Printed in China
C/05

Contents

Foreword

Increasingly, we as nurses are taking responsibility for managing patients with minor injuries, giving us the opportunity to develop a new specialty of minor injury care. For years, nurses in many Accident & Emergency (A&E) departments, in the UK, have informally managed the complete care of patients with less serious injuries; however, since the mid-1980s a more formal nurse-led minor injury service has been emerging in a growing number of these departments. Today nurse practitioners are to be found in the majority of A&E departments across the UK as well as in Minor Injury Units, NHS Walk-in Centres, GP surgeries and many health centres.

Whilst emergency nurses have so often been responsible for advising junior doctors on how to treat many minor injuries, they have officially lacked the authority to manage these patients themselves. With the introduction, in 1992, of the UKCC's document *Scope of Professional Practice* and the withdrawing of previous guidance from the UK's Chief Nursing Officers on certification for extended role, nurses have been given increased freedom to reach their full potential. The profession has grasped this opportunity, and recent research has shown a large increase in the number of nurse practitioner roles. This revolution began in the UK in the 1980s, but has a longer history in the USA.

The birth of the nurse practitioner movement began in the USA in the 1960s as an initiative to meet the shortage of medical staff in many areas. Loretta Ford and Henry Silver began the first paediatric nurse practitioner training programme at the University of Colorado in 1965. This new concept of the nurse practitioner soon spread. In the UK the role first developed in general practice with the pioneering work of Barbara Stilwell, and very shortly after, in A&E with the first 'Emergency' Nurse Practitioners at Oldchurch Hospital in Essex. Early pioneers of the nurse practitioner role, both here and in North America, have shown the potential of such services. Nurse practitioners now work in many different specialties including paediatrics, general practice, community nursing, neonatal care, ophthalmology, gastroenterology and emergency care. Most nurse practitioners in the UK who work in emergency care settings predominantly manage minor injuries. Minor injuries are also being managed by nurse practitioners in a growing number of other countries around the world including Canada, Australia, Ireland and Denmark.

A number of randomised controlled trials have been undertaken in North America, the UK and Australia which show that nurse practitioners working in primary care settings (including A&E departments) can provide high-quality care to patients who present with undifferentiated health-care problems. All this research evidence is helping to support the role's development. Currently in the UK the majority of minor injury care in emergency departments is provided by junior doctors and emergency nurses working together. As junior doctors tend to change every 6 months this potentially means that the quality of any particular minor injury service may fluctuate. One benefit of nurse practitioners managing these minor injuries may be to ensure a more-consistent quality of service. Medical staff may also gain more time to spend with patients who are more acutely unwell, and nurse practitioners could become more involved with the training of junior doctors in managing minor injuries.

The role of the nurse practitioner provides the opportunity to unlock the potential of nursing, allowing nurses to deliver better and more-integrated health care. Nurses are team players and the role of the nurse practitioner is very much as one member of the larger health-care team. Whilst we continue to contribute new knowledge, in the form of research findings, to support our practice we still have a great deal to learn from our fellow professionals. However, our educational backgrounds are not the same and our learning requirements differ.

Even amongst nurse practitioners there is often considerable variation in scope of practice, educational preparation, and even role title. In the UK there is no nationally recognised educational preparation for the nurse practitioner who manages minor injuries. Training can vary from what is learnt from experience alone, to what is taught at Master's degree level. However, whichever level of preparation an individual practitioner chooses, the knowledge and skills relating to musculoskeletal assessment will be new to any nurse embarking on managing minor injuries for the first time. It is important that as minor injury nurse practitioners we start to set educational and practice standards to ensure that we can continue to provide the very best quality of care for our patients.

We must not rest on our laurels. If we are to continue to manage minor injuries and develop the specialty of minor injury care, we must not only ensure that we continue to provide high-quality care, but we should strive to examine ways of improving care. Taking on responsibility for managing patients with minor injuries means that we also take on the responsibility for ensuring that not only are we properly prepared and kept up to date, but together with nurse practitioner colleagues we should also strive to undertake appropriate research into improving the provision of minor injury care, and that we base our practice on sound research-based evidence.

In this book, Dennis Purcell has drawn together knowledge from several different professions. He has combined his skills as an artist with his experience as a nurse practitioner and teacher of nurse practitioners, in order to produce an invaluable textbook which nurse practitioners managing minor injuries have been waiting for. Anatomy is combined with practical clinical assessment and discussion of the management of commonly seen minor injuries. Clear, precise diagrams help consolidate understanding of important anatomical structures, together with simple clinical tests to assess their function. The book is not and does not purport to be the only textbook minor injury nurse practitioners will ever need; however, it will undoubtedly be the first one they will want to read.

Glasgow, 2003 Mark Cooper

Preface

I work in a stand-alone minor injuries clinic in Edinburgh treating a variety of injured patients and assessing any other self-presenting patients whose problems bring them to our door. I have been doing this for 8 years, and have seen, on average, about 2,000 patients each year. My job title is 'nurse practitioner'.

Before I took this job I was a staff nurse with a background in acute work, A&E, coronary care and intensive care. I was not attracted by a career in management and I was pleased to see doors opening to clinical careers for nurses which included the idea of a degree of autonomy.

Once I had passed through one of those doors I found myself doing work which suited me very well. However, I had no formal training course or qualification and a job title which some people said did not exist. Those who felt that it might exist were unable to agree upon its meaning. Others said that although it did exist, I might not be qualified to claim it. This was a situation which could not continue.

From the start, I have had the pleasure of working with managers and colleagues who represented the best of the new dispensation. We were aware, in particular, of the need for nurses to provide the infrastructure to support a nursing endeavour. We developed a training course for nurse practitioners in minor injuries. Through this course we met nurse practitioners from all over the UK. Many of them were thinking along similar lines to ourselves, and we have begun to make common cause. At the same time, national initiatives, governmental and professional, are beginning to bring us out from the shadows of stinted recognition and improvised training, but there is still a lot to do. Even the title 'nurse practitioner', one which has a public image almost as successful as Florence Nightingale's lamp, is still not recognised by our statutory bodies.

This book is a contribution to the process of developing education for nurse practitioners by nurse practitioners.

Nurse education has shifted from its old hospital training-school base to the universities. This process has thrown up new problems to replace those which troubled the old system. One of these is that it is difficult to teach anything as practical and dynamic as nursing away from the area where it is practised. If the universities are asked to teach advanced clinical practice in a field which is so new that the only people who understand the job are all still based in their clinical areas, there are bound to be problems. At the same time, it is not adequate for nurse practitioners to set up hospital-based courses without reference to national standards for education, and without academic validation and teaching expertise. It is clear that the two sides must get together and that a joint approach must evolve. A strategy to achieve this kind of cooperation is being implemented in Scotland, and something similar will have to be at the heart of developments elsewhere.

This book is written from the clinical point of view. It does not pretend to cover all of the material which a university degree course would include. It is written to meet a need which I experienced when I started work, for information, not only about the tasks which arise, but also about the underpinning principles which lead to clinical actions. It gives priority to material with two considerations in mind, the types of problems most commonly seen by nurse practitioners in minor injuries, and the areas in which nurse practitioners are most likely to lack knowledge from their previous training and experience. The subject which comes first when these criteria are applied is musculoskeletal examination, especially for the diagnosis of closed soft-tissue injuries.

I remember well, when I started my job, standing with a senior colleague in front of a patient who had an injured knee, staring at the uninformative swelling, and wondering how I was supposed to work out what was happening in there. Or sitting at a lecture on examination of the knee, and being told that this manoeuvre or that one would lead to this or that result, which would imply this or that diagnosis. No one seemed to know why, or to be able to reason beyond the point where these simple generalisations let them down. I discovered that the kind of teaching that junior doctors tended to receive in A&E was no better, but I suspected that their medical training, with its detailed emphasis on anatomy, supported by dissection, gave them a large advantage. I think that doctors who teach nurses do not always realise that we lack this background.

Clearly, all of the information which was needed was available somewhere. There are no new clinical facts in this book. I sifted the literature, looking for the information a nurse practitioner would need, knowing what *I* had needed to find out to do my job properly. I also realised that sources other than doctors' textbooks would be useful, because doctors are taught in a way which is not always helpful to nurses. The anatomy drawings in this book, for example, are not dissection-based, but based on the more dynamic approach of the Kendalls and their successors in physiotherapy, who enhanced our understanding of function by showing the muscles in movement.

I have an aspiration, for the days beyond the present struggle to become established, nurses will become not only the main source of care for minor injury, but that we will turn it into a specialty. At present, patients with minor problems are given a low priority, and are often treated by inexperienced doctors in busy departments where other patients are seriously ill. This environment is not conducive to detailed examination and accurate management. Yet patients with so-called minor injuries may suffer prolonged disability and pain, often avoidable with good advice, or treatable if well diagnosed. There is much to play for here, both for ourselves and for our patients.

Edinburgh, 2003 Dennis Purcell

Acknowledgements

It is a pleasure that life rarely offers to be able to give public thanks to those who have given help and support. I have an uneasy feeling that it is a cheap way to pay your debts, but my gratitude is real.

Carol Crowther and Jan Lumley started the minor injury clinic at the Western General Hospital in Edinburgh. Later, they led the setting up of our minor injury course and encouraged us to develop our teaching skills. It is more than 8 years since the clinic opened, but it is still unique in Scotland in its independence and range of activity. It was not at all clear at the start that it would succeed, and it took a lot of imagination and commitment to take the idea to completion.

I have used ideas from every nurse practitioner in the clinic, past and present, at one time or another, and my view of what our job can be has been formed by our joint experience. They are Louise Davidson, Christine Lawson, Jan Lumley, Eileen Marshall, Stephen McGhee, Fiona Murdoch, Catherine Ross, Linda Stark, Fiona Watts and Lynne Willis.

I am particularly in debt to Eileen for permission to make use of her teaching materials on the eye.

Stephen was kind enough to pose for the photographs of knee and shoulder examination, and my daughters Jude and Rebecca lent themselves for photographs of hip examinations and wound care. Fiona Watts demonstrated wound-closure techniques and Liz Harris made the make-up skills of the army available for us.

Fiona Lowe is a senior physiotherapist at the Western General Hospital, Edinburgh. She has been involved with us since the beginning. She has offered support not only to our patients but also to the nursing team in the form of excellent teaching and, in this book, her demonstration of the examination techniques in the photographs. She has a gift for making things clear and she has added a lot to this book.

Thanks to Mark Cooper for his Foreword.

At Elsevier my particular thanks are due to Alex Mathieson, Mairi McCubbin and Joannah Duncan.

1

Part 1
GENERAL ISSUES

1 DEFINITIONS

CONTENTS

This book is written for nurse practitioners (NPs) in minor injuries and it opens by discussing what a NP is and what is a minor injury. The chapter goes on to discuss the important question of discrimination between patients who are injured and those who are ill and closes with a discussion of the difficulties which minor injury clinics, especially in stand-alone settings, face with 'inappropriate attenders'.

What is a Nurse Practitioner?

The title Nurse Practitioner along with others, of which consultant is the most ambitious to date, is the subject of a good deal of political and professional interest. There are two issues:

- defining the qualifications and the range of activity of the NP
- dealing with the problems that arise from the fact that NPs concentrate on clinical work: there is no pathway for them to develop their careers or improve their salaries.

These discussions are beyond the scope of this text.

At present, many nurses assume the title NP without having any formal qualification for that title. This is a situation which should not continue and is being addressed. It is, however, an inevitable result of the way that the role has evolved. In the meantime, nurses rely upon two supports. The first of these is the guidance offered by the NMC (Nursing and Midwifery Council) to nurses who take on new tasks. They are also supported by local agreements, in the form of protocols or guidelines.

For the purposes of this book, it is assumed that the NP will be a senior registered nurse who has taken on a new role. The NP will have relevant clinical experience, most of which will have been gained in Accident and Emergency (A&E). The NP may, or may not, hold a postregistration qualification as a NP and may hold other, relevant, postregistration certificates. The NP treats patients who present with minor injuries.

The NP acts in accordance with the provisions of the NMC Code of Conduct and Scope of Professional Practice documents. The guidance in these documents on the links between the development of NP practice and the tenets of safety, competence and accountability is of particular importance.

The activity of the NP is also regulated in the workplace by agreement between the NP, the nurse managers, local doctors and other interested people, including those who commission services and oversee standards. This agreement covers matters such as the training and qualifications for the job; the extent, nature and limitations of practice; mechanisms for referral of patients; the nature of liability in cases where there is complaint; and issues, such as nurse prescribing, where there is, as yet, no definitive professional code. The agreement is likely to be written in the form of clinical protocols or guidelines which will enable NPs to act, will limit their actions and will protect or expose them in cases where they are called to account.

The role has several distinctive features. Activities are mainly clinical (this includes activities such as health promotion) and there is limited autonomy in a field where, until recently, responsibility lay with the doctor. The NP may offer a diagnosis of the patient's problem and may discharge a patient whose treatment is completed. The NP must also learn other, new skills to meet the needs of the local situation, such as suturing and the requesting and interpretation of X-rays.

This definition of the role of a NP is no more than a stop-gap in a time of transition. It establishes a context for this book. Also, it does not touch upon areas such as research and teaching, which are implicit in the NP role, and which will develop as a career structure evolves for clinical nurses.

What is a Minor Injury?

There is no definition of the term minor injury. It is a blanket term which covers different things in different places, and a list of the problems which come under that title does not settle the issue. It is also difficult to imagine a definition of clinical features which make a problem invariably 'minor'. Generalized definitions like 'self-limiting problem' do not enclose the subject, as anyone who has had tendinitis of the shoulder for years can testify. Nor are there any convincingly 'minor' bits of the body. Even a circular definition that 'a minor injury is an injury which can be managed in a minor injury clinic' does not apply consistently. Some fractures can be categorized as minor but still require orthopaedic follow-up, and many patients with minor problems are referred on for practice nurse care, physiotherapy and so on.

Factors Contributing to a Definition

A working definition of 'minor injury' is implicit in the conditions under which individual units operate. The limits which are placed on NPs, what may be treated and what must be referred, define minor injury for that practice. The guidelines or protocols to be followed, and the professional obligations which are spelt out in the NMC Code of Conduct and the Scope of Professional Practice documents, mark out this territory. A minor injury is whatever it has been agreed it will be in an area. This is hardly a satisfying definition for those who wish to establish universal standards for the NP, but it allows things to move on in the meantime.

Certain restrictions (which vary from place to place) constitute a negative definition of what may be regarded as minor. For example, it might be decided that drunk patients, infants and ambulance cases should not be treated at stand-alone minor injury sites.

In spite of all the problems which surround 'inappropriate' attendances, patients themselves are very good at deciding whether their problem is an injury and whether it is minor. More than 80% of attendances at my own unit fall within our definition of minor injury. Of those who are referred on, some have medical problems and others have injuries which were not classed as minor in this particular clinic.

Breaking the term minor injury into its parts, it is clear that *minor* is the word which frustrates definition.

An injury is a mechanical event. A part of the body is stressed by an excessive force, and tissue is damaged. There are many practical situations where this definition does not help in understanding the patient's problem. The main difficulty is that it does not always allow discrimination between patients who are ill and patients who are injured, especially in cases where patients are injured by overuse rather than sudden violence. This will be discussed at length in the text.

The term minor, applied to an injury, is subjective. It must, to some extent, reflect the NP's facilities and abilities for dealing with injuries, but certain things can be said.

1. The term represents one end of a continuum. Severe injuries are designated *major*.
2. Usually, a minor injury will be to the musculoskeletal system or the skin and subcutaneous tissues. There are exceptions. Patients may, for instance, be discharged with mild, concussion-type symptoms, such as headache, and you may be expected to deal with some minor eye and ENT (ear–nose–throat) problems.
3. There will be no threat to the patient's life, no collapse, no need for resuscitation. There will be no neurological deficits, the patient will be alert and able to give a history. If the mechanism of injury raises the possibility of a serious injury, threatening life or limb, that possibility must be excluded.
4. There will be no injury to organs. There will be no risk of a disability as a result of the injury, no elements of nerve or major blood vessel damage, no tendon injury, no displacement or instability of bone.
5. There will be no potential for large, troublesome or cosmetically significant scars.
6. The diagnosis of minor injury will be clear, with no risk that an illness is being missed. Any complication which calls for further referral will be excluded. The patient will not suffer from any medical problems which will complicate the management of the injury.
7. There will be no severe symptoms or signs, the patient will not be in agony, the wound or burn will not be very large or deep, ligament damage will not destabilize the joint.
8. The treatment which the injury requires will fall within the competence of the NP.
9. The assessment of certain groups, children, the elderly, the mentally ill, people with learning difficulties, people with non-accidental injuries, people who have taken alcohol or drugs, may include factors other than the injury itself which will lead to the decision that the injury is not minor.

Aspects of Minor Injury and Illness

The most important distinction which the NP must make is between patients who are injured and those who are ill.

The argument for the existence of the NP depends, in part, on the assertion that a person who is not a doctor, but who has a suitable alternative training and skill, can practice safely within a small part of the medical field. This concept is not fully tested by a challenge to the basic competencies of NPs as they will surely become skillful in the treatment of patients with minor injuries if they are properly trained and if that is what they do every day. The test arises when the patient has a different kind of problem, one that the NP has not been trained to treat. The important part of that test, and the part which it is most easy to fail, is that the NP must be able to recognize that patient when the patient presents.

The importance of a history of injury

The taking of a history from a patient, of the problem and matters which are related to it, is a part of the process of **clinical examination** (Ch. 3). It is important to ensure, when a patient claims to be injured, that the history is really one of injury and not illness. There is a tendency for patients to describe a problem as an injury, whether or not they have suffered any such event, perhaps to relieve the worry which unexplained symptoms cause. Some patients are unaware of the difference between injury and illness, or that it can be important. In other cases, language may cause muddle and the NP may be at cross- purposes with the patient. Finally, some presentations will be difficult to assess, and the NP will not know, even after a full history and examination, whether the patient is injured or ill.

It has already been said that an injury is a mechanical event. Often, it is a sudden and violent exposure of a tissue to an overwhelming force. This event will be memorable. There will have been happenings, a fall, bleeding, pain, and the patient will be able to describe them. Also, because the event was mechanical, the patient's account of how it happened, direction of force, duration, speed, height, the part which suffered violence, collectively called the **mechanism of injury**, will allow prediction, before the patient is examined, not only that the patient is injured but also the likely and possible injuries which may have occurred. This is a reassuring situation for the NP. A convincing history of injury goes more than half way to a diagnosis, and the NP can be sure that a patient with such a clear tale is not mistakenly presenting with an illness which is thought to be an injury.

Things are not always so smooth. There are two main types of force which cause injury. Injury can be caused, as described above, by a single overwhelming event which causes the tissue to fail in an instant. It can also be caused by a series of slight injuries, **submaximal stresses**, which inflict damage in small, incremental ways; consequently there is no single moment of injury and there may be just a slow onset of worsening pain or a sudden, unexplained rupture of a tissue. The factors which may lead to this result include excessive repetition of a movement, poor technique in performing a habitual action, poor equipment or conditions for performing the action, the repeated lifting of loads which are slightly too heavy, and so on. Injuries of this type are sometimes called **overuse injuries**. They are common in certain workplace and sport situations.

It will be harder, in such a case, for the NP to be sure that the patient has an injury and not an illness. The history will be less conclusive. However, there should be a history of repeated use of the painful part, and telling symptoms and patterns of pain. The examination should confirm this by exposing a loss of function of the overused tissue. Where it is impossible to decide whether or not the patient is injured, it should not be assumed that it is an injury. The range of possible diagnoses should be assessed and an appropriate referral made to a doctor.

Inappropriate Attenders

A mismatch between the service which a unit offers and the service which the patient demands is often described by health professionals as a failure on the patient's part to use the service properly. The patient is labelled an inappropriate attender.

There are problems about the use of this label. It reduces a complex question about how services and demand should be matched to a matter of blame. It creates a dangerous distance, which can become outright conflict, between the NP and the patient. It predisposes the NP to underestimate the patient's problem, to fail to offer help when it is needed and perhaps to commit an act of negligence.

The fact is that a problem cannot be wished away regardless of how poorly the NP is equipped to deal with it. Patients cannot be returned to the street until it is established that they are well enough to leave the safety of the clinical area. The question then moves on to its real ground, which has nothing to do with whether or not a patient is appropriate. The question is, what is the appropriate course of action a NP should take to help the patient? The NP is obliged to evaluate the situation and come to an understanding of the type of problem the patient has, and its urgency, so that the patient can be redirected in an appropriate and safe manner.

A junior doctor in A&E is expected to treat emergency illnesses as well as trauma of all degrees of severity. Such a doctor is, at least in theory, trained to confront any type of medical problem, whether or not the patient's attendance is regarded as appropriate. NPs are not in that position and must confine their attention to minor injuries. So what is the correct thing to do, especially in a stand-alone minor injury clinic, when a patient turns up who is not injured but ill? The situation is not really very different from that of the junior doctor or any other nurse. Doctors are often confronted by problems which they cannot deal with. When a doctor is inexperienced, this may be more often than not. A trained nurse has the capacity to make accurate assessment of the general condition of *any* patient who presents and to keep that patient safe until the proper place is reached. It is important to document the patient's attendance fully, to take a history and to show evidence of the patient's condition by recording relevant vital signs and other observations. In some cases, the NP may have to begin basic life support and summon help.

Once a patient has been fully assessed, the NP will have an idea of the best course to take. Very often it is to recommend a visit to the GP. Sometimes an urgent referral to a medical specialist is required. The mechanisms will be in place for doing that. The decision made will be supported by the written record of the whole process, and a copy of this will probably be sent with the patient to the next place of treatment.

2 THE BACKGROUND TO CLINICAL PRACTICE

CONTENTS

Triage

This is a discussion of particular difficulties facing the NP in a stand-alone minor injury clinic, and a brief description of the recommendations of the Manchester Triage Group.

Triage in the Minor Injury Clinic

Triage is a word which comes to us carrying a whiff of the battlefields where it was coined, where the rationing of care was a necessity too stark for any denial. It means the accurate allocation of a clinical priority (Manchester Triage Group, 1997) to a patient by a professional who is competent to make that assessment.

Nowadays, triage is not only about clinical priorities. The concept has been integrated into the modern drive to provide quality service which can be measured. However, this consumerist gloss does not completely disguise a simple fact. Triage is about putting the patients' notions of their priority beside a professional assessment of those priorities, and comparing them with the other demands which are being made on the service at that moment. There is bound to be something uncomfortable about that process for everyone involved. It is important, both for the safety and effectiveness of the process and for the demonstrable fairness of the system, that there are rules for that process. Those rules must be seen to be implemented on every occasion. They must be safe and sensible. They must be explained to the patient as the basis for decisions.

It is important that other factors (such as the pressure to meet target times for triage and treatment) do not distort the process of giving the patient safe and effective care.

If a NP works in an A&E department, there is a larger system which incorporates triage into which the NP clinic will fit. In a stand-alone minor injury clinic, there may be greater difficulties. The clinic will probably have a small staff, and patient numbers will not justify the allocation of one person exclusively for triage. This could lead, at least in some cases, to a delay in making an initial assessment of the patient.

A good answer to this difficulty is hard to find. It is not ideal that a NP who is treating a patient is constantly interrupted to triage every new arrival, but it is even less acceptable that patients are allowed to sit for long periods without an assessment. The allocation of the task to a colleague who is not a NP can only be allowed if that person has enough training and experience to carry out triage properly and is readily available. It is also difficult, in that situation, to implement a system of triage which conforms to modern standards of care, where triage is seen as an ongoing process rather than a one-off encounter at the time of arrival.

Certain aspects of the situation will ease the problem for a minor injury clinic. Patients who are in a serious condition will not tend to walk into a minor injury clinic very often. Waiting times will often be so short that patients can be seen on arrival. Nevertheless, these advantages will not apply on every occasion, and they do not eliminate every concern. Patients who are in a serious condition will sometimes present themselves at the nearest medical service, whatever it is. Factors such as severe pain, or extreme youth or age, are also important considerations for triage, which weigh just as heavily in a minor injury clinic as elsewhere. There will also be days which are busy, when the waiting time will run into hours. A solution to these problems must be sought in the light of the particular conditions.

The Manchester Triage Group

The Manchester Triage Group is a group of senior doctors and nurses from A&E who have worked together to develop a systematic method of implementing triage. Their aim has been to provide a tool by which triage can be carried out effectively, in the same way and to the same standards, with results that are reproducible throughout the whole of the UK. Work of this kind has already been carried out in Australia and Canada. The group has provided lectures in different parts of the country and has published a text, Emergency Triage, which explains the system and provides a complete set of flow charts for different patient presentations. These charts are the instrument by which patients can be assessed consistently.

The NP must turn to that text for full information on the system. The discussion here is a general one on some aspects of triage which the group have felt to be important.

The group set itself the task of producing common terminology and definitions, a method of performing triage, a package for training others to perform triage, and a guide to audit. A National Triage Scale, incorporating categories which are defined by number, colour, name and target time for treatment, is given in Table 2.1.

The purpose of triage is *not* diagnosis. The process does not allow a diagnosis in most cases. The diagnosis might not decide the priority which is given to the patient, even if it were known at the time of triage. At triage, the NP will discover the signs and symptoms which characterize the patient's problem and will use these as **discriminators**. A patient can then be assigned to one of the five categories described in Table 2.1. The pathway which the patient follows arises from that allocation.

The system of flow charts has been developed from a list of **presenting complaints**, the chief signs or symptoms which bring the patient to the treatment centre. These are listed in flow charts. Each chart is organized from the most urgent possibilties to the non-urgent. The triage nurse takes a brief history from the patient and selects a chart. The list of presenting complaints is not necessarily a list of possible diagnoses. It includes such categories as 'apparently drunk', 'back pain', 'crying

Table 2.1 The National Triage Scale

Number	*Name*	*Colour*	*Target Time (min)*
1	Immediate	Red	0
2	Very urgent	Orange	10
3	Urgent	Yellow	60
4	Standard	Green	120
5	Non-urgent	Blue	240

With kind permission from the Manchester Triage Group, 1997.

Triage

baby', 'diabetes', 'head injury', 'headache', 'limping child' and 'shortness of breath'.

Once the flow chart has been chosen, the patient is assessed by testing the presentation against the discriminators which indicate the urgency of the problem. Some discriminators are general to all presentations, while others are specific to the selected chart. General discriminators include 'life threat', 'pain' and 'haemorrhage'. Specific discriminators for a patient with a fall include 'abnormal pulse' and 'focal or progressive loss of function'.

Priority is determined by a patient's condition at the time of triage. This situation may change at any moment and every encounter between a nurse and the patient is an opportunity to reassess. The fact that the system is intended to be reproducible should mean that any appropriately trained nurse who uses the flow chart should be able to decide whether a change has occurred.

The Manchester Triage Group gives special attention to the problem of measuring the patient's pain, and to the effect that variables (such as extremes of age, anxiety levels and cultural background) may have on the patient's perception of pain. These aspects of triage are as important in a minor injury clinic as in the A&E department. A fractured wrist, sprained ankle or superficial scald may cause the patient extreme pain and anxiety. Triage is a vital part of the work in any open-access, emergency centre both for the patient's comfort and safety and for the quality of the service. At a time when national standards for practice are being developed, every NP must be proficient within a system which meets those standards. This is difficult in some settings, but the problems must be solved.

Radiography

X-ray examination is the main investigation available to the NP in the minor injury clinic. There is no general agreement on the guidelines or protocols that permit the NP to request X-ray scanning, if at all. This debate will continue and, hopefully, universal standards of practice will be laid down. At the moment it is a matter of local policy.

It is usual for the NP to be restricted to requesting views of the limbs, or parts of the limbs. It has not been fully explored whether or not it makes sense for NPs to X-ray a given joint, for example the knee, when they are not able to manage the problem which has prompted the request. Another difficult area is the question of X-ray scanning for children. Practice develops partly in response to local conditions and resources, and the solutions to such questions may always be subject to variation.

Training on the interpretation of radiographs is beyond the scope of this book, and guidelines on the what and when of requesting X-ray films is very much a matter of local policy. This section will simply take a brief look at some general principles on the use of X-ray as it affects the NP in a minor injury clinic.

Requesting and Reporting Radiographs

Three people, at least, are involved in the sequence of requesting, taking and reporting the findings from a plain X-ray film. These are:

- the person who treats the patient
- the radiographer who exposes the film
- the radiologist, a doctor with postgraduate training in diagnostic radiology.

Usually, each of these people will offer an interpretation of the film. The person who requests the X-ray film will have training in the interpretation of radiographs, and will also be able to compare the film with the patient's signs and symptoms. The radiographer sees the patient and provides the views which seem to be appropriate and offers a provisional interpretation of the film. The final report is issued by the radiologist. The Royal College of Radiologists (1998) 'takes the view that a referral for a radiological examination is . . . a request for an opinion from a clinical radiologist in the form of a report to assist in the management of a clinical problem'.

A radiologist will not normally be present for the taking of a plain X-ray film in a minor injury clinic and will not report on the film until the patient has left the department. Therefore, responsibility for the patient's immediate treatment and safety must rest with the person who has requested the X-ray. Furthermore, the radiologist's report will not be based upon a clinical assessment of the patient. It will be based upon the information in the written request, and on the film itself. The report which comes out will only be as good as the information which has gone in. Radiographers supply additional protection in this system. They are obliged by their code of professional conduct not to perform unnecessary radiographs and to perform both standard and additional views when they are appropriate. However, the only person who performs a full clinical examination of the patient is the person who requests the radiograph. It may be that a flaw at that stage of the process, either in the examination or in the writing of the request, will generate errors which neither the radiographer nor the radiologist will be able to detect. The result may be a wrong diagnosis.

Guidelines on the Use of X-rays

There is a division of responsibility for the care and safety of the minor injury patient who receives an X-ray. The person who treats the patient sees the clinical picture, and the radiologist is the final authority on the interpretation of the X-ray film. This division has always, in medicolegal terms, been founded on the fact that both parties were doctors and both qualified and accountable within the structures of that profession. (The Royal College of Radiologists regards the radiographer as a person who carries out a delegated task on behalf of a radiologist, while the radiologist retains responsibility for the patient.) The NP is stepping into this arena, without a medical qualification, to assume the clinical role. It is clear that a NP cannot progress to requesting and interpreting X-ray films without the agreement of the radiologists who will report on the films. In addition to clinical skills, the NP must be trained in requesting and interpreting X-ray films and in the regulations and hazards associated with the use of ionizing radiation. The NP must work within limits which have been agreed with local radiologists and other relevant clinicians such as A&E and orthopaedic doctors. Elements which are important in this area are:

- that a system is in place for requesting and interpreting X-ray films which is accepted as safe by the responsible doctors
- that the scope and the limits of the NP's activities are defined by protocols or guidelines, validated by the relevant doctors, and that these are reviewed regularly
- that a system of clinical audit is in place.

A NP dealing with minor trauma will request an X-ray when a fracture, dislocation or radio-opaque foreign body is suspected. In this, as in every other professional issue, the NP is guided by the NMC Code of Conduct and Scope of Professional Practice documents, and by local protocols or guidelines.

There is some tension for any person who requests X-ray between the medical and the legal aspects of the situation. On the one hand, attempts are made to reduce unnecessary X-ray

Radiography

exposure using clinical guidelines (e.g. the Ottawa ankle rules [Stiell et al 1993]) to identify the patients who have a high risk of fracture. On the other hand, doctors in A&E tend to be aware that no system of clinical assessment is foolproof, and a missed fracture may well lead not only to difficulties for the patient but also to litigation. Policies differ and the NPs must follow their own guidelines.

This situation can be made more complex by the pressure which patients apply to have an X-ray. Many patients do not feel that they have been properly treated until they have received such a scan, whether or not it is required for treatment of the injury.

The Royal College of Radiologists (1998) has published a booklet of guidelines for doctors, Making the Best Use of a Department of Clinical Radiology. Adams and Yates, in their foreword to ABC of Emergency Radiology, recommend that readers use that text in conjunction with 'guidelines of good practice', such as those offered by the Royal College, to ensure that X-ray films are being requested appropriately.

A few points from Making the best use of a Department of Clinical Radiology will be discussed here in the context of patients with minor injuries. Avoid, where possible, the overuse of X-ray examination. It wastes time, money and other resources and exposes the patient to unnecessary radiation (although the doses absorbed during plain X-ray of the limbs is relatively low). Consider the following questions:

1. Is a positive finding likely? If the X-ray film is positive, will this change the treatment of the injury? Many of the X-rays which patients ask for in a minor clinic, for example of the ribs and of the toes, are not justified by this standard.
2. Has an X-ray film been taken, in another hospital, of this injury? If so, try to obtain the existing film rather than request a second one.

Nurse Prescribing

Nurse prescribing is an issue which has taken wing in recent times, and the pace of change makes it unlikely that a text of this kind will be up to date on this matter when it reaches the reader. This discussion will therefore be brief.

The argument for nurse prescribing springs from two notions. First, there are areas of clinical practice where most of the skill and knowledge belongs to nurses rather than doctors. Second, a patient's care should be carried out by the best person, in that specific situation, to give that care. It would seem to be a perversion of the notion of professional accountability, as well as a waste of time and resources, to have a doctor assume nominal responsibility for a nurse's activities in areas where the doctor's assent is no more than a rubber stamp. This debate began in the community, where nurses have always had to work in a more autonomous fashion than their hospital-based colleagues. The early initiatives in nurse prescribing have also been community based, with district nurses and health visitors in England and Scotland receiving special training and participating in pilot projects at chosen sites.

The terms of reference for the Cumberlege Report team, in 1986, which led to the adoption by the UK government of nurse prescribing in the community as a policy, included questions of the best use of resources and the improvement of services to the patient. There is no difference between hospital and community in the need to pursue those values.

Dr June Crown has chaired two reviews for the government, with reports issued in 1989,

1998 and 1999, and her recommendations have been the basis for the transition, which is still occurring, to a system of nurse prescribing that will hopefully allow specialist nurses, in hospital or community, to prescribe medicines for their patients as part of their care.

Crown recommended the use of group protocols for the dispensing of medicines, and legislation was enacted in August 2001 to allow prescribing by protocols known as **patient group directions** (PGD).

A PGD is a written instruction sanctioned by a senior clinician (and also by a pharmacist and by the relevant health trust or other body). It lays down the conditions for a named health professional to treat an easily identified class of patients (i.e. patients who have similar medical needs) with prescription-only medicines without the patient being seen by a doctor and issued with an individual prescription.

Patients with minor injuries are not so simple a class as, for instance, patients who require foreign travel vaccinations. However, if the case is accepted, as it has been, that nurses can see and treat such patients without recourse to a doctor, then it seems clear that the conditions exist to include prescribing for them within the range of activities performed by the nurse. Again, in practice, this has occurred already for years against the unsatisfactory background of an unresolved legal position, and it has worked perfectly well. Hopefully, the time has arrived when proper structures are being put into place to protect and support nurse and patient alike.

What Medicines Should the NP Prescribe?

The recommendation that a nurse should prescribe medicines must be based on the fact that this is the best person in the particular situation, with the knowledge, skills and contact with the patient, to deal with the patient's needs. It is not an acceptable departure, for instance, that a patient should be treated at a minor injury clinic where the staff have no training in the treatment of minor ailments and be given a bottle of antibiotics for an earache because the patient could not get through to the GP.

It is, therefore, fairly straightforward to draw an outline of the NP's range of competence and supply a formulary which covers the main situations that are likely to arise. The patient who has some specific problem, such as allergy or intolerance, or a medical complication, can be referred to a doctor.

There is a role for the use of a simple oral analgesic, **paracetamol**, for adults and children. In addition, **ibuprofen** for musculoskeletal pain is a part of management of many injuries.

Localized wound infections (Ch. 8) may require an oral antibiotic such as **flucloxacillin.** Given the large number of patients who claim, rightly or wrongly, that they are allergic to penicillin, a substitute such as **erythromycin** is useful. The use of prophylaxis for animal bites is a matter for local discussion, but a suitable antibiotic such as **co-amoxiclav** (amoxicillin plus clavulinic acid, and a substitute for those who are allergic to it) is valuable for patients who have clinical signs of infection.

A patient with a wound may need to be immunized against tetanus (Ch. 8). **Adsorbed tetanus** vaccine and, on occasion, **human tetanus immunoglobulin** are required.

Effective wound management, in the stages of cleaning, exploration and closure, can only be achieved if the patient is calm and comfortable. An infiltrated, plain, local anaesthetic such as **lidocaine** 1% is needed.

This list of drugs is restricted to the core activities of the NP and takes no account of variations in local policy, which are particularly marked in the use of antibiotics.

3 CLINICAL EXAMINATION AND DOCUMENTATION

CONTENTS

This chapter deals with communication. Nurses should be equipped in this area and may feel that they need no lessons here. Nurses may feel that they are already able to talk to and observe patients so that they can learn what they need to know, and are used to writing these findings down. However, the new role of NP requires a tool with which nurses are largely unfamiliar, **clinical examination**, to achieve a purpose which nurses have not had to attempt, **diagnosis**. This requires the reshaping of traditional skills and the addition of some new ones, so that the NP can approach a new patient ready and able to help. Clinical examination is a large subject. This chapter focuses on how to obtain a history from the patient, which is the first part of that process, and the method of recording the clinical examination in writing. The later stages of the process are dealt with in other chapters. This chapter also discusses the use, and misuse, of technical language, the use of diagrams in written records and the general shape of a clinical history.

Clinical Examination

When a doctor, or other therapist, offers a **clinical** impression of a patient's problem, that impression has been formed during a personal meeting with the patient and has been obtained by observation, discussion and examination. This process is called clinical examination. Clinical examination is divided into two parts: taking a history and physical examination.

Clinical examination is a rigorous routine, or rather, a sequence of routines, to find out what is wrong with the patient. If the 'thing' that is wrong with the patient is found and named, a diagnosis (from Greek, meaning, 'knowing one thing from another') has been reached. The information from the clinical examination may lead to further actions. These may include **treatment**, **investigations** to clarify the diagnosis or **referral** to another specialist.

A NP sees patients whose complaints have not been diagnosed. Treatment is completed by the NP, in most cases, during the first visit. There is a very limited menu of investigations which can be performed and the NP depends almost exclusively on a sound clinical examination for the right outcome.

The term clinical examination has come to have rather impersonal associations. It evokes the idea of an objective process carried out upon a passive agent, the patient, by an expert, the doctor. Indeed, there is an alternative terminology for the history-taking and physical examination phases. They are often called the subjective examination and the objective examination. That terminology seems to underline the unreliable nature of the patient's perspective and the cool detachment of the clinician.

This is not an accurate picture. The Greek word *klinikos* means bed, and clinical activities are bedside interactions with patients. They depend upon communication skills which are highly valued in nursing as well as in medicine. Clinical examination requires empathy, skilled listening and keen observation.

Physical examination does employ standardized techniques, but they cannot be performed without the trust and cooperation of the patient. Interpretation of the findings is a matter of skill and experience. In all of this the *relationship* with the patient is the lynch-pin.

It is not the case that clinical examination is a field which belongs only to doctors. Many doctors are complaining that the advance of technology, which gives them increasingly sophisticated means of investigating patients' complaints, is robbing them of their clinical skills. Meanwhile, professions like physiotherapy are breaking new ground in the field of clinical examination.

Nurses can feel perfectly comfortable about entering this field. It offers a new discipline to tackle, skills which can deepen throughout life and the rewards of a patient-centred, *clinical* career.

Clinical Records

A separate but indispensible part of the process of clinical examination is writing down a formal record of the findings. This written record has two important functions:

1. It is essential for continuity of treatment for the patient. The person who has ultimate responsibility for the continuity of the patient's medical care is the GP, and a report should be sent to the GP outlining any treatment.
2. It provides evidence, acceptable in a court of law, of what happened during the examination. Patients who are treated for acute trauma often come to the civil or criminal courts. Patients may come to court to sue *you*, or your employers, if they feel that there has been negligence in their treatment. The court will be inclined to accept the nurse's account of events only if a written record, made at the time of the episode, supports what is said. This slogan should be engraved on your heart: *if it is not written, it did not happen.*

The written record has other uses. It carries data which can be used for audit, and a record of details may be requested purely for that purpose. It is written to a template, which imposes an order on thoughts and work that becomes habitual. This makes it less likely that something important is forgotten.

The double status of the written record, as a medical and as a legal document, means that it must conform to certain standards.

1. The patient should be identified by full name, date of birth and address. If continuation sheets are used, the patient's name and date of birth should be recorded on each sheet.
2. The date and time of attendance, as well as the time of triage and the time of starting and ending the consultation, should be noted. If the patient is seen more than once, the date and times of each visit should be written down.
3. The NP must sign the notes and write name and designation in capitals below the signature. Anyone who writes on the sheet should sign it. This may be a nurse who has checked a prescription, or a radiologist who has recorded an X-ray report.
4. If the treatment sheet is handwritten, it must be legible. It should be written in black ink and abbreviations should only be used if they are widely understood and unambiguous.

Technical Language

Nurses, at least on the acute side of hospital work, are equally immersed with their medical colleagues in a stream of jargon and abbreviation: Us and Es, ST elevations, ABGs, Po_2 and all the rest. It can come as a surprise to the NP that there is a new jargon to master, one relatively unknown to nurses, the language of the clinical examination.

Technical language is a polite term for professional jargon. It refers to words which are either not in common use or are common but are used in a special way. The medical profession outshines even the high churches in its adherence to musty old Latin formulations. It also enjoys annexing parts of the body, as well as various deformities, injuries and diseases, no matter how unappetizing, and labelling them with a doctor's own name instead of using a descriptive term which would guide the student to its meaning. Modern branches of study, such as sports medicine, are innovaters in the creation of clunking new jargon. Much of this language seems to obstruct rather than enhance understanding, and it is hard not to suspect that much of it is unnecessary. However, NPs will have to grapple with it if they wish to study these subjects.

They will also have to use technical terminology, which does have an essential function. Ordinary words are often not sufficiently precise, are too ambiguous or do not exist for our special needs when we write records of patient consultations.

This creates a conflict. The medical profession turns to an obscure language in order to communicate more clearly. For professional contacts, this is necessary. The problem is that not all of our communications are with other professionals. Patients do not understand our jargon. Detailed advice to patients on management of injuries and health promotion is a vital part of our work. A lot of the medical language which causes problems (words like trauma, fracture and sprain) inhabits a middle-ground where many patients understand it, but others do not. We must assume nothing and we must ensure that we are understood.

The technical language used belongs to one of five categories:

- anatomical terms for parts of the body
- terms which describe the movements of parts of the body
- terms which describe the position of one part of the body in relation to another
- Names given to parts of the body surface in order to describe things in relation to them
- types of injury.

Anatomical names are not always necessary. The everyday equivalents are often just as precise as the Latin (knee-cap for patella, collarbone for clavicle, shoulder-blade for scapula and so on), and many Latin names are widely known, especially among sportsmen. However other everyday words such as stomach are often used vaguely, and it is not clear whether the patient has chest pain, or a problem in the abdomen. Shoulder, as the word is commonly understood, describes a group of joints, and a more exact description is sometimes needed.

Everyday language is not good at describing positions and movements of the body. To say that an injury lies just below the wrist, when the hand can be held above or below that joint, is unclear. The outside of the hand can be any surface, depending on how the arm is rotated. To say that the patient's finger, wrist or ankle hurts because he twisted it, does not give a picture of the exact movement. That picture is needed to narrow down the range of injuries which might have occurred.

In an effort to be clear, pay attention to simple matters. Record whether the right or left side is affected, whether an injured digit belongs to the hand or the foot, and which joint of a finger is painful. The standard to aspire to is that a person who reads the account can reconstruct every important fact without seeing the patient. In a court of law, this may include the position of a wound to the centimetre, and its exact length, depth and direction.

Diagrams

A treatment sheet will probably contain a space for a diagram, and certain injuries, especially wounds, lend themselves to pictorial representation.

It is not necessary to be a master artist to do this. It is fine to draw a bunch of bananas, but it must say whether these are hand bananas or foot bananas. Label the diagram, even if it appears to be totally clear, saying left or right, front or back, naming the body part and sketching the injury (and labelling it too). There are rubber stamps available, illustrating all parts of the body, and these can be used.

The terminology which is necessary for describing injuries will be included at the appropriate places in the text.

Clinical History

The taking of a history is a social act, a conversation, and it calls for the skills which mark the conversationalist: warmth, empathy, listening and a grasp of the nuances of unspoken communication. However, it is not a casual conversation. It occurs in a very unequal situation. The medical contributor is in control, on his own territory and has professional status. The patient needs help and is vulnerable.

The conversation has an agenda. It is the job of the NP to pursue it. A rapport should be established with the patient quickly, and the conversation should be directed to elicit the information needed.

The patient should be asked who they are, how the injury happened, what effects it is having and the medical history, especially any aspects which have a bearing on the present situation. Ask open questions. Listen and observe. Once the broad outline is clear, there will be an indication of possible problems and clarifying questions, inviting brief factual replies, will be needed. This should help to make a **differential diagnosis**: a list of the problems or diagnoses which the patient's story suggests but has not eliminated.

This is an ideal picture. It is only possible to direct the process skillfully if the NP has some idea where it is going. This takes knowledge and experience. Some patients are so talkative, or so monosyllabic, that it is a struggle to get useful information out of them.

The exact method of taking a history depends on the patient's problem. The NP is interested in the recording of the history of an injury. Even this is too broad a category. Different kinds of injury raise different concerns. The history of different types of minor trauma, including musculoskeletal injuries, wounds and head injuries, will be discussed in more depth at the relevant places in the text.

The History of an Injury

An injury is, as a rule, a sudden interruption of the patient's normal routine. Look ahead and anticipate any problems which the injury might provoke in daily life.

The patient's age, gender and occupation should be recorded. If there is an arm injury, is the patient right or left handed? Ask about hobbies. Depending on the context, ask about the home situation. Is there anyone at home, are there stairs in the house, and so on? Did the patient drive to the clinic; if so, is the patient alone? Always record who is present with a child.

Ask about any treatment which has been used so far by the patient, and any impression of its success or failure.

The fact that an injury is a mechanical process dictates the approach to the history. Establish the **mechanism of injury**, the physical facts which the patient knows about the way that the injury occurred. *When, how, where, what, who* and *why* are Kipling's 'six honest men', trusty questions, which will get to the facts in every situation. Some will be more important than others in a given case, but three are always relevant: when, where and how.

When

Always establish the time of an injury. Healing occurs in stages and the same injury requires different treatment at different times. Similarly, the same symptoms, such as pain or the inability to bear weight, are of different significance if the injury is 2 hours, 3 weeks or 6 months old.

Test all the links *within* the patient's account of the timing of the injury, for two reasons. First, the time that it takes for certain signs and symptoms to emerge after injury, such as swelling or inability to walk, gives an indication both of the diagnosis and the severity of the injury. Second, it is not unusual to hear a patient assert that the injury occurred on a given day and that the pain is a result, and then to discover that the pain did not come on until days, or weeks, after the so-called injury and that it has no connection to the incident.

The time elapsed since an injury is important when the patient has a wound. Policies for wound closure and the assessment of infection risks, including tetanus, are partly based on the age of the wound.

How

The central question about an injury is 'how did it happen?'. The answer to this question contains the facts about the mechanism of injury. It will help in understanding what injuries the patient may have suffered. The question is so important that, when a patient cannot say how the injury happened, you must keep an open mind about whether or not an injury *has* happened.

Questions will relate to mechanical factors, speed, height, duration, direction and any other element which may have contributed to the injury.

In an ideal situation, the patient's replies will provide a reconstruction of the whole incident, so that the event can be 'seen', as in a video replay.

Do not press too hard. The patient may have no idea of how the injury happened but may offer an answer anyway if you seem determined to have one. Do not lead the patient to describe the mechanism of injury which you think fits with the presentation.

Where

The place where a patient is injured matters because it contributes to the mechanism of injury. Whether a patient falls on grass or concrete, down a flight of stairs or out of a tree will influence thinking about the possible range and severity of injuries.

When the patient suffers a wound, the place where that has happened is important. If a patient's hand is cut on waste ground where there is broken glass then there may be glass in the wound. The site will also influence an assessment of the risk of tetanus and other infections.

There may also be health promotion and legal issues around the question of where an injury happens; for example, an employee could be injured in a dangerous workplace, or a child could find a syringe in a play park.

What

What caused the injury tells about the possible extent of the damage. A craft knife with a 2 cm blade will not cause a deep wound. This information can be related to the anatomy of the area injured to decide what underlying structures may be harmed. If the patient has an abdominal wound inflicted by a long, narrow-bladed knife then, regardless of how well the patient looks, an urgent surgical review is needed.

If the 'what' is a piece of broken glass or torn metal, a soft tissue X-ray can be used to look for a foreign body.

Who

Sometimes, the question 'who?' is actually about the identity of the perpetrator of an injury. This may arise if a non-accidental injury to a child has happened. Sometimes it is a question about the other person's medical status, if, for instance, the patient has suffered a human bite wound. On other occasions, the question is an extension of the search for the mechanism of injury. How big was the person who fell on the patient?

'Who' may also cover other concerns. Was anyone present who can give an account of how the patient suffered a head injury? Who is at home to look after this patient if discharged?

Why

'Why' is the lever that the health promoter presses to extract a useful conclusion from an unhappy event. Some accidents are caused by events which are not likely to be duplicated. In other cases, an equipment flaw, a poor workplace practice, a bad lifting technique, someone else's carelessness, an overindulgence in alcohol or some other factor has made the injury. The injury is not just a random event but an 'accident waiting to happen'. In those cases there are three considerations. It could happen again; steps could be taken to prevent it happening again, and there may be litigation.

'Why' can also be important if the answer to 'how' is in doubt. A common scenario is the elderly person who has had a fall. The patient may indeed have tripped, but there may be something else going on. The patient may have collapsed, and the cuts and bruises may be the least of the troubles. The first question is 'why did you fall?'. If the patient does not know, or if the answer suggests a medical cause, this must be pursued.

The Past Medical History

Once the patient has given an account of the injury, the general medical history should be established, particularly aspects of the history which may influence treatment.

TAM is a useful acronym when you are taking a medical history from an injured patient. It means tetanus, allergies, medicines.

Tetanus

If the patient has a wound (and this includes burns, splinters and eye injuries), always ask if tetanus immunizations are up to date (Ch. 8).

Allergies

The patient should be questioned about any allergic response to any medication or skin tapes such as elastoplast. Find out what the allergic reaction was (the patient may not know if it occurred in childhood). Many patients who have difficulty tolerating a medicine for some reason believe that this is an allergy. Advise the patient to talk to the GP if there is doubt.

Medical history and present medications

Many of the questions which you would ask a sick person (for example, family medical history) are superfluous when a patient has suffered an injury. However, major illnesses, such as diabetes, heart disease, stroke or epilepsy, should be elicited. Certain problems may be worsened by treatment (such as using ice on the hands of a person who suffers from Raynaud's disease).

Always think carefully about the patient's presentation if there is a history of cancer (is there a clear history of injury, is the pattern of pain consistent with injury, is the apparent severity of the injury consistent with the violence of the mechanism?).

Ask about past orthopaedic, neurological and rheumatological problems when a patient has joint pain of uncertain cause. Ask also about recent and present infections, and there can be connections between skin problems and arthritis.

Does the patient suffer from gastric or renal problems, or asthma? This is relevant if ibuprofen could be prescribed. Is the patient taking any medicines just now? Corticosteroids and anticoagulants should be specifically mentioned. Corticosteroids can cause decline in bone, soft tissues and skin; they can mask serious infections and cause dangerous complications if the patient should need a general anaesthetic. Anticoagulants, commonly warfarin, can trigger excessive bleeding after an injury, particularly dangerous in the case of a head injury.

Recording the Examination

In this section, the layout of the written record of a clinical examination will be shown. It will close with some fictional written records. These are workaday samples of common presentations, and no claim is made that they are flawless (in fact, the reverse can be guaranteed). The examples may include some terminology which is new. Those terms are all defined at the appropriate sections of the book. The important thing to grasp at this stage is the general method of presenting the information.

The way of writing the record (succinctly) is determined by limitations placed on the NP in the clinic. The record is a contemporary one, written at the time of treatment, and the working day is busy. In fact, if notes are not written *during* the consultation, there may be problems. Most A&E nurses can recall doctors going round casually asking whether the woman who left a minute ago injured her left ankle or her right, and NPs are not likely to do any better. In addition, if the sheet is not written during the examination the benefit is lost of the structure which it imposes on the examination. Sitting in front of the patient and writing what is more or less a summary of the whole interaction can also help to put ideas in order and to reach a decision about how to proceed.

Layout

There are variations on the recommended layout, and it has to be adapted for different problems, but the basic pattern of the notes should be as follows. The first two items are based on things that the patient relates, which is also called the subjective examination. The rest of the notes record the findings and actions, the objective examination.

1. The history of the presenting complaint (sometimes labelled as HPC; the abbreviation C/O, meaning 'complains of' is also used). This part will begin with some bare details about the patient and the present situation. This is what the patient relates edited to what is considered relevant, but still, essentially, the *patient's* words. These may be quoted directly (in quotation marks).
2. The patient's past medical history (PMH), any current medication, any history of allergies and, in the case of a patient with a wound, current tetanus status.
3. The examination (O/E meaning 'on examination' is often used). The structure of the examination depends on the type of problem (often a NP will follow the orthopaedic method, 'look, feel, move', which is discussed in Ch. 5). All general observations, all examination techniques and any significant findings, positive *and* negative, are recorded.
4. An impression (Imp) or provisional diagnosis.
5. Investigations (most commonly X-ray).
6. The results of investigations.
7. A final diagnosis (if one is reached).
8. Plan. This may include treatment, discharge, referral, review by NP, advice and any other steps needed to complete the process.

The NP should let each patient's GP know, in writing, the important details of the patient's visit. The simplest way to do this is to send a copy of the treament sheet. Give the patient a copy of the notes or a letter if a referral elsewhere is made. Case studies 3.1 and 3.2 are examples of records for patients with two similar situations for injury but differing results. The similarity between these two examples underlines the two crucial differences, mechanism and diagnosis, and the relationship between those differences. In Case study 3.1, the *likely* diagnosis, with that mechanism and that presentation, is a fracture, while a sprain is much more likely in Case Study 3.2. Injuries tend to fall into patterns, and most injured, swollen ankles are caused by an inversion mechanism. The patient can be vague in the description of the incident and lull you into overlooking something important. In these two cases, a NP would have been likely to arrive at the correct diagnosis regardless of the assessment of the mechanism, because an X-ray would probably be requested. That will not always be the case and the NP must get the whole story. Two further case studies (3.3 and 3.4) illustrate the use of records to reach a diagnosis.

Case Study 3.1

A 20-year-old man, who works in an office, is playing football. He jumps up to head the ball and collides in the air, shoulder to shoulder, with another player. He falls on his left side. The other player falls heavily across his right ankle as the foot lies, outer side up, on the ground. The man hears a crack and feels sickening pain in the outer ankle. He is unable to walk. His team-mates carry him off and put an ice-pack on the ankle within 10 minutes. He is brought straight to the hospital. He is in a wheelchair. He looks pale and there is a large, bruised swelling over the outer ankle.

Written record

HPC: 20 yrs man, office worker.
Brought by friends in a car.
Lives with partner, ground floor flat.
Football, 1 hour ago.
Pt on ground on left side. A player fell across his right ankle. Heard 'crack'. Immediate pain. Swelling at outer ankle. Non-weight bearing since. Has used ice. Can feel/wiggle his toes.
PMH: No allergies, no medications. No asthma, gastric, renal problems.
O/E: Right lower leg/foot
Pt looks pale.

- large, bruised swelling over lateral malleolus
- no deformity
- sensation and circulation to foot intact
- tender distal fibula; no tibial tenderness
- all ankle movement restricted by pain at lateral ankle.

Imp: Fracture of distal fibula.
Investigation: X-ray lower leg and ankle.
X-ray: Fracture distal fibula.
Plan: Orthopaedic review.

Case Study 3.2

A 20-year-old man, who works in an office, is playing football. He jumps up to head the ball and collides in the air, shoulder to shoulder, with another player. He lands awkwardly on his right foot and feels it twist inwards at the ankle. The man hears a crack and feels sickening pain in the outer ankle. He falls. He is unable to walk. His team-mates carry him off and put an ice-pack on the ankle within 10 minutes. He is brought straight to the hospital. He is in a wheelchair. He looks pale and there is a large, bruised swelling over the outer ankle.

Written record

HPC: 20 yrs man, office worker.
Brought by friends in a car.
Lives with partner, ground floor flat.
Football, 1 hour ago.
Pt jumped 2 to 3 feet, came down on right foot, 'went over on it' (shows inversion). Heard 'crack'. Immediate pain. Fell and was carried off. Non-weight bearing since. Swelling at outer ankle. Has used ice. Can feel/wiggle his toes.
PMH: no allergies, no medications. No asthma, gastric, renal problems.
O/E: Right lower leg/foot
Pt looks pale.

- large bruised swelling over lateral malleolus
- no deformity
- sensation and circulation to foot intact
- tender inferior aspect lateral malleolus. No tenderness at base 5 MT
- all ankle movement restricted by pain at lateral ankle.

Imp: Sprain, but exclude fracture to base of lateral malleolus.
Investigation: X-ray ankle.
X-ray: No fracture.
Further examination: Anterior drawer test; pain but no obvious ligament laxity.
Diagnosis: Sprain, grade two.
Plan: Has transport.
Home on crutches to partner.
Has ibuprofen – full advice on dosage and side-effects.
PRICE (double tubigrip, PRICE advice sheet explained)
Physio tomorrow 1100 h, full ligament assessment and treatment.

Case Study 3.3

A 45-year-old man, an engineer, married with two grown-up children living at home, is working in the boiler room in the bakery where he is employed. He ducks under a metal pipe to reach the boiler. He forgets the pipe and bangs the top of his head (he is wearing a cap) on a sharp-edged pipe-bracket as he stands up. The pain makes him dizzy, he sees flashing lights for a moment and his ears ring. He sits down for few minutes. He starts to feel better, but his head is throbbing where he hit it. He puts his hand up to his head and feels blood. He gets up and goes to his first-aider, who bandages his head and brings him to hospital.

Written record

HPC: 45 yrs, man, engineer in a bakery.
Brought from work in a van, work-mate still here.
Lives with wife, 2 adult children. Wife home now.
1 hr ago stood up under a sharp, dirty metal pipe bracket (Pt wearing hat), painful blow and laceration to top of head.

Brief dizziness, 'flashing lights and ringing in ears' all resolved now, headache local to injury only, 'throbbing'. No LOC (loss of consciousness), neck stiffness, vomit, amnesia, vertigo, nose/ear discharge. Walking well, no loss of power/sensation in limbs.

Wound is bandaged, has not been cleaned.

PMH: Tetanus – booster 2 yrs ago. No allergies. No medications.

O/E: Head

1. Neuro
   - GCS (Glasgow Coma Scale; see Ch. 9) 15 Looks pale but fully mobile and responsive.
   - PERL (pupils equal, react to light), FROEM (full range eye movements), no diplopia or nystagmus,
   - FROM neck (full range movements), no paraesthesia or weakness in limbs.
2. Wound
   - 2 cm transverse lac, in left parietal area.
   - Not full thickness, no haematoma, bone smooth and firm.

Imp:

1. Minor head injury.
2. Wound for clean and closure.

Plan:

1. Phone home. Pt home to wife (has a driver). Discussed HI (head injury) advice sheet with her. Return if problems.
2. Wound toilet with saline. No dirt.
3. Staples to close. Staple advice sheet. GP if any infection signs.

Practice nurse in 5/7 for ROS.

Case Study 3.4

A 23-year-old woman, a right-handed, self-employed picture framer who runs her own shop single-handed, is carrying a sheet of picture glass when she trips and falls, breaking the glass and pressing her right palm onto the shards. She has a cut over the muscle pad of her thumb. It looks deep and is bleeding very freely. She wraps a scarf tightly around her hand and calls a taxi to take her to hospital.

Written record

HPC: 23 yrs woman, right-handed picture framer, self employed, works alone.

1 hr ago, carrying picture glass, fell on top of it, cut right palm on broken glass.

'Heavy' bleeding, not spurting. Pressure dressing improvised, bleeding controlled. 'Could be' glass in wound.

PMH: Tetanus – booster at school, ? seven years ago. No allergies, no problems with lidocaine, no medications.

O/E: Right hand

- diagonal 1 cm cut in middle of thenar area
- sensation intact
- bleeding, moderate oozing
- penetrates to fat, no visible deeper structures.

Imp: ? Glass in wound.

Investigation: Soft tissue X-ray.

X-ray: no radio-opaque foreign body.

Further examination: Resisted movement intact in thenar muscles and flexors of the thumb and index finger.

Imp: No structural injury. Wound for closure.

Plan:

1. Local anaesthetic
2. Wound toilet with saline
3. 2 × 4.0 prolene sutures to close. Dry dressing.
4. Suture advice sheet discussed. GP if infection.
5. ROS in 10/7 by practice nurse.

Note: the local anaesthetic prescribed would be recorded in a separate part of the record.

4 THE INJURED CHILD

CONTENTS

This chapter is for the NP who deals with patients of all ages, adult and children. It will look at those ways in which the care of children differs from that of adults. The notional 'patient' in the rest of this book is an adult, a simplification which is acceptable in most cases when discussing injuries.

It is not possible to cover the full range of injuries to children in a text of this kind, but some broad generalizations will be offered on the types of injury which children suffer. Further information is included in the sections on specific types of injury.

This chapter does not deal with paediatric emergencies, but attention is drawn to the recommendations, discussed below, that minor injury clinics which treat children should have a nurse who is trained in paediatrics on every shift, and that all nurses should be routinely updating in emergency care of children.

Facilities and Resources

There is acceptance, in central and local government (enshrined in the Patient's Charter for children) and in the bodies representing doctors and nurses, that separate provision should be made for children (people under 16 years of age) when they attend an A&E department or a minor injury clinic.

The document Emergency Health Services for Children and Young People, a Guide for Commissioners and Providers by Christine Hogg (1997) offers advice on the standards which minor injury services for children must meet. Some of her points are offered here.

Training

There should be a NP who is qualified in the care of sick children on every shift in a minor injury clinic. The illnesses and injuries which children suffer, and the ways in which they react to them, are different in many ways from those of adults. A child can become seriously ill very quickly. If the signs of non-accidental injury (NAI) are present, these must be recognized. Staff should know their local child protection procedures. They should also be skilled in health promotion and accident prevention, and they should have literature which can be given to parents on those subjects.

NPs should be trained in emergency care for children and should rotate to A&E departments to retain their skills.

There should be a doctor available who is trained in chidren's emergencies.

The protocols or guidelines which govern the practice of the NPs should be agreed with the local clinicians who are responsible for the care of sick and injured children. There should be clinical supervision by, and access to, a consultant paediatrician.

Triage

The patient should be triaged by an appropriately trained person as soon as the child arrives in the unit. Children who are under 10 years of age and who have a complaint which has the same triage priority as that of an adult should be seen before the adult. Children who are under 5 years should not wait more than 1 hour for a full assessment.

The management of pain is a high triage priority for adults and children. This may involve the use of paracetamol, or the application of a broad arm sling. Covering a wound can reduce distress.

The triage system (Ch. 2) should be explained to the patient.

Facilities

There should be a separate waiting area for children, and treatment should be offered in a room decorated and designed to be safe and reassuring for them. Children should not be mixed with adults who are ill or injured.

Consent

In England, Wales and Scotland, children who are under 16 years of age may consent to medical treatment on their own behalf if a doctor is satisfied that the child understands the meaning of the decision in the fullest sense of the term 'informed consent'. English law, however, allows a child to consent to treatment but may not allow the child not to *refuse* it, if the High Court, or even the parents, decide to overrule this decision. The child may both consent to and refuse treatment in Scotland if the conditions for an informed consent are met. Morton and Phillips (1996) offer an interpretation of this situation from the viewpoint of senior doctors working in A&E in England.

When an adult who is the parent or a carer brings a child to A&E for treatment, the consent of the adult to treatment, on behalf of the child, is implicit provided that the treatment has been explained. If the child needs an anaesthetic, written consent should be obtained.

If a child of 12 years or older comes to A&E alone for treatment, every effort should be made to contact a responsible adult to obtain consent for treatment. However, if no adult is available, and the child understands the situation, then minor treatment, not including the taking of radiographs or the giving of medicines, might be performed. At the other extreme, in a dire emergency, life-saving measures can be undertaken without consent if the child is alone.

The situation should be documented, continuing efforts made to locate the parents and the parents should be informed in writing of the action taken.

The legal situation depends, in part, on the *medical* qualification of the person giving care to assess the competence of the child to give consent.

In a dire emergency, a NP will be acting under the supervision of the medical team. Given that a NP should not do anything extensive for a child who presents alone for minor treatment, it seems illogical to give *any* treatment without parental consent. If the problem is small, it can wait until consent is available. If the problem is more urgent, consent becomes important. However, it does not seem to be in the patient's interest, for example if the child appears alone in the unit with a filthy graze on the knee, that a NP fails to reduce the risk of infection by cleaning a minor wound. This kind of situation does arise. It calls for common sense, but it is important for the NP to remain within the permitted scope, for the sake of both the practitioner and the patient. A NP should have a protocol or guideline, developed with the senior clinician in the local children's A&E, to deal with it. Where there is doubt, a doctor should see the patient.

A Child's Rights

There are two areas, well recognized by all professionals who deal with the welfare of children, where values may come into conflict: the child's immaturity and a conflict of interest between the child's and the parents' rights.

Immaturity

Children are immature dependents, but they are as complete in their humanity and their rights as an adult. The child's immaturity imposes a greater burden, not a lesser, on carers to protect the child's rights.

The principle which emerges from the UN Convention on the Rights of the Child (1989; ratified in the UK in 1991) is that children who can understand the issues involved have the right to consent to treatment on their own behalf.

Medical treatment is often imposed on young children against their stated desire. The child's refusal is based on fear and an inability to weigh the consequences. However, the child's will should not simply be overridden. The completeness of the child's rights must be respected as well as the limits of a child's understanding. The heedless use of force may cause more harm than a physical injury. Consent for the treatment will come from the parents. If a NP intends to treat the child, the parents and the child should have an appropriate explanation, and the method of delivering the treatment must reduce the fear as well as address the injury. A children's A&E department has options (such as sedation and general anaesthetic) for dealing with these problems, and the child should be referred *at the outset* if there is any doubt.

Conflict of Interest

There are always cases in the public eye, arising from matters such as adoption and suspected child abuse, where the conflict between the rights of parents and the rights of the child emerges as the central problem. The difficulty is increased by the fact that a simple assertion that the rights of the child must always come first does not deal with the fact that any disruption of the family will hurt the child.

The law, in The Children's Act of 1989 and The Children (Scotland) Act 1995, recognizes this complexity. The preservation of the family, the prevention of problems and the continuing involvement of the family if problems have occurred are emphasized. However, the safety of the child is the first concern.

Non-accidental Injury

The responsibility to report, usually to police or social services, the suspicion that a child is being abused belongs to us all. However, a NP in a minor injury clinic will be certain to meet children who have been injured deliberately by their carers. Non-accidental injury (NAI) is the term used to describe this form of abuse. A NP should be able to identify the known patterns of injury and presentation and know how to proceed if there are concerns.

The other forms of abuse which are recognized are sexual abuse, emotional abuse and deprivation, and neglect. There are a number of indicators that can assist in assessing whether child abuse is occurring.

1. Certain external factors are recognized as presdisposing to child abuse (which includes NAI):
   - poverty
   - a single parent, especially if young and isolated
   - a stepfather living in the house
   - a parent who has suffered abuse, has mental health problems or is of low intelligence
   - a parent who has unreasonable expectations of a child and is angered by failure
   - an unwanted or difficult pregnancy
   - postnatal depression, or any other problem which causes difficulty with parent–child bonding
   - a child who is difficult or disabled
   - a previous history of abuse of the child or a sibling.
2. Certain aspects of the child's appearance are indicators of possible abuse:
   - failure to thrive, looking malnourished, not meeting milestones in speech development
   - dirty, not properly dressed for the weather (although this can be misleading and should be interpreted in context)
   - neglected physical disorders; severe nappy rash or 'cradle cap'
   - a child who does not interact normally, especially with the parents: 'frozen watchfulness' is the precocious, subdued demeanour of a child who expects violence
   - a child with disturbed, hyperactive behaviour.

   Great care has to be taken in the interpretation of predisposing factors. They are ambiguous.
3. The following signs should raise concern about the specific possibility of a NAI:
   - a delay bringing the child to hospital, especially if the injury is of a severity which calls for immediate treatment
   - the injury does not seem consistent with the story; concern should be greater if the injury is consistent with known patterns of deliberate harm (see below)
   - the parent (or carer) is aggressive, uninterested or evasive when asked questions
   - the story of how the accident happened changes.
4. Types of injury which suggest NAI (the following list is not definitive):
   - grip-mark bruises on the limbs or trunk, showing the imprint of fingers and fingertips

- signs of violent shaking (including neurological signs and intraocular bleeding) or skull fracture caused by being dashed against a wall combined with grip marks on the legs
- bruised, hand-prints on face or buttocks; marks on the cheeks or swollen ears
- bruises caused by pinching
- bite marks, which may be bruises or wounds, or both (a forensic odontologist may be able to match the marks to the attacker)
- scratch marks
- hair pulled out
- clearly defined, patterned or rectangular bruises (caused by hitting with a heavy implement)
- welts from hitting with a belt or similar
- ligature marks on the limbs, caused by tying
- choke marks, contusions on the neck, with pin-point haemorrhages on face, neck, behind ears or in the conjunctivae
- two simultaneous black eyes (although this appearance can follow an accidental nose injury); there may be a base of skull fracture
- eye injuries with loss of vision
- mouth injuries, especially with a tear of the frenum of the upper lip, which can be caused by pushing a bottle into the mouth
- injuries, bruising and bleeding around the genitals (may indicate NAI or sexual abuse)
- burns and scalds; burns on the feet, back of hand or buttocks are suspicious because these are unusual sites for accidental injury
- cigarette marks, sometimes in clusters
- immersion burns with a clearly defined boundary, often at the buttocks; splash marks (although these are often innocent)
- deep brand marks on parts which the child would not injure accidentally, such as the buttocks, from an iron, a hot poker
- old fractures, multiple fractures of different ages, skull fractures, rib fractures, fractures in the first year of life, avulsion and epiphyseal fractures (especially in the upper arm), spiral fractures of long bones
- signs of injuries of different ages and/or types.

There are a number of conditions which can be mistaken for NAI:

- accidental bruises and head bumps caused by being active, or injured by other children (these are likely to look more random and will not have the features listed above)
- impetigo can resemble cigarette burns
- some bleeding disorders may result in bruising, and some bone disorders may cause pathological fractures
- 'Mongolian spots' are found on the skin of some Asian children; they can be mistaken for bruises.

If NAI is suspected medical advice must be sought. Child abuse is not a purely medical issue, but physical injuries require examination, investigation and diagnosis. The responsibility for the diagnosis of abuse may be shared, depending on the circumstances, between paediatricians, the police surgeon, genitourinary specialists and others. The child's safety will be a main concern, and a child may be admitted to hospital in the first instance. The broader management of the problem is a multiagency affair, including the police and social work departments.

A NP should know the local child protection measures and initiate them when it is appropriate.

Certain documentation must be created if NAI is suspected.

1. Any episode where NAI is suspected must be documented with detailed descriptions and drawings of any injuries.
2. The filing system in the department should flag up children with a history of previous attendances.
3. The law allows for an Emergency Protection Order, to take a child who is thought to be in danger to a place of safety until the immediate problems are resolved. The

police would enforce this order. A hospital may be deemed a place of safety.

4. The social services department in each region of the UK maintains a **child protection register**, listing the names of children who are currently assessed as being at risk of abuse. Access to the register is restricted to 'authorized enquirers', and these will normally include all doctors, and selected senior nurses.

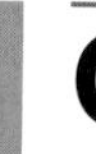

Communication

When an injured child is brought to a minor injury clinic there is distress and anxiety, both for the child and the parents. The initial task is to assess and calm the situation. The injured child should be triaged at once, and enough time should be spent to convince not only yourself but also the patient and the parents that the problem is under control.

Triage and the hospital environment have already been discussed. Communication with the child has to be adapted to both age and development. There should be some toys and pictures on the wall for young children, and the child should have easy access to parents, whether the child sits on the parent's knee or plays around the room.

The skills to be shown with a young child are the same skills which are called for socially. Talk to the child. Use the child's name a lot. Be flattering. Take your time and keep your distance at the start. Ideally, the room should be safe enough for the child to roam about. Tune into the child's level of development, show warmth and interest. There is a good deal to be learnt about the child's general well-being and the function of the injured part from observation at this stage. If the child is listless, ask yourself why. The child may be tired, may be ill, may have a significant head injury, or there may be deeper problems in the family.

There may not be an adequate history of the injury if the child is too young to tell you. It is common to meet a harassed mother who has been phoned at work by a nursery to collect an injured child, which she does in such haste that she arrives at hospital with only the vaguest idea of what has happened. Questions like 'was he knocked out?' are unanswered. A small child is sometimes injured when the parent is out of the room. The history may be based on an inaccurate assumption. A parent of a child who has a pulled elbow may present the child as having an injured hand. The danger is that you will miss something. If there is doubt, keep an open mind and assess the child from head to foot. A NP who has concerns or cannot assess the child should refer to the A&E department.

For a more detailed examination, the child should be close to the parent, preferably on the parent's knee. Be gentle. You may have to negotiate, divert the child, or you may be able to make a game or a joke out of the process. If you win the child, the parent will be with you too. Do not lie to the child and do not collude with the parent if the parent uses that route to persuasion. Explain what you are about to do and, without causing anxiety, let the child know if something will hurt. Do the painful thing last, it may be the last thing you get to do.

It can be difficult to strike the right note with an adolescent. A brash or sullen manner often covers a high level of anxiety or embarrassment. There is often a need for information and advice, and the patient should feel comfortable about asking questions. Health promotion is important but has to be offered in a sensitive way.

There can be considerable conflict between parent and teenager. In cases where a NP is treating the child in the presence of the parent, there may be pressure from either party to enlist the NP to browbeat the other.

Social problems, difficulties with drugs or alcohol or criminal offending may be part of the background to the injury, and other agencies may be involved.

Referrals

The setup of a minor injury clinic which sees children as patients must be overseen by the local children's consultants, and guidelines or protocols must be agreed for the referral and the transfer of the patient if that is needed.

Few patients at minor injury clinics are admitted to hospital. For most, any continuing care will be carried out by the primary care team. Direct referral can be made by giving the parents a letter for the practice nurse or GP, but there should also be a routine system for sending the GP a letter by post. Health visitors are an important part of the support system for children and families and do a good deal of work in accident prevention, health promotion and parenting skills, matters which may arise out of an attendance at your unit. A NP may contact a health visitor directly or may have a liaison health visitor for community contacts in the hospital.

Giving Medicines to Children

Calculation of the dosage of medicines for a child is usually based upon the child's weight, and this should be recorded on the patient's treatment sheet. It is easy to give a child an overdose of medicine.

It is likely that the only medicine which a NP in a minor injury clinic will prescribe for young children will be paracetamol elixir. Oral paracetamol in a child liquid suspension, such as Calpol, at a dosage of 15 mg/kg is very effective for the pain of minor wounds, burns, and musculoskeletal injuries.

Special Features of Children's Injuries

Pain

It is easy to overlook the need for analgesia in an injured child. Distress is often interpreted as fright, and silence as calm. Pain may be influencing either presentation, and the need for analgesia should be assessed rapidly. Other measures, such as the use of a broad arm sling to support a fracture, or cooling for a burn, should be offered at triage.

Musculoskeletal Problems

The clinical presentation of a child with a musculoskeletal problem, where the differential diagnosis includes fracture, should define the approach. A NP may be restricted in the X-ray films that can be requested. The film may show no abnormality. It may be difficult to interpret. Sometimes the demeanour of an injured child suggests that there is a fracture. As with the ill child, the patient may catch your eye by passivity rather than by any loud complaint. The child may be pale and quiet, and guarding the injured part. If this impression that there is something amiss is supported by a clinical appearance of a fracture, this should be the guide, rather than the radiograph. It will do no harm to ask for a medical opinion.

This section looks at musculoskeletal injuries to the limbs in general terms. The protocols or guidelines in a particular clinic may not allow X-ray of these injuries, and the patient will be referred after a clinical assessment.

Aspects of children's fractures are discussed in Chapter 5. Children's fractures (depending to some extent on their proximity to the epiphysis) heal much more quickly than those of adults. This means that the time when any realignment can be performed is shorter. Always refer for prompt review.

Children with open fractures are at a particular risk of osteomyelitis.

It is important to make an accurate assessment of fractures around the epiphyseal plate, because the more severe injuries may not heal well and may affect the growth of the bone. The Harris–Salter classification (Fig. 4.1) is widely used, with the injuries increasing in severity from I to V.

When callus develops around a fracture of the clavicle, the prominent swelling may alarm the patient and the family.

Upper limbs

Interpretation of a radiograph of a child's elbow is made difficult by the elaborate way in which ossification proceeds, at separate times, from six different focal points around the joint. The usual order of this process must be known in order to judge the significance of the apparently detached fragments of bone seen on the X-ray film of a child's elbow. Ossification starts at 6 months and continues until the child is 12 years of age; its pace varies but the order is usually the same. The acronym CRITOL, is used (**c**apitellum of the humerus, **r**adial head, **i**nternal (medial) epicondyle of the humerus, **t**rochlea of the humerus, **o**lecranon process of the ulna, **l**ateral epicondyle of the humerus). The most important clinical application of this information relates to fracture of the internal epicondyle of the humerus (Raby et al., 1995). The flexor muscles of the forearm, which are attached to the medial epicondyle of the elbow by a common tendon, can avulse the epicondyle and may displace it so far from its attachment point that it cannot be seen, or

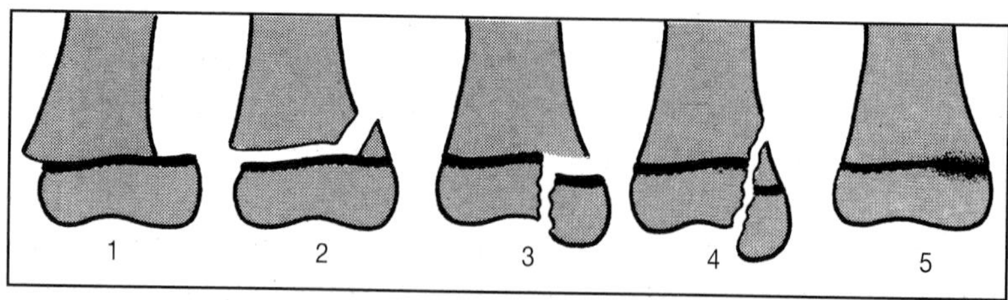

Figure 4.1 Harris and Salter classification of epiphyseal injuries. 1, epiphyseal slip only; 2, fracture through the epiphyseal plate with a triangular fragment of shaft attached to the epiphysis; 3, fracture through the epiphysis extending to the epiphyseal plate; 4, fracture through the epiphysis and shaft crossing the epiphyseal plate; 5, obliteration of the epiphyseal plate. (Reproduced with kind permission from Dandy and Edwards, 1998)

is misinterpreted on the X-ray film. The order of ossification can vary from person to person, but the trochlea always starts to ossify after the medial epicondyle. If the trochlea can be seen on the radiograph, but not the medial epicondyle, a displaced fracture has occurred. A lesser avulsion, where the medial epicondyle is pulled a small distance from the attachment, can be difficult to diagnose from the X-ray film, and the patient should be reviewed at A&E. The ulnar nerve passes behind the medial epicondyle and it should be assessed distal to the injury.

A supracondylar fracture at the elbow (Ch. 6) with anterior displacement of the distal part of the humerus is a threat to the circulation to the hand. The lack of a radial pulse is an emergency. The pulled elbow is also described in Chapter 6.

Fractures of the forearm can occur in combination with dislocations, and there may be combined elbow and wrist injuries. Make a full assessment of the forearm and wrist. Request X-ray films that will show all possible injuries.

Lower limbs

A child with an unexplained limp, and one who complains of pain at the hip or knee, should be assessed with care. If the knee is painful but there is no history of injury and no local findings to explain the symptoms, referral of pain from the hip should be excluded. There are various hip problems which are common in children, including irritable hip, osteomyelitis, septic arthritis, Perthes disease and slipped femoral epiphysis. Other systemic problems can also express themselves through pain at the hip. The history should include any recent injuries or illnessses. The patient's movement at the hip should be examined, the child's temperature and pulse documented and the child should be referred to a doctor.

A child (usually a girl) in the years before and during adolescence may suffer an acute dislocation or a traumatic partial dislocation of the patella. The dislocation is outwards, with stretching and trauma to the vastus medialis and associated soft tissue, and there may be a fracture at the patella. The patient will sometimes reflexively reduce the dislocation herself, or it may reduce spontaneously, and the event will have to be deduced from the history and clinical examination. This event may recur and may happen on the other knee. There are different reasons why the patella may dislocate, including an abnormality of tracking of the patella in the groove of the femur during movement. Physiotherapy to strengthen the vastus medialis sometimes helps, but some patients need surgery.

An active adolescent may present with no history of injury but pain at the front of the knee (sometimes both knees) over the insertion of the patellar ligament at the tibial tuberosity, brought on by exercise. The child will have tenderness and swelling at the painful place. This is a stress injury. Traction on the apophysis into which the patellar ligament is inserted causes it to avulse. The problem usually settles with a reduction in the most stressful forms of exercise.

Wounds

The same standards for wound care apply to children as to adults, although the difficulties in implementing them can be much greater. Dirty wounds must be cleaned thoroughly. A child with a wound will suffer great distress if prolonged or painful treatment is carried out unless the child has been properly sedated or anaesthetized. Refer if there is any doubt.

Many of the small lacerations which are seen in minor injury clinics are to forehead and chin. Children injure these areas more often than adults. If there is no concern about fracture, foreign body or dirt, these wounds are usually suitable for closure with steristrips. On the odd occasion when a laceration is longer or is gaping, think about the cosmetic implications and refer. Warn the child's parents that any laceration will leave a small scar, which will improve with time.

A staple closure of a scalp laceration will cause a few moments of pain, but it can be done quickly and it is a useful treatment for children. The patient can be reassured that removal of the staples, which should be done 5 days later, is painless.

If a freshly closed wound lies over a mobile site, such as a joint, precautions may be required with a young child to prevent reopening. Splinting for the first few days may be needed, and it may be necessary to review the patient to remove the splint and assess the wound. It is possible that children with wounds at such difficult sites should be referred, and NPs should not apply splints unless they know how to do so, and know the possible complications at any particular joint.

The question of tetanus immunity is discussed in Chapter 8. Children are usually protected but check on any who may not have been included in the system, such as travelling people and those from abroad.

Burns

The criteria for admission to hospital of a child with burns (Beattie et al., 1997) are:

- a burn greater than 5% of the total body surface area
- a full-thickness burn
- burn affecting 'difficult' area (Ch. 8)
- complications present (e.g. smoke inhalation)
- social circumstances poor.

Admission is always a possibility where a NAI is a possibility (see above).

A child's skin is thinner than that of an adult, and deep injuries are more easily achieved. There is a high correlation between burns and NAI.

Children with burns are especially at risk of **toxic shock syndrome** after a burn, from *Staphylococcus aureus* infection of the site. The burn may be small. Key symptoms are a systemic illness, high temperature and rash. This is an emergency, and you should warn parents to seek immediate help if symptoms develop.

Head injuries

Small children's heads are proportionately larger than those of adults, and this can cause overbalancing and injury to the head.

Repeated vomiting after a minor head injury will cause a child fluid-loss problems, regardless of the seriousness of the underlying condition, and a child may need admission for intravenous fluid replacement.

A child who is discharged after presentation with a minor head injury must go home to a responsible carer. The carer is given a sheet of written advice (Ch. 9) on complications which may develop. The child must be brought back to hospital, or see the GP, if there are any problems.

The indications for skull X-ray examination for a child with a head injury (Beattie et al., 1997) are:

- loss of consciousness
- large laceration/wound
- scalp haematoma
- clinical fracture
- focal signs/seizures
- altered level of consciousness
- suspected NAI
- difficult assessment
- severe mechanism of injury, e.g. hit with a hammer, fall greater than 5 metres.

The indications for hospital admission for a child with a head injury (Beattie et al., 1997) are:

- skull fracture
- altered level of consciousness
- decreasing level of consciousness
- focal signs/seizures
- suspected non-accidental injury
- social.

Two scales are in common use for the assessment of the level of consciousness in a child, the modified Glasgow Coma Scale and **AVPU** (in this acronym each letter signifies a lower level of consciousness than the preceeding: A, awake, V, responds to voice, P, responds to pain, U, unconscious). For the purposes of the NP in a minor injuries clinic, AVPU is much the more useful tool. It is simple, easy to remember, and sufficient for the initial assessment of the patient.

There are a number of important differences between adults and children with head injuries (Wrightson and Gronwall, 1999):

- children under 7 years of age have a large head, with relatively weak neck muscles
- the skull is more elastic
- the meningeal arteries can be torn without a fracture
- extradural haemorrhage can occur with no loss of consciousness, bruise or fracture
- those under 5 years of age may have a delayed systemic response, of up to 3 or 4 hours, to injury
- status epilepticus is a possible complication of head injury in young children.

Neck

The flexibility of a child's spine may permit a serious injury to the spinal cord with no fracture, a phenomenon named SCIWORA (spinal cord injury without radiological abnormality). The mechanism will usually be severe: a road traffic accident or a fall from a height of 5 metres. If a child has suffered a mechanism which could produce neck injury, such as a significant head, trunk or spine injury, leg fractures, or if the patient has neck pain, radiating pain or neurological deficits, the neck should be immobilized in a hard collar with sandbags to position the head until a full assessment can be carried out.

A child with torticollis should be seen by a doctor. A local infection (such as tonsilitis) should be ruled out. Atlanto-axial rotatory fixation (AARF) is a traumatic, fixed spinal rotation at C1 and C2, which requires early treatment. Other reasons for torticollis include congenital problems and minor injury.

5 BASICS OF MUSCULOSKELETAL INJURY AND EXAMINATION

CONTENTS

This chapter discusses musculoskeletal injuries in general. It offers the information which is needed to assess, diagnose and treat a minor, musculoskeletal injury. Part 2 deals with injuries to particular areas of the body. Limb injury forms the largest part of the work of a minor injuries clinic, but it makes little sense to look at the arm and the leg without relating them to their central origins. Therefore, in Part 2 the chapters look at the neck in relation to the arm, and the lower back in relation to the leg. Minor rib injuries are discussed along with the back.

With all but the most minor of problems, musculoskeletal injuries are slow to heal, sometimes taking more than a year for complete recovery. Many patients will receive medical attention more than once during that time. It may be that the patient will be reviewed in the minor injury clinic or may be referred to a GP, physiotherapist, orthopaedic specialist or other agency. However, the main task of someone working in an emergency service is to deal with the injury at the time it happens, and this section will focus on the problems of early management rather than the details of later rehabilitation.

The process of looking after patients with acute musculoskeletal injuries can be divided into triage, taking the patient's personal details, taking a history, examination, investigation, diagnosis and treatment.

The NP often works in a busy clinic, with pressure to see patients quickly. The NP must examine the patient, a task which first level nursing training does not cover. A NP is restricted in the investigations that can be ordered. The injuries are often acute, and the examination is made difficult by initial distress, pain, swelling and disability, which can mask the underlying injury. It is not always certain that the patient is injured. The patient may be ill; therefore, it may not, at this stage, be possible to make a diagnosis and an examination would be confined to a broad assessment to rule out severe problems. The NP begins the patient's treatment but may refer to someone else if the problems are medical, if there are complications or if further help is needed with treatment.

In this situation the role of the NP is to take a history (Ch. 3) and perform an initial assessment. The technical skill needed above any other is clinical examination. The NP should develop a routine of thorough, basic examination and will need a knowledge of anatomy and the principles of examination which will allow interpretation of any findings. These chapters will provide that information.

Terminology

The language of anatomy is used when writing patient records and making referrals. Some general terms are defined in this part. Additional new terms are introduced in bold type at the relevant parts of the text.

Anatomical position (Fig. 5.1) This is the pose upon which anatomical description is based. The body is standing, symmetrical, feet together with hands at the sides, palms to the front. The terms which follow should be read with this position in mind. A medical professional who reads examination notes will assume that the descriptions are based on that image.

Right and left Always means the patient's right and left, not the examiner's.

Axis and plane (Fig. 5.1) An axis is an imagined line (which sometimes corresponds to the line of a real structure) around which movement happens. A plane is a flat surface. The idea of the body divided by imaginary planes is useful for describing the direction and angle of movement. Three basic planes are described, each at right angles to the others. A **sagittal plane** is vertical, passes from front to back and divides the body into left and right parts. A **sagittal axis** is a horizontal line passing from front to back on a sagittal plane. Movement about this axis (e.g. abduction and adduction of the hip) happens on a coronal plane. A **coronal plane** (also called **frontal**) is vertical, passes from side to side and divides the body into front and back parts. A **coronal axis** is a horizontal line passing from side to side on a coronal plane. Movement about this axis (e.g. flexion and extension of the hip) happens on a sagittal plane. A **transverse plane** is horizontal and divides the body into upper and lower parts. A **longitudinal axis** is a vertical line about which certain movements (e.g. lateral rotation of the shoulder) occur on a transverse plane.

Anterior (ventral) and posterior (dorsal) Anterior (or ventral) means to the front and posterior (or dorsal), to the back.

Superior (cranial) and inferior (caudal) Superior (or cranial, 'towards the head') means above and inferior (or caudal, literally 'towards the tail') means below.

Lateral and medial Lateral means away from and medial means closer to the midline of the body.

Proximal and distal Proximal means closer to and distal further from the origin of a limb or other structure (e.g. the elbow is proximal to the wrist, and the wrist is distal to the elbow, both in relation to the origin of the arm, which is the shoulder).

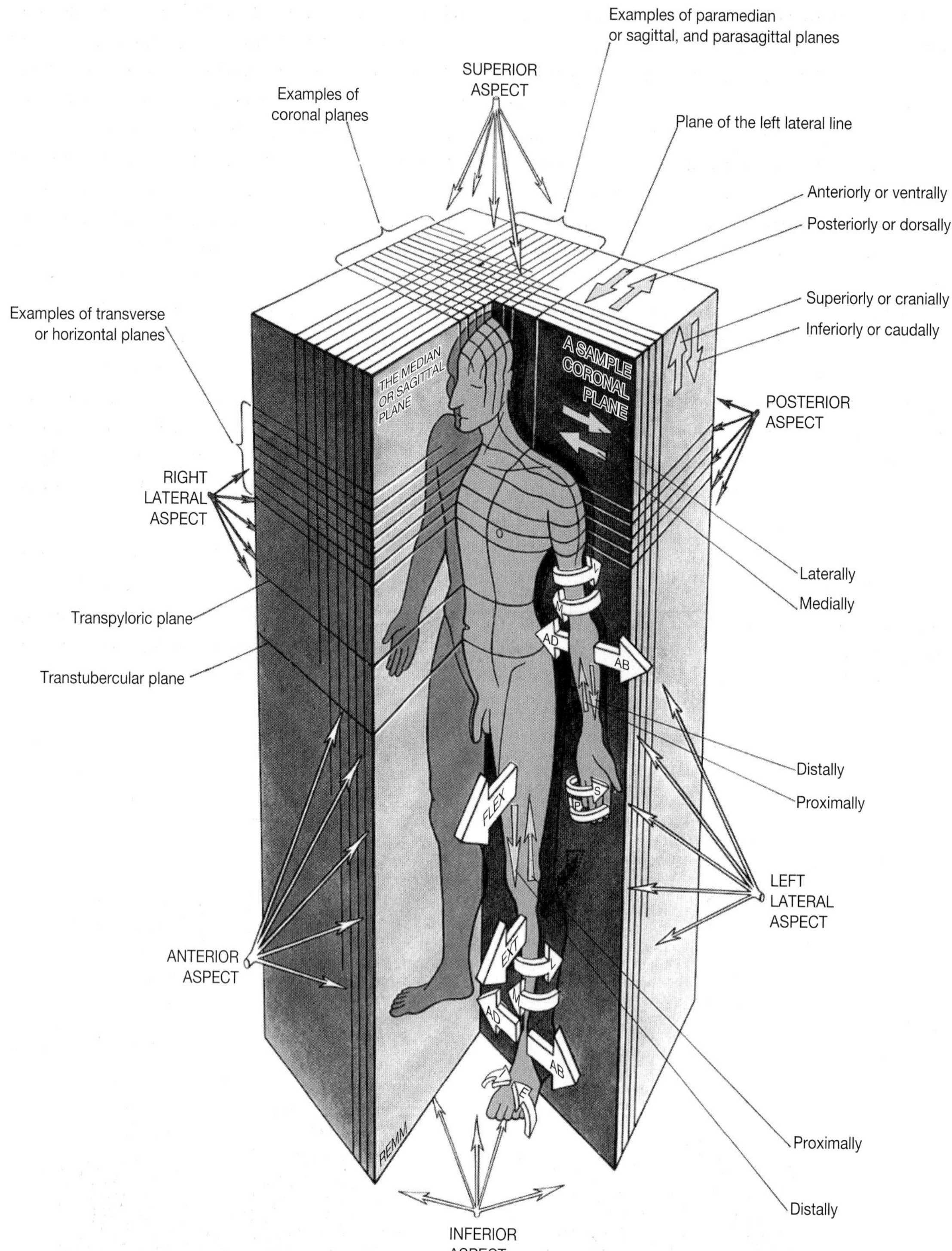

Figure 5.1 Terminology of anatomical position. AD, adduction; AB, abduction; FLEX, flexion; EXT, extension; M and L, medial and lateral rotation; P, pronation; S, supination; I, inversion; E, eversion. (Adapted with kind permission from Williams, 1995.)

Flexion and extension Flexion is movement at a joint which reduces the angle between the bones on the sagittal plane. Extension is the opposite movement at the same joint (e.g. the elbow flexes to bring the hand nearer to the shoulder and extends to bring upper arm and forearm into a straight line). Note that flexion occurs in an anterior direction at the elbow and in a posterior direction at the knee, but both movements occur on the same plane. Special terms are used for flexion and extension at the ankle (Fig. 5.2). The foot joins the leg like the crosspiece on an upturned letter T. The angle between foot and leg is reduced by movement in either direction, which makes a distinction between flexion and extension difficult. Therefore, movement of the foot towards the shin is **dorsiflexion** and pointing the toes is **plantar flexion** (the sole of the foot is called the **plantar** surface and the opposite surface is the **dorsum**).

Abduction and adduction Abduction is movement away from the midline of the body on a coronal plane, for example at the shoulder when the arm is lifted away from the side (Fig. 5.3). In the hand, abduction is movement of the fingers away from the midline of the middle finger. In the foot, the toes abduct from the midline of the second toe. Adduction is movement towards the midline. Certain movements on the coronal plane cross the midline and combine abduction and adduction; consequently, these words are not useful. Movement to the side at the cervical and lumbar spine is **lateral flexion**, or side flexion, to right or left. Side-to-side movement of the hand at the wrist is called **deviation**, and its directions are named for the forearm bone that the hand moves towards, **ulnar** and **radial**. In other words, movement of the hand, at the wrist, towards the little finger is ulnar deviation and towards the thumb is radial deviation.

Circumduction This is a fluent sequence of four movements, flexion, abduction, extension and adduction, at one joint, to make a single circular movement. Hip, shoulder, wrist and base of thumb are all capable of circumduction.

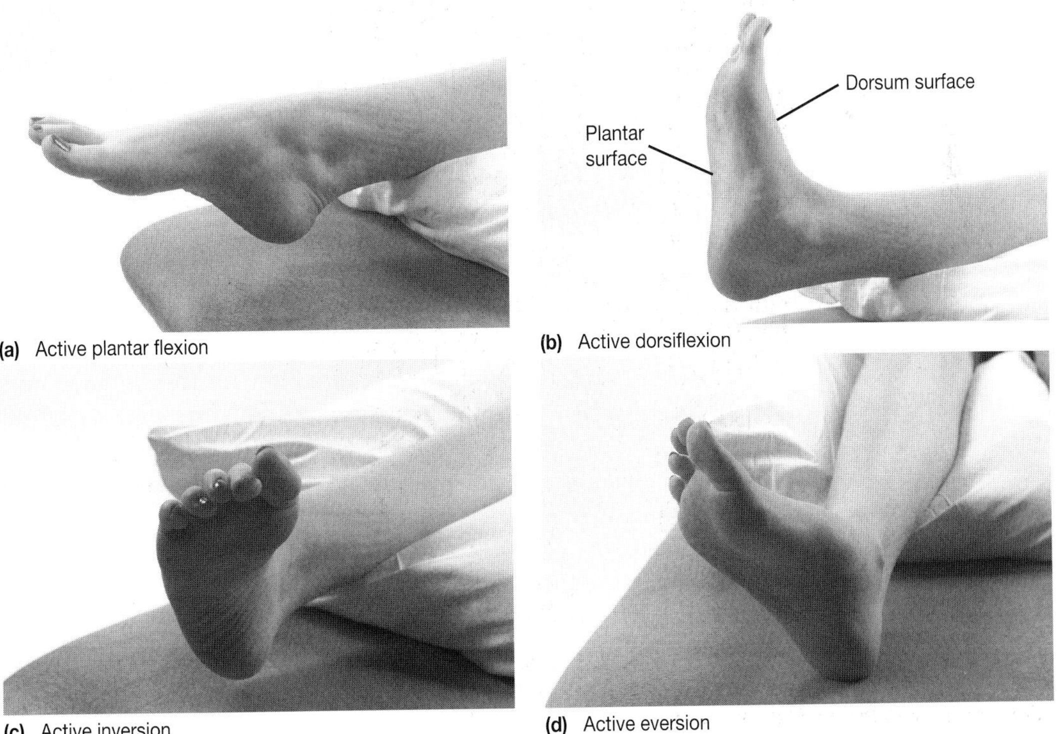

(a) Active plantar flexion

(b) Active dorsiflexion

(c) Active inversion

(d) Active eversion

Figure 5.2 Movements at foot and ankle.

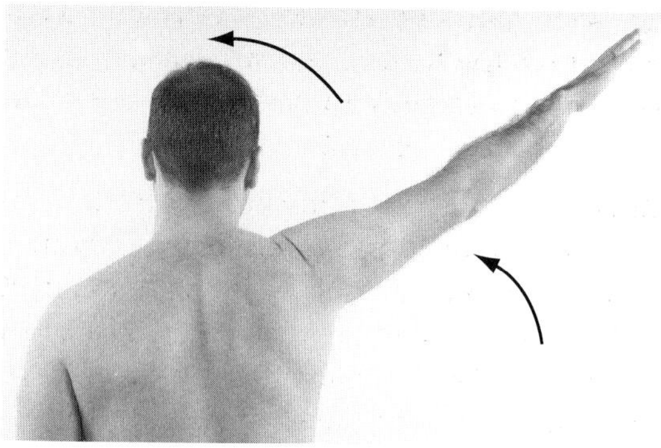

Figure 5.3 **Abduction of the shoulder.**

Rotation A movement of a bone around a longitudinal axis (e.g. at the neck, shoulder and hip) is known as rotation; towards the midline of the body is **medial** or **internal** rotation and away from the midline is **lateral or external** rotation.

Supine and prone Supine means face up and prone face down. **Supination** of the hand is movement to the palm-up position by lateral rotation of the forearm. **Pronation** of the hand means turning the palm down. Supination of the foot means raising its medial edge, a movement more commonly called **inversion**. Similarly, pronation of the foot, lifting its lateral edge, is usually called **eversion** (Fig. 5.2). (This is simplified. Foot and ankle movements are complex, multijoint combinations.)

Valgus and varus These terms describe direction, often of an abnormally angled bone. They always refer to the direction of the distal part of the deformity. Valgus means angulation away from the midline of the body (e.g. knock knees). Varus means an angulation towards the midline (e.g. bow legs).

The Musculoskeletal System and Healing

This part introduces musculoskeletal anatomy and contains general information on the healing process and the principles of treatment of injuries. This is followed by a survey of anatomy, types of injury and healing and treatment of each of the tissues of the musculoskeletal system. Particular injuries are described at the appropriate places in Part 2.

The Musculoskeletal System

The musculoskeletal system is a frame made of segments of hard connective tissue, **bone**, held together by various softer connective tissues (skeletal muscle, tendons, cartilage, ligaments, synovium, bursa and fascia). Connective tissue is characterized by large amounts of extracellular material, mainly the proteins **collagen** and **elastin**, which give it strength and resilience. The frame is moved, at its **joints**, by the contractile skeletal **muscles**. The functions of the musculoskeletal system are protection of the organs, movement and stability.

Movement and stability are conflicting priorities. Stability is easily attained by lying down and doing nothing. In our waking lives we stand erect, we move around, we reach out with our hands, we give up absolute stability so that we can interact with the world around us. Stability becomes relative and dynamic, subordinate to movement but indispensable.

Our stability may be challenged by the forces which we meet in the world beyond our bodies. Internally, the forces generated by our own muscles and the alterations caused by our slightest movements require an endless stream of stabilizing adjustments.

The structure of different parts of the musculoskeletal system, and the problems to which they are prone, reflect, in part, this trade-off between movement and stability. The shoulder is highly mobile but prone to dislocation. The knee will accept heavy loads but can be injured by slight abnormal movements.

Severity of Injury

Various labels are used for the severity of soft tissue injuries, and certain aspects of description are peculiar to individual tissues. There is a general tendency to assign injuries, especially tears to ligament or muscle, which make up the bulk of acute soft tissue injuries, to one of three categories. These may be called grades 1, 2 and 3, or minor, moderate and severe.

In the minor clinic, these distinctions are made by assessing the severity of the mechanism of injury, the appearance of the injury, and the pain and disability it has caused. It is suggested, for the NP, that this grading system can be used to clarify documentation and the pathway for managing the patient's injury.

Grade 1 A grade 1 injury will typically damage only a small number of fibres, perhaps 5% in the case of a muscle (although this figure is meaningless in the clinical setting, where only examination findings are useful). It will cause pain when the part is used or stressed, and perhaps some visible swelling and bruising, but the patient will not be disabled and recovery should be uncomplicated. Severe signs such as deformity, heavy bruising, inability to walk will be absent. The NP will discharge the patient with clear advice on the care of the injury, and advice to seek further help if it is not improving.

Grade 2 A grade 2 injury will have been caused by a more severe mechanism and there will be a larger number of damaged fibres. The bleeding and the disability will be greater; there may be some abnormal laxity in the case of a ligament or a painful loss of function in the muscle. There will not be a complete division of the whole structure (if there is doubt about this, the NP will treat the patient as having a grade 3 injury). The patient will, if resources are available to match the best management pathway, receive advice and treatment from the NP for the first stage of care and will return promptly to have the injury managed by a physiotherapist.

Grade 3 A grade 3 injury is a complete division of an injured tissue, most commonly ligament, tendon or muscle belly. The most notable clinical finding will be a complete loss of function in the injured part. Pain may or may not be present, depending on other factors such as inflammation. It will not, however, hurt to stress the torn tissue, simply because it will not be possible to put stress on a divided structure. Clinical findings, such as deformity, absence of the structure in its normal position, visible and palpable gaps in the structure, abnormal laxity of movement, will support the suspicion of a grade 3 injury. The NP will refer patients in whom there is a suspected grade 3 injury to a doctor.

Tissue Healing

The various tissues of the musculoskeletal system have different capacities to heal and renew themselves. However, it is possible to describe the process of healing in general terms and to propose some basic principles for the treatment of injuries.

Scarring

The optimum form of healing is replacement of injured cells with identical new cells, so that the tissue looks and functions exactly as before. Skin has a high, but not absolute, capacity to regenerate itself in this manner, and it tends to heal relatively quickly. Other tissues, including some in the musculoskeletal system, heal slowly and replace injured tissue with an inert, tough, fibrous tissue which forms a scar at the injury site. Ligament can take more than a year to heal and cartilage may not heal at all.

Scar tissue in a moving part such as ligament or muscle causes problems. The scar cannot reproduce the functions of its host. It is strong but inelastic. It shrinks as it forms, distorting the balance of the surrounding tissue. It may block nerve impulses. It may give rise to adhesions and be the site of complications such as chronic inflammation, pain and calcification of muscle or ligament. The host tissue will probably not return to full function and may be prone to reinjury.

Many patients arrive in a minor injury clinic with acute injuries such as muscle tears and small sprains. These tend to be seen as 'self-limiting', not serious, but they may have a better outcome with treatment which minimizes the problems caused by the scar.

Cyriax & Cyriax (1993) declare the aim of recovery, when moving parts are injured, to be 'the formation of a strong and *mobile* scar'. This means that 'healing must take place in the presence of movement'. However, healing of a soft tissue occurs through several phases, each requiring a different approach. A premature return to exercise can be as damaging as prolonged inaction.

The healing of soft tissue injuries is normally described in three phases, with graduated changes in the treatment of each phase.

The inflammatory phase

Inflammation is a non-specific response of the body to injury or infection. Its chief signs are **redness**, **heat**, **swelling** and **pain**. When inflammation affects a moving part it will also cause **disability**, a fact which matters if the injury is to heal 'in the presence of movement'. Injury damages blood vessels and cells. These release chemicals which cause a momentary **vasoconstriction** followed by a prolonged **vasodilatation** at the site of the injury. Blood fluids full of clotting factors and antibodies swell the area, causing the signs of inflammation. These substances form a clot from which the construction of healing tissue will begin. **Macrophages** begin to remove waste material from the area.

The inflammatory phase, in the patient's experience, is dominated by pain, swelling and disruption of normal routines and sleep. It usually lasts for 2 to 7 days. The first aim of treatment is to reduce the severity of these symptoms and to ensure that inflammation is banished as early as possible. Regeneration is yet to begin. Recommend rest rather than movement.

Some complaints, such as supraspinatus tendonitis (Ch. 7) show a non-infective, chronic inflammation which can last for years. Inflammation then becomes the main problem, rather than a stage on the road to healing. It may cause pain and disability with degeneration, scarring and the risk of rupture of the tissue. In these cases, a more active treatment of inflammation is required.

The Proliferative phase

The proliferative (or organization) phase begins as the period of acute inflammation ends.

Fibroblasts synthesize collagen; macrophages remove the haematoma, and a frail network of new capillaries begins to grow. The new scar is developing.

At this stage, a certain amount of movement will improve the organization of the scar and its ability to cope with the loads that normal use will place on it. However, heavy exertion will damage the delicate new tissues. Prescribing the correct type and degree of exercise is important. If the injury is more than minimal, early advice from a physiotherapist is invaluable.

The maturation phase

The last stage of healing, known as the maturation or remodelling phase, is prolonged, lasting for up to 2 years.

The tissue combines regeneration and fibrosis and develops new tissue or a mature scar. A developing scar becomes stronger in response to the stresses placed on it, loses vascularity and shrinks. Excess tissue produced around the wound during the earlier phases is reabsorbed.

The patient will gradually return to full activity during this phase.

Treatment of Acute Injury

The treatment of broken bone is dealt with below. This part will cover the treatment of acute injuries to the other musculoskeletal tissues. These are often classed together as **soft tissue injuries** and discussed as one category. This is a generalization. There are a variety of soft tissues, and they suffer different injuries which require different treatments.

Holistic Care

It is essential to assess not only the physical effect of a patient's injury but also the effect it will have on the patient's life; treatment should be modified to help with any problems.

The history should bring out the necessary information. Patients who have injured their hands need also to be asked if they are right or left handed, what their jobs are, what are their hobbies. Patients who are unable to walk should be asked about where they live and whether they have stairs. Elderly patients should be asked their circumstances and whether there is someone who can lend a hand at home.

Patients who are injured at work may have problems related to their jobs. They may be casual workers, or self-employed, and feel unable to take time off to rest an injury. The patient should be advised on the best management of the injury and reminded that safety at work must not be endangered. However, nothing is achieved by rigidly advocating a course of action which cannot be achieved. Discuss available options. Are light duties available? Can schedules be reorganized? It may help the patient in dealing with the employer to give a copy of the treatment sheet, bearing clear advice to rest. (The patient should not normally go to a GP for a sickness certificate until after a week's absence from work.) The NP may also be able to speed recovery by referral to a physiotherapist.

The treatment of sports injuries is becoming a separate specialty. Young, growing athletes often need counselling on safe levels of training and the dangers of recurring injury and overuse. They feel pressure to achieve and they may be impatient of the restrictions caused by injury. Young athletes are also prone to patterns of injury, such as growth plate injuries and bone avulsions, which are specific to their stage of development. Do not ignore a complaint because the history is vague. Seek advice when a problem is not settling down in the expected way.

Treatment in the Inflammatory Stage

Treatment of a fresh soft tissue injury in the minor injury clinic is basically the management of the inflammatory stage of healing. This is normally a period of 2 to 3 days but may, depending on the severity of the problem, be as little as 1 day or as much as a week.

Inflammation is a source of pain and disability and, if prolonged, inhibits healing and may worsen scarring and other complications. The aim of treatment is to minimize the period of inflammation and reduce swelling. The method of doing this is known by the acronym PRICE, which means **protection**, **rest**, **ice**, **compression** and **elevation**.

Surprisingly, although some approximation to this method of treatment is found everywhere, there has been no consensus on whether or how it works and its optimum application. The Chartered Society of Physiotherapy has tried to address this by issuing a set of guidelines, based on a review of the evidence, for the management of soft tissue injuries during the first 72 hours. This section is based upon that work.

Protection

The idea of protection is to prevent tension on a freshly injured tissue. There are two reasons for this.

1. The tissue will become weakened, over a period of days, in proportion to the severity of the injury, while the inflammatory phase progresses. It may not be clear at the outset how severe this weakness will become.
2. The new fibres which will appear at the site of the injury when healing begins will be frail, and undue stress on the tissue will disrupt them.

Methods of protection are many and are adapted to the part of the body affected, the severity of the injury, the lifestyle of the patient and other factors. They may include bedrest, crutches, plaster casts, strapping, splints and slings.

It is desirable to minimize the intervention as much as possible while still achieving the aim. Complete immobilization of the injury, or of the patient, will have adverse results.

Swelling is a feature of the fresh injury, and any treatment should allow for it.

Rest

There is a conflict between the need for rest and the benefits which healing tissues gain from movement. Overuse of a fresh injury may lead to more severe scarring and poorer muscle regeneration, but prolonged immobilization causes new fibres to be weak and badly organized, and patient recovery is slower.

A middle-ground approach, tailored to the severity of the injury, is required.

Patients are often reluctant to rest. Some people are simply impatient, and others have difficult lives. The problem is at its worst when a leg is injured and the patient is asked not to walk.

Nevertheless, rest is the cornerstone of early treatment. Deterioration in the cells and fibres of injured tissues can continue for up to a day after the incident. This can be aggravated by use of the injured part. Swelling will worsen, increasing pain and reducing mobility. The second stage of healing will be delayed and prejudiced.

Rest means not using the injured part, usually for 2 days but in more severe injuries, for up to a week. This time should be spent on the other parts of the early treatment, ice, elevation, compression and elevation. Emphasize that time invested now in healing may save time later and lead to a better outcome.

Ice

Putting ice on an acute injury (sometimes called **cryotherapy**) has multiple benefits. The cold reduces nerve conduction, and this is the probable reason why it relieves pain after a brief period when it may feel uncomfortable. The metabolism of oxygen is slowed down at the injury site. This reduces the rate of cell death caused by lack of oxygen, with a beneficial knock-on reduction in the inflammatory process.

The ice pack causes local vasoconstriction, which helps to stop bleeding.

Ice is thought to reduce swelling, but it is hard to assess this in the clinical situation because ice is normally used in combination with elevation and compression, and the contribution of the different components of the treatment is unclear. There is experimental evidence which suggests that ice alone may actually increase swelling.

It is noticeable that the guidelines urge the value of ice in the first few hours after injury and are less emphatic about its use in later days. This seems to be because the claimed benefits from ice which research actually confirms are all most useful in the early hours. The main reason for continuing use, the reduction of swelling, is not upheld by current research.

Certain risks and contraindications, with greater or lesser degrees of evidential support, apply to the use of ice.

There is some evidence that prolonged use of ice may trigger a reflex vasodilatation (the so-called **hunting response**, a reflex which is thought to prevent tissue damage in cold conditions). An increase in blood flow would be counterproductive.

Ice should not be put directly against skin or left on for too long. There is the potential for an ice burn, a frostbite injury, if it is overused or applied without a suitable barrier.

Peripheral nerves which lie near the skin can suffer injury from ice. Thin people are more susceptible to the effects of ice than those who have plentiful subcutaneous fat, and the recommended times of application should be adjusted accordingly.

Certain patients should not use ice. Ice should not be placed over a cut, to an area of poor circulation or reduced sensation, in the case of increased or reduced sensitivity to cold, and where a skin condition exists. Be wary with patients suffering from diabetes, peripheral vascular disease, peripheral neuropathy, sickle cell anaemia and Raynaud's disease.

The Chartered Society of Physiotherapy recommends the following:

- Apply ice to a fresh injury
- Crushed ice on top of a wet cloth seems to have the best penetration
- Cover the whole area which is injured
- The bigger the circumference of the part which is injured, and the thicker the layer of subcutaneous fat, the longer it takes for ice to cool the deep tissues. Thirty minutes is the maximum recommended time to leave an ice pack on, and this should be reduced where there may be complications. The treatment can be repeated 2 hourly.

Compression

A compression bandage discourages bleeding and swelling by exerting circumferential pressure on the limb. It offers benefits during the first 3 days after injury.

Misapplication of pressure, or poor timing of its use, may have undesirable effects. It may cause an *increase* in swelling.

Compression should not be used in combination with elevation or when the patient is lying down, because it can compromise the circulation to the area.

For the same reason, the bandage should not be applied while the limb is raised, must not be tighter at its proximal end than its distal, and should be applied in a distal to proximal direction. The standard compression bandage is the double-layer tubigrip, applied, in the appropriate width, from the joint above the injury to the joint below the injury. (The guidelines state that tubigrip is regarded as an effective compression agent but are unclear about the fact that tubigrip tends to apply greater proximal than distal pressure because it is not graduated in width, while limbs taper to ankle and wrist.) It offers gentle compression only, if correctly fitted and is unlikely to restrict the circulation. Patients generally report that it gives comfort and some ease to the injury. It is easy for the patient to put it on himself, a factor which makes crepe bandage impractical if the compression is to be removed and reapplied often.

The chief hazard of a compression bandage is that it may restrict the circulation too much. Give the patient a few minutes to assess the comfort of any bandage, check the capillary refill yourself. The patient should remove the bandage if it becomes uncomfortable.

Elevation

The drainage of swelling from the limbs is easier if the patient can reverse the burden of gravity on the venous circulation by raising the injured part above the level of the heart.

The arm needs comfortable support on cushions or pillows so that the hand can be raised to head height or higher and kept there. The ankle will only be raised above the level of the heart if the patient lies down and props the feet above the level of the chest.

Compression should not be combined with elevation.

Other aspects of treatment

Exercise

The prescription of exercise for the injured patient is a task for the physiotherapist. However, not every patient can be sent to a physiotherapist and patients with mild injuries should be given simple advice on exercise after injury. When the problem is more severe, the patient should be advised on the management of the injury until the physiotherapy visit.

This section offers an outline of the use of exercise, during the three stages of soft tissue healing and the thinking behind the advice offered to patients. Beware: this is not a blueprint for action. These techniques should only be used by appropriately qualified people. Advice to the patient should be based on the individual, the injury and other circumstances, and it should be simple and cautious. Consult the local orthopaedic and physiotherapy services and make advice compatible with their practice and policies.

The purpose of exercise in the treatment of an injury is to maintain those parts which are not affected by the injury, to restore the parts which are damaged and to allow the patient to return to normal function.

Exercise treatment is used to improve **flexibility**, **strength**, and **coordination**.

Exercise in the inflammatory phase

During the 2 days after injury, the patient will experience pain, swelling and loss of function of the injured part. There may be muscle spasm. The priority of treatment at this stage is rest and protection of the injury, and the reduction of swelling.

There is no role for active movement or stretching of the injured part. In the case of a muscle injury, this could increase bleeding and separate the torn fibres. If the injury is to a joint, it could increase pain and swelling. If pain is too severe for comfortable exercise, or if exercise triggers pain, it should not be attempted.

Adhesion of an injured ligament to bone is a complication which very gentle passive movement of the joint, without stretching, may help to prevent. Massage of the ligament fibres may also help.

The muscles around the injured joint are prone to wasting and progressive weakness. **Isometric** exercise, a contraction of the muscle maintained for 6 seconds without changing its length, can help to maintain tone without disturbing the joint. A gentle form of isometric contraction, called **muscle setting** (contraction without external resistance), is used at this stage, with the joint in a comfortable, neutral position. It is sufficient to increase circulation and delay wasting, and it can reduce spasm. It can also be valuable for injured muscle, provided that the muscle is in a relaxed position. It can reduce shrinkage of the scar. However, it will be counterproductive if the muscle contracts in a stretched position, or too forcefully, and tears the healing fibres.

When muscle is torn, it is difficult to keep mobility in the surrounding joints because the muscle should not be stretched. **Joint play** exercises allow some mobility to be maintained without stress on the injured tissue. These exercises form a passive exploration of the joint's range of **accessory movements** (see below), by **distraction** (pulling apart the joint surfaces), **compression** of the joint surfaces, **gliding** (moving the joint surfaces across each other) and **rotation**.

The patient should maintain parts not affected by the injury by active movements, taking care not to involve the inflamed area.

Exercise in the proliferative phase

The new tissue which is laid down during the healing phase aligns its fibres in the direction of the stresses which it experiences. In other words, it develops its strength to cope with the tasks which are imposed on it. The forming scar is more elastic and less shrunken if it develops in the presence of movement. Collagenous fibres which are laid down at an immobile injury are badly organized and weak, and the scar is shrivelled. There may also be other complications such as adhesion and contracture.

However, the new tissue is very frail, and violent exercise can damage it, reignite inflammation (sometimes in a chronic cycle) and worsen scarring.

In the proliferative phase, there should be less pain, less swelling and an increased range of movement. If the exercise programme is too heavy, there may be a return of earlier symptoms, and the aim is to avoid this and make improvement at a pace which is comfortable.

There can be some resumption of active and weight-bearing exercise, using aids such as splints, strapping and walking sticks (see below). Isometric exercise, below the intensity which causes pain, can continue.

Specific difficulties can be addressed, joint restriction and shortness of muscle, by combinations of stretching, passive joint play and isometric exercise, depending on the features of the problem.

Exercise in the remodelling phase

As the new collagen strengthens, the exercise programme should, in a graduated programme, subject it to the types of stress which it will face in normal life. Attention must still be paid to any adverse symptoms. If the new tissue is injured, the risks of regression, chronic inflammation, restricted movement and poor healing are still there.

The difficulties of reintegrating the injured part into the body's overall activity must be addressed. If the injury has involved sensory nerves, it may be that there is a loss of **proprioception**, the capacity of the brain to control movement in that part of the body. The aim of rehabilitation must be to regain full coordination of healthy and injured tissues. The programme will progress from uncomplicated to multidirection movement, and to movements which challenge the patient's coordination. The intensity and nature of such a programme will depend upon the activity the patient is returning to, whether an office worker, a builder, an athlete or a couch potato. The target is to restore full function as the patient knew it before the injury.

Problems such as weakness in the muscles around an injured joint, or restriction in the joints around an injured muscle, together with any other complications such as adhesions must be addressed by the means already described. Splints and other devices may still be required until any imbalance between joint and muscle has been rectified.

Heat

The effect of heat on an injury is to increase the blood flow and stimulate cell activity. Its benefits include a decrease in muscle spasm, a reduction of pain and a spur to the healing process. It may also help to prepare tissues for a session of exercise.

Heat should not be used in the first stage of healing, when the objective is to reduce swelling and inflammation.

A simple way to warm injured tissue, and to relax muscle which is in spasm, is to use a hot water bottle – take care to avoid burns. There are various packs and rubefacient rubs which are more or less effective.

The patient must avoid painful levels of heat, prolonged use of heat and irritant and allergy-provoking substances.

Any person with a tendency to bleed or a restricted circulation, poor sensation or malignancy should avoid the use of heat treatment.

Ultrasound

Ultrasound is a treatment normally used by physiotherapists and has several applications for musculoskeletal injuries. It sends high-frequency sound waves, through the medium of gel on the skin, directly into tissue.

Its effects are described as **thermal** and **non-thermal**. The thermal effects are similar to those of other forms of heat therapy. Non-thermal effects improve the healing environment by stimulating tissue renewal and reducing swelling.

Ultrasound is helpful for the reduction of haematoma, swelling, spasm, certain kinds of pain, myositis ossificans, adhesions and contractures.

Walking aids

The walking aids which are commonly available in a minor clinic are walking sticks and wooden axilla crutches.

Patients often resist the idea of using a walking aid. For those patients who need one, it is a part of their treatment. Emphasize that it is not regarded as optional.

A patient who needs a walking aid probably also needs review, either by the NP or the physiotherapist. This can be a good time to reclaim the walking aid. Failure to retrieve walking aids is an expensive problem which is well known in all emergency departments. The usual indication for giving axilla crutches is that the patient is completely unable to walk.

The indications for giving a walking stick are that walking is painful, that the patient has a severe limp or that the patient's gait is unstable and unsafe. Explain the need for a normal walking pattern. First, healing tissues should organise new fibres for their intended purpose. The scar must be formed 'in the presence of movement' (Cyriax & Cyriax, 1993), and the movement should be as close as possible to normal movement. Second, a patient walking for any length of time in any manner other than normal will stress other parts of the body, and this will lead to more trouble.

Elderly patients will rarely cope with crutches, which require strong arms, balance and agility, and judgement in hazardous places such as roads, kitchens and stairs. A zimmer frame is sometimes useful for the injured elderly, but it requires some ability to bear weight on the injury and is not a substitute for axilla crutches. Treatment may have to be directed primarily to the patient's immobility rather than the injury itself. This may involve crisis community care or hospital admission.

Splints, strapping and slings

Splints, strapping and slings are used to prevent movement around one or more joints. The immobilization of fractures is discussed below. Some of the devices mentioned here are also used for bone injuries.

Devices used in the minor injury clinic for immobilizing injured parts include the wrist brace, the thumb spica, buddy strapping for fingers and toes, the soft collar and the collar and cuff sling for the shoulder. Plaster of Paris is sometimes used for severe soft tissue injuries.

The degree of immobilization varies depending on what is possible at the particular joint, on the device used and on the intended effect of the treatment. There are different indications for the use of these devices, and some of these will be discussed throughout the book.

Splints should be used with care. Restriction of movement can lead to complications, such as stiffness, contracture, wasting, weakness and adhesion. Certain joints, notably in the hand, can suffer permanent contracture if they are splinted in an unsafe position. Strapping at a fresh injury can restrict circulation if the swelling increases. A splint should only be used for a clear reason based on accepted principles of treatment and the particular patient's condition. Advice should be given, preferably written, on how it is to be used, any possible complications and an appropriate exercise routine.

Rest is the foundation of the PRICE programme, and a splint or similar device will certainly rest a joint. However, complete immobilization is not necessarily the same thing as rest. In the case of a bleeding muscle, a patient may need to rest completely, whereas one with a ligament tear may be advised to perform gentle movement to prevent adhesions. PRICE is usually recommended for 2–3 days only, after which movement is gradually introduced. The advice on the use of the splint should be consistent with the rest of the treatment.

Relief of pain and other symptoms

Random movement of an injured joint may be the main source of a patient's pain. The muscles in an injured neck may go into spasm. Support might do more than any other measure to make the patient comfortable. The most painful phase of an injury may only last for a couple of days. The patient should be advised to wean off the splint and on to gentle exercise after this time.

Supported movement

Physiotherapists will sometimes use strapping to stabilize a painful joint so that the patient can begin to exercise it. Sportsmen often use strapping to stabilize an injury while they play. Application of this kind of strapping is a specialized skill.

Safety

In cases where complete examination is deferred to a later day, or where a patient is to be transferred with an unstable injury, a splint may be of value in preventing any worsening of the problem.

The decision to immobilize a joint may have more to do with the severity of the patient's symptoms than the exact type of injury. Guiding factors are the patient's posture (torticollis, cradling the arm, holding the head to prevent neck movement), the range of movement at the affected part, the ability to use the injured part, the level of pain and signs such as swelling and bruising.

Bone

Bone is a hard connective tissue, made of collagen and mineral salts, especially calcium. There are two basic bone tissues, **cortical** (also compact, or dense) and **cancellous** (also spongy, or trabecular) (Fig. 5.4). Cortical bone is smooth and dense and forms the outer shaft of the long bones. Cancellous bone is porous and its tiny calcium struts absorb and channel weight like a buttress.

Bones are classified into various types.

1. **Long** bones: the main group represented in the limbs. These bones have a cylindrical **shaft** or **diaphysis**, made of cortical bone on the outside and spongy bone within, with a hollow core, the **medullary cortex**, where yellow marrow is produced. The diaphysis is covered in a membrane called the **periosteum**, which has a lavish nerve and blood supply and which provides attachment for tendons and ligaments. The ends of the bone are called the **epiphyses** (singular, epiphysis). In children there is the **physis**, or **epiphyseal plate**, between the epiphysis and the diaphysis, made of cartilage, where growth occurs in the bone. This plate closes when growth is complete. The articular ends of the epiphyses, the parts which form joints with other bones, are coated in **articular** or **hyaline cartilage**.
2. **Flat** bones (the scapula and sternum).
3. **Short** bones (the carpals and tarsals).
4. **Sesamoid** bones, which lie within tendons apparently to increase the mechanical efficiency of the tendon

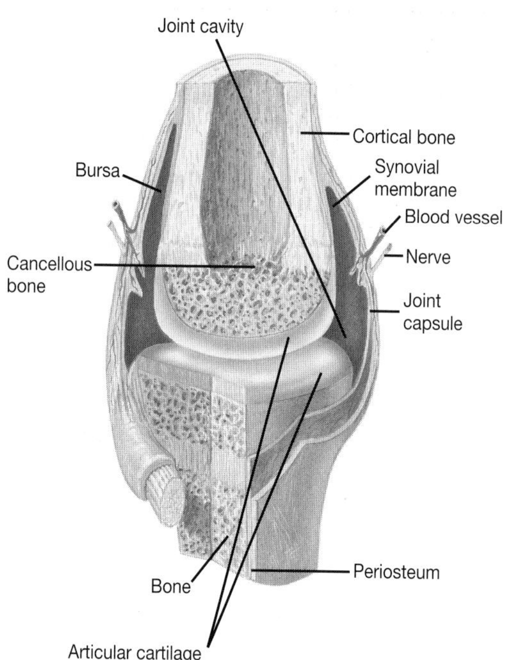

Figure 5.4 The structure of a synovial joint. (Adapted with kind permission from Thibodeau and Patton, 1999.)

(e.g. the patella and pisiform, with others in hand and foot).

5. **Irregular** bones (the bones of the pelvis). These bones all have an outer layer of cortical bone, with spongy bone inside. They may be cuboidal, plate-like, oval or irregular.

Bone Injury: Fracture

A **fracture** is a break in the continuity of a bone (Fig. 5.5). It can be caused by direct violence or by indirect, transmitted force, with injury at a distance from the point of contact. Injury may be transmitted by an **axial** force, often along the shaft of a long bone (e.g. the head of the radius is fractured by a fall on the outstretched hand), or by twisting or leverage. **Traction** (or **distraction**), a pulling force which separates joint surfaces, can cause **avulsion**, when a soft tissue such as tendon or ligament pulls off a piece of the bone to which it is joined (and it can cause dislocation). **Crush** force, the compression of the part between two surfaces, may break bone, often with soft tissue damage and the complications of swelling. Areas of cancellous bone, such as the vertebrae, are subject to crush, but the commonest crush injuries seen in a minor injuries clinic are to the tips of the fingers.

Stress fracture is caused by the cumulative fatigue of overuse, rather than a single violent event, and **pathological fracture** by disease which weakens bone.

Types of fracture

Fractures may be **open** (**compound**) or **closed** (**simple**). An open fracture has a wound at the site of the injury. If the injury is closed, the skin is intact. An opening in the skin over a broken bone, or the protrusion of the bone through the skin, exposes the bone to infection. Bleeding may be severe in such injuries.

A fracture may be **transverse**, with a break at approximately a right angle across the shaft of a long bone, dividing it into two pieces. This happens after a direct blow or bending force to the shaft. The separated surfaces are horizontal and usually keep good position and unite without shortening. However, the broken areas are small and poised one on top of the other, like two pencils balanced end on end. They need support until healing is well advanced.

An **oblique** fracture is one where the bone is broken diagonally along its shaft. This is caused by a blow to the site or indirect force. A twisting force may cause an obliquely angled **spiral** fracture. The broken areas are larger than is the case with a transverse fracture. This makes union easier, but the angle of the broken surfaces and the action of the muscles attached to the bone, may encourage slippage, angulation and shortening. The bone is sharply pointed and wounding of soft tissue, nerve and blood vessel is possible.

Fractures in which the bone is broken into more than two parts are called **comminuted**. Injuries of this kind are usually caused by direct force, sometimes by crush. There are

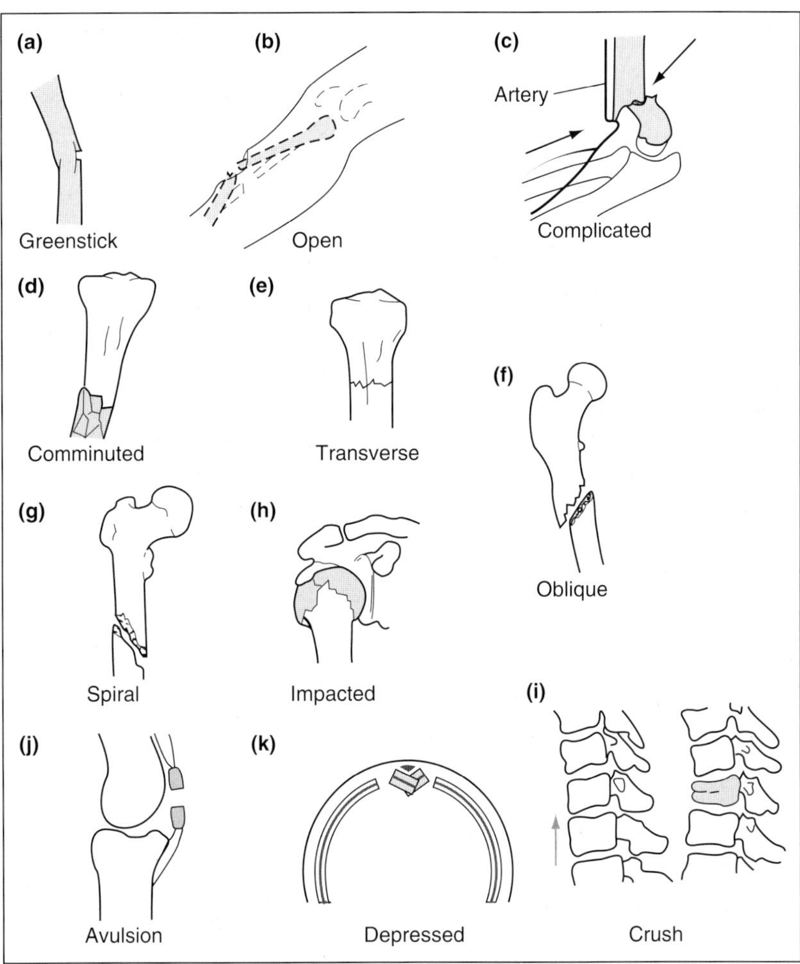

Figure 5.5 Types of fracture. (Reproduced with kind permission from Walsh 1999.)

various classifications of these fractures, depending on the number of fragments and their potential for union. They tend to be unstable and difficult to treat. The violence of the injury is usually severe and soft tissue damage and impaired blood supply, at least to some of the fragments, are common.

Impacted fractures are those in which the broken ends of bone are driven together by a force along the axis of the bone. Shortening and displacement coexist with an unreliable stabilizing of the broken ends. Sometimes the position will obstruct normal function. Fracture in which bone is punched out and deposited in the underlying soft tissues is called **depressed**. This type of injury occurs in the skull.

In children, the bones are soft and **greenstick** fracture is common, with incomplete separation of the injured surfaces and some degree of angulation. A **buckle** fracture is one where a small bulge in the outline of the bone is seen on X-ray film, on the margin opposite to the side which has suffered the force of the injury. There is minimal damage to periosteum and other soft tissues. These injuries heal quickly. Severe angulation may need correction. Fractures to the child's **growth plate**, sometimes involving the near joint, may arrest the growth of the bone and need expert assessment and, in a few cases, surgical reduction. The Harris–Salter classification of growth plate injuries is widely used (Fig. 4.1, p. 32). It is a quick guide to severity, treatment and likely outcome of the various types of injury.

Bone Healing

Broken bone can renew itself completely and heal without fibrous scarring, the only tissue in the body which can do this.

A **haematoma**, a blood clot, forms at the site of the fracture. The ends of the broken bone suffer a small amount of necrosis. Inflammation occurs. New blood vessels, fibrous material, collagen and mineral salts appear in and replace the haematoma. A **soft callus** forms, joining the injured ends, with **osteoblasts** (bone-producing cells) and **osteoclasts** (absorbing and removing dead and unwanted bone). The new bone material is spongy rather than cortical, and mixed with cartilage type material.

The callus appears in response to movement at the broken bone ends, to stabilize them and to provide the environment for healing. It is not found where bone is immobilized by surgical pins. It sometimes does not appear at impacted injuries. These heal in a different manner. If the bone ends are well opposed, the bridging process called **union** takes place. Union is a temporary state on the way to healing. The broken ends of the bone are joined but not strong enough for normal use. This part of the healing process takes 3 to 4 weeks.

Non-union may happen if the broken ends are separated by displacement or because muscle or other soft tissue is caught between the broken ends, if the ends are excessively mobile or if they have a poor blood supply. Comminuted injuries are particularly prone to problems with blood supply. The failure to unite can result in a fibrous union, a grossly distorted union, a complete separation of the bone ends or a false joint called a **pseudoarthrosis**.

From union, the fracture progresses, over a period of months, to **consolidation**. A **hard (bony) callus** of woven bone replaces the soft callus. The injured ends fuse and become stable and strong enough to withstand normal use.

Over a much longer period, up to 2 years, **remodelling** takes place. The bone is restructured in response to the loads which are placed on it. Excess materials left over from healing are absorbed, and cortical bone reforms along the shaft. The bone slowly assumes its former shape.

All stages of bone healing happen more quickly in children. Remodelling is a more active and perfected process, which can even adjust some degree of angulation in a preadolescent. However, rotation needs active correction at any age.

Treatment of bone injury

Certain fractures (e.g. toe injuries without deformity) will heal without special treatment (i.e., treatment which is different from that for a soft tissue injury at the same site). Some centres do not request an X-ray to find them. However, this text will assume that the NP has protocols for the referral to a doctor of every fracture that is found or suspected.

The patient may be referred to a casualty officer or orthopaedic surgeon in the same department or may be transferred to an A&E department elsewhere. A NP may have access to a fracture clinic for an agreed list of uncomplicated injuries and will be responsible for ensuring that more urgent cases are properly assessed and transferred. The common thread running through these scenarios is that treatment of fractures in a minor injury clinic is temporary and contingent upon decisions that will be made later, in another place. The priorities are to ensure the patient's safety, relieve immediate discomfort as much as possible and stabilize the injury for the short term.

Emergencies

Among patients who present to a minor injury clinic with a fracture, the emergency which does arise from time to time is loss of the blood and nerve supply distal to a displaced fracture, most commonly in the wrist or ankle. This threatens the limb and the patient requires the most urgent access to help. If the patient needs transfer to another hospital, call an emergency ambulance. Do not begin any procedure which delays transfer. Lie the patient down and stabilize his injury as much as possible, possibly by using padded splintage, pillows or sandbags. This emergency can arise at any time while the patient is in the minor injury clinic. It is important, especially with displaced injuries, including dislocations, to review the nerve and blood supply constantly.

A displaced open fracture requires sterile dressing. If bleeding is severe it may also need compression. If the bleeding is not coming under control, transfer the patient urgently. Record vital signs and obtain intravenous access if you can.

Routine treatment

The treatment of a fracture depends on many variables. The main considerations are the age of the patient, the site and severity of the injury, the severity of pain and complicating factors such as an open injury. Other factors, such as an elderly person living alone and non-accidental injury, may also influence management.

The NP should not try to reduce a displaced injury. If the patient needs transfer, the injury is stabilized in its given position with padding, splintage and bandaging, leaving fingers or toes exposed to assess circulation and sensation. The aim is to prevent further displacement in order to avoid circulation or nerve damage and to minimize pain.

The affected part should be elevated as soon as possible to reduce swelling. This may be done by using a high sling or propping the injured part on pillows.

Certain fractures are difficult to immobilize because of their anatomical position, such as so-called boxer's fractures at the head of the fifth metacarpal of the hand and injuries to the collar bone, proximal humerus and toes. It is often judged unnecessary to immobilize other fractures such as avulsions from the base of the fifth metatarsal of the foot. In these cases the agreed treatment protocol should be followed, such as the use of collar and cuff for the shoulder, tubigrip and crutches for the foot, buddy strapping, tubigrip and high sling for the hand, and buddy strapping for the toes. The NP should be alert for any complications which make these injuries worse than usual and in need of urgent orthopaedic assessment.

Certain fractures are difficult to diagnose on X-ray film and may have to be treated provisionally as fractures, on clinical grounds alone, on indirect evidence of fracture, such as raised fat pads on the radiograph, or after assessment by a specialist. Common occasions for these problems are when treating children, when treating injuries to the elbow and knee and, most common of all in the minor clinic, with wrist injuries which produce clinical signs at the scaphoid. Particulars of these injuries are found at the appropriate place.

A reverse problem often arises with the elderly. An old person with arthritis may have severe symptoms after an injury, and a radiograph shows an appearance of bony disintegration, sometimes combined with dislocation of the joints. A radiologist's report is probably required to decide whether these appearances are caused by degeneration or trauma. Management of these injuries must take social factors into account. The NP may have to contact the primary care services, crisis care providers, the hospital care of the elderly or orthopaedic teams.

Immobilization

The decision on the method of immobilizing fractures is, in part, a local one. It depends on the policies, routines and preferences of local A&E departments and orthopaedic consultants.

For short-term immobilization (for transfer or until a fracture clinic appointment) of undisplaced fractures in the distal forearm and wrist, it is possible to use ready-made splints of the type which is often used to rest soft tissue injuries. They are adjustable to accommodate swelling, easy and quick to apply and there is no mess. There is a type available with thumb support which can be used for patients who need repeat scaphoid X-ray after 10 days. Whether or not these splints are regarded as acceptable is a matter of local policy.

Plaster of Paris for orthopaedic use is available in impregnated rolls of bandage and in lengths of bandage known as slab. When it is soaked in water an irreversible chemical reaction, which produces heat, occurs, and the plaster and bandage bond to form a hard, brittle shell.

The plaster bandage can be moulded around the limb to form a splint during the first minutes after it is wet. When it dries, further wetting degrades the plaster so that the splint softens and falls apart. The warmer the water that is used to immerse the bandage, the more quickly the plaster will dry. Lukewarm water is normally used.

Plaster is very messy, travelling around the room in its dry dusty form and as quick-drying splashes when wet. It marks clothing and blocks sinks.

Plastering is slow and requires separate facilities if it is to be done routinely. Some plasters require two staff for proper application. This makes it less useful for stand-alone clinics with small numbers of staff.

It is preferable to the ready-made splint for patients whose injuries are very painful, and for those who may not comply with a splint, which can be removed.

Soft Connective Tissues

The soft connective tissues of the musculoskeletal system comprise muscles, tendons, cartilage, ligaments, synovium, bursa, fascia and joints.

Skeletal muscle

Active movement of the skeleton is achieved by coordinated contraction and relaxation of groups of skeletal muscles. These movements can be **voluntary** or **reflexive**.

A skeletal muscle has an upper **origin**, a central **belly** and a lower **insertion**. Origins and insertions are usually formed by the attachment of tendon to bone (Fig. 5.6). The belly is the **contractile** area. Belly and tendon have different functions but work as one unit. The place where they meet is called the **musculotendinous junction**.

The muscle crosses at least one joint. The **muscle fibres** are **irritable**, which means that they **contract** in response to a stimulus. When the fibres contract, the overall length of the muscle shortens forcefully (individual fibres can shorten by up to half of their length) and movement of the skeleton occurs around the affected joint. The muscle which contracts is the prime mover or **agonist**. Muscles which assist the agonist are **synergists**. Other muscles, **antagonists**, with action opposing that of the contracting muscle (i.e. they move the bones at that joint in the opposite direction), cooperate with the contraction by lengthening to allow the movement. They are **extensible** and can relax and stretch. They are also **elastic** and can return to their normal length after stretching.

Muscles work in harmony, not only as movers of the joints but also as stabilizers, both to prevent and to control movement. In this, they form a partnership with the ligaments, the muscle action being termed

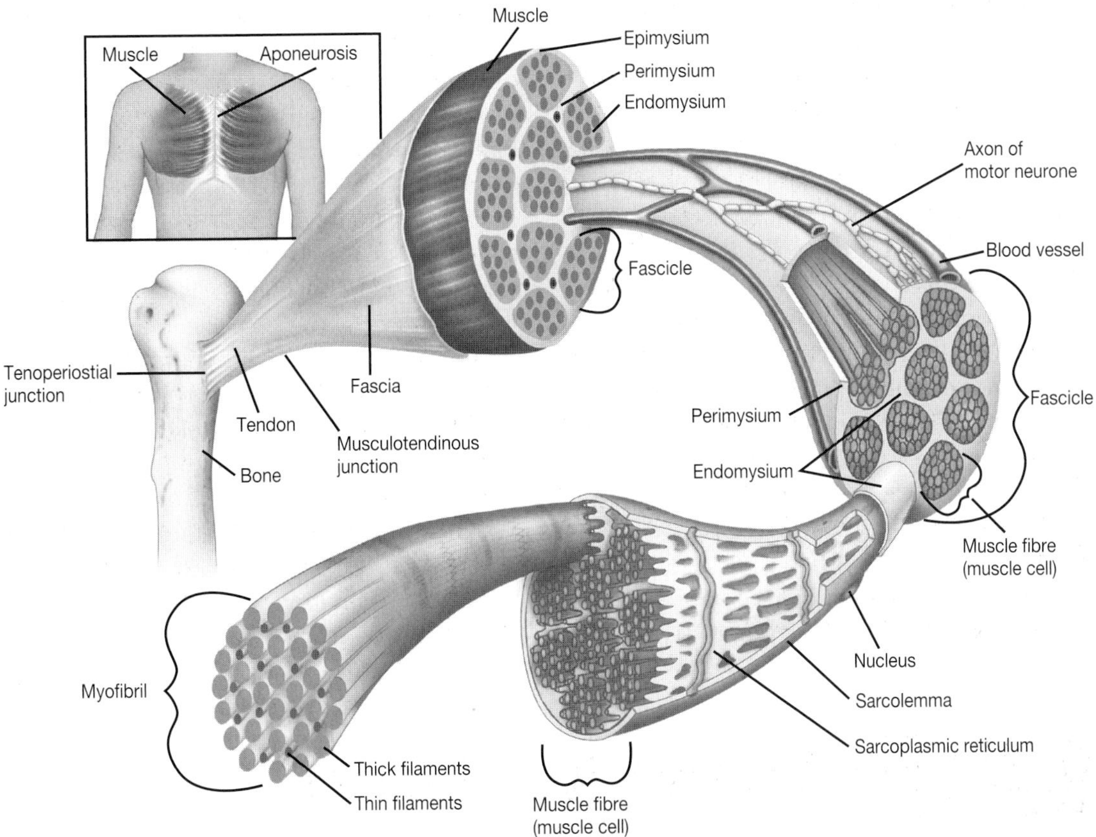

Figure 5.6 Musculotendonous anatomy. (Adapted with kind permission from Thibodeau and Patton, 1999.)

Soft Connective Tissues

contractile, **active** or **dynamic** and the ligament action being termed **inert** or **passive**. This distinction is basic to clinical examination of the soft tissues. The terms contractile and contract can confuse. They are often used to describe action which does not involve a reduction in the length of the muscle. Contraction which shortens the muscle is called **concentric** (e.g. in the biceps when the elbow is flexed). Muscles can contract without changing length: this is **isometric** contraction (e.g. a straight leg raise requires isometric contraction of the quadriceps to keep the knee straight and immobile). Contraction combined with lengthening of the muscle is called **eccentric** (e.g. the quadriceps contract while stretching to control knee flexion when you walk downstairs).

Muscles contract most powerfully if the fibres lie parallel to the axis of the muscle, and the fibres of many muscles, such as the biceps, are arranged in this **fusiform** manner. However, it is also true that a muscle increases in strength in direct proportion to the number of fibres it contains. The fusiform arrangement limits the number of fibres in a muscle, and many, such as the rectus femoris of the quadriceps, have a **penniform** arrangement. The fibres lie diagonally to the axis of the muscle, like cars parked diagonally to a pavement, increasing their number without unacceptable bulk. This is a trade-off. The length of each fibre (and, therefore, the length of its contraction) is reduced and the direction of its pull is oblique, which is less effective than the direct pull of the fusiform.

Skeletal muscle has a huge number of capillaries to meet the demands of heavy activity. At rest, these vessels can close down to 5% of maximum capacity. The degree of engorgement of a muscle with blood at a time of injury is important because the amount of bleeding, and subsequent haematoma, is a major factor in healing.

Muscle fibres are long cells made up of **myofibrils**. Myofibrils contain groups of filaments, of different types. The movement of these filaments in and out of a position of overlap with each other gives rise to contraction. The **sarcomeres** are the repeating units of contraction along the myofibril.

Muscle cells are successively wrapped, individually, in small bundles, in single muscles and in groups of muscles, in layers of collagenous membrane called **fascia**. Individual fibres are wrapped in **sarcolemma** and **endomysium**. Bundles of fibres, called **fasciculi**, are wrapped in **perimysium**, and a single muscle is enclosed in **epimysium** (Fig. 5.6).

Muscle fibres are divided into two types. **Type I**, also called **slow twitch** or **red**, takes its energy **aerobically** from blood-borne oxygen and has high endurance. **Type II** (subdivided further into types IIa and IIb), also known as **fast twitch** or **white**, takes energy **anaerobically** by breaking down muscle glucose. It has less endurance but greater power than type I. Both fibres are found in each muscle. The proportion varies from muscle to muscle and person to person but an equal distribution of the two types is normal. During exercise, these fibres become active in numerical order according to demand. Light activity may only involve type I fibres, with harder work needed to stimulate type II. This has implications for training of muscle and for rehabilitation of injured tissue.

Injury to muscle may be caused by two forces, impact and stretch. These forces often coexist, and the presence, position, extent and treatment of bleeding is a key factor in the recovery of full function.

Injuries to muscle

Rupture

Overload and **compression** injuries cause **rupture**, which may be partial or complete. A rupture is also called a **strain**. Rupture occurs when muscle fibres are torn.

Overload is often the result of the patient's own action, stretching the fibres beyond their limits. Factors such as failure to warm up before activity, previous injury, old scarring in the muscle, tiredness, poor technique or misjudgement of the load may contribute to the injury. Muscles which cross two joints, such as the calf muscles (the gastrocnemius), may suffer contradictory demands during a movement, or demands which exceed their capacities; this type of muscle is particularly prone to rupture.

Compression is the tearing of muscle fibres by a direct blow, which crushes them against bone and causes deep bleeding.

Swelling, induration, bruising and local tenderness may be found with all degrees of rupture, although a very minor tear may only cause localized pain on exertion, with minimal loss of strength and no visible swelling or bruising.

Partial rupture may cause pain on active and resisted contraction, and on passive stretching of the muscle (see below). Spasm may be present.

A complete rupture may not be painful on examination. Total division of the fibres means that the injury cannot be stressed by contraction or stretching. Absolute loss of function is the key sign, perhaps accompanied by a palpable gap across the muscle or a visible deformity caused by retraction and bunching of part of the belly. The loss of function may be concealed by the action of another muscle which can perform the same active movement. Palpation during movement will show the lack of contraction in the injured muscle, and a resisted test, or other tests specific to that muscle alone, should reveal weakness or incapacity.

Bleeding

Muscle injuries cause bleeding, which may be inside a single muscle, **intramuscular**, or between adjacent muscles, **intermuscular**. The amount of bleeding will be determined, in part, by the blood flow to the muscle at the time of injury, which is determined by the level of exertion of that muscle at that moment.

Intramuscular bleeding is contained within the fascia of one muscle. This means that the bleeding may create pressure within the sealed unit of the muscle, which closes the vessels and ends the haemorrhage. In cases where swelling continues, the increase in pressure within the muscle can lead to the complications of **acute compartment syndrome**.

The pressure caused by acute compartment syndrome may cause ischaemic injury to the muscle. It may also compromise the circulation and nerve supply to parts which are distal to the injury, often the hand or foot. Acute compartment syndrome causes severe pain in the muscle, especially when it is passively stretched, and it may swell to the point of rigidity. If it appears that swelling is not resolving quickly after a muscle injury the situation must be monitored carefully. **Pain, pallor, paralysis, pulselessness** and **paraesthesia** are the signs which indicate this potential emergency, but do not wait for a certain diagnosis. Refer the patient on suspicion.

Intermuscular bleeding is more visible, with superficial bruising which can be vivid and alarming to the patient, but recovery should be quick with correct treatment.

Blood at the site of injury separates the torn ends of muscle fibre and inhibits healing. This can result in scarring and **myositis ossificans**, where calcification occurs in fibres which have not been able to heal because of deep haematoma. These problems cause continuing pain, failure to recover strength, and a tendency to further injury.

Another form of compartment syndrome, where there is painful swelling within the fascia compartment which is *not* caused by bleeding, is called **chronic compartment syndrome**. This usually affects athletes who have been training the muscles of the lower leg so that they enlarge beyond the elastic capacity of the fascia during exertion, causing pain and reducing circulation to the muscle. The reduced oxygen to the tissues in the compartment leads to oedema, which adds to the problem. Pain is felt during exercise and settles at rest.

Healing of muscle

Bleeding is the major cause of complication in muscle injury. Haematoma is an important agent in the healing process in all soft tissue injuries, but muscle is enormously vascular. If it is injured during heavy activity it may bleed disproportionately and repeatedly. Normal healing is prevented by a large, deep clot which separates torn fibres and does not disperse, recurrent bleeding and bleeding which increases the pressure inside a muscle compartment. This gives rise to severe scarring and may go on to troublesome complications.

A tear may be mild, moderate or complete. All tears separate some contractile fibres, and the torn ends shrink away from each other. The clot occupies the gap.

Muscle healing is a combination of regeneration of new fibre and scarring, with both types of tissue combining in the same fibres. If there is a lot of scar tissue mingled with the contractile fibres, the function of the muscle, which depends on the coordinated action of many small parts, may be compromised. The scar will be a weak spot, prone to reinjury.

Treatment of muscle injuries

Correct advice about when to rest and when to exercise the muscle is vital for recovery. Without exercise, the muscle will waste and its healing fibres will not organize themselves for a return to function. A premature return to heavy use can lead to further bleeding (with the risk of acute compartment syndrome in some cases), excessive scarring and myositis ossificans.

The core treatment of a new muscle injury is PRICE. Treatment will be dictated by the severity of the tear, the extent of bleeding and whether the haematoma is intramuscular or intermuscular. In mild cases, the patient can be discharged with advice on rest, ice and return to activity (see above). Moderate injuries need ongoing treatment, preferably by a physiotherapist, and the patient should be warned against activity while the injury is swollen. In cases where an intramuscular haematoma is worsening or a complete tear is present, the patient should be referred to a doctor.

There are specific forms of treatment for injuries at different sites, and these are discussed at the appropriate places.

Tendon

Tendon is a connective tissue, containing collagen and some elastin. Its shape depends upon the size and position of the muscle it serves, but it is often a flattened sheet with an oval cross-section, or round and long like a cable. It connects muscle to bone and relays the power of the muscle contraction so that movement can occur or force be transmitted. Consequently it is very strong. It has only a minimal capacity to stretch, but a great capacity to resist a stretching force.

The tendon joins the muscle at the **musculotendinous junction** and the periosteum of the bone at the **tenoperiostial junction** (Fig. 5.6). It also continues into the cortex of the bone as **Sharpey's fibres**.

Some tendons lie, along a part of their length, inside a double-layered **tendon sheath**, which secretes synovial fluid to lubricate the tendon and guides its movement. These are found at points where the tendon is subject to stress as it passes over a joint, through a bony channel or is restrained by a ligamentous or fibrous band.

Injuries to tendon

There are two main classes of injury to tendons (see also Ch. 8 for open injury): division or rupture, and disability caused by overuse injury.

Rupture of tendons

Tendons tear when they are stretched to 5% or more beyond their normal length. They may also be divided by blunt force or a cut. Tendons weakened by chronic inflammatory disease, such as rheumatoid arthritis, may rupture under normal load without an injury. Tendons or parts of tendons with poor blood supply, such as the distal part of the Achilles tendon, may also be prone to rupture. Tendons lose their resilience with age, and a burst of unaccustomed activity by a middle-aged person may lead to injury. An overwhelming external force or a sudden and sustained muscle contraction may cause a tear.

The damage can be partial, with pain but no obvious loss of function, and the sufferer may not realise that the tendon is torn. There is a history of injury, local tenderness and pain on resistance and passive stretching of the tendon. Sometimes a bruise is seen, and a defect may be seen or felt at the site of injury. A failure to treat this injury properly, with the correct balance of rest and graduated exercise, can lead to chronic problems. The healing tendon develops scar tissue, which is repeatedly reinjured by the action of the muscle. Inflammation becomes established and difficult to treat.

Complete rupture of a tendon, particularly common in older manual workers (at the rotator cuff of the shoulder), and older sportsmen (at the Achilles tendon), annouces itself in various ways. There is usually a crack and a sudden pain at the back of the heel when the Achilles tendon ruptures. Rotator cuff tears are described as causing a brief pain at the time of injury, then a period of relief and then a later onset of more severe pain. The rupture of the extensor tendon of the distal phalanx of the finger, the **Mallet** finger, is often painless, and the patient is chiefly aware of deformity and loss of function. It is true of all cases of complete rupture that the function of the muscle attached to that tendon will cease completely. There may be a gap felt at the tendon, and there may be bruising and tenderness.

Painful tendons

There are a number of difficulties when assessing and treating a patient suffering from painful tendons with no history of violent injury. The symptoms are frequently caused by subtle factors, often unknown to the patient. There is no clear history of injury, and no immediate guarantee that the problem is not medical. Tendons are exposed to stress at joints, and the symptoms are often felt there. It may be hard to tell whether the problem arises from the joint or the tendon. Some cases are caused by a one-off burst of unusual activity, such as redecorating or moving house, and these usually settle when the cause is removed. More difficult are the cases which are caused by prolonged overuse, at work or in following a sport or hobby. Failure to diagnose and treat these patients properly can contribute to permanent disability, affecting a key part of the patient's life. Healing can be slow and the problem can recur. Patients who are committed to a sport, or who depend upon an activity for their livelihood, are often reluctant to rest and may not comply well with treatment.

Inflammation is a feature of any injury and is a part of the healing process. It becomes a problem in its own right when it is prolonged. It can contribute to scarring, adhesion and contracture. It may be the chief source of symptoms and cause prolonged and worsening disability.

The signs of inflammation are swelling, redness, local heat, pain, tenderness and disability. When the mobility of a lubricated tendon within its sheath is impaired by inflammation, **crepitus** is often felt at the site.

Overuse injuries are caused by repetitive wear rather than a single violent incident. The injured part is not being used properly but can sustain the accumulation of injury for a time. Damage follows when either the load or the frequency of action (or, in some cases, both) is beyond the endurance of the injured tissue. The patient may be predisposed by physical makeup, and external factors such as bad technique and poor working conditions may add to the problem.

Tendinitis is inflammation of the tendon itself. A small tear in the tendon may cause the problem, creating a permanently painful, chronically inflamed scar which never heals because movement of the tendon provokes it. Tendinitis can occur anywhere in the length of the tendon, and also at the musculotendinous and the tenoperiostial junctions. Tennis elbow is an example of the latter.

Tenosynovitis is caused by a roughening of the tendon and the inner layer of its synovial sheath; as a result, there is pain and crepitus when the tendon moves in the sheath.

Tenovaginitis is a thickening of the tendon sheath which causes pain on movement of the tendon but does not cause the crepitus which is found in tenosynovitis.

Trigger finger or **thumb**, also called **stenosing tenosynovitis**, causes locking of a finger in flexion. The patient makes an unusual effort, against resistance, to extend the finger. It straightens suddenly, which is called triggering. This happens because the flexor tendon has thickened and may have developed a palpable node. The enlarged tendon can pass through the tendon sheath during flexion but will not return. This problem worsens and can result in a permanent flexion deformity of the finger.

Tendon healing and treatment

Injuries to tendons may be characterized by any of various features which make healing prolonged, difficult or impossible without specialist treatment.

Inflammation, often ascribed to overuse, may become chronic in a tendon and its sheath and not respond to rest. It may also be associated with rupture or calcification of the tendon. Scarring on a tendon may set up a source of long-term pain and inflammation, and it may prevent the movement of the tendon in its sheath. Nodal swelling on a tendon may prevent smooth passage through the sheath, a mechanical problem which will not heal.

Tendons may break (or be cut). They can heal as other soft tissues do, slowly and with scarring, but there is considerable difficulty immobilizing them until they heal. Mallet injuries are usually treated conservatively, with prolonged splinting, but success is not guaranteed, and this method is not always suitable for other injuries. Surgical repair is often necessary, but very difficult in places where the tendon lies in a fibro-osseus sheath, and where postoperative scarring may obstruct the tendon's glide. Patients often underestimate tendon tears because the defect causes little discomfort and does not look bruised or swollen. They will occasionally present with a finger in an established boutonnière deformity, which has developed slowly but painlessly to a point where the contractures are too severe for effective treatment.

None of the resources needed to treat the more intractable tendon problems is found in the minor injury clinic. The GP may use cortisone injections; the physiotherapist may use massage and other techniques, or the orthopaedic surgeon may operate.

The patient who presents with a mild, acute tendon inflammation caused by a recent bout of unaccustomed activity should be advised to rest. This means avoidance of any movement which causes the pain. A splint or strapping may be used to immobilize the part. The symptoms will usually settle in less than a week. The patient can then return slowly to normal activity.

Cartilage

Cartilage is a connective tissue. It is strong and resilient. Its chief limitation is that it has no blood supply and it does not heal well.

There are various types, each performing some variation on the role of buffer. They all contain collagen and elastin, in differing proportions according to function.

Hyaline cartilage (**articular**) is the type which lines the synovial joints (Fig. 5.4). It prevents friction between the articular surfaces of the bones. It is rich in collagen, which holds water like a sponge, and it obtains nourishment from the synovial fluid. An increase in pressure inside the joint squeezes water and waste products out of the cartilage, and a decrease allows it to draw water and nutrients in. Inactivity or a reduced range of movement in the joint lessens the ability of the cartilage to nourish itself. Age causes deterioration, and the cartilage becomes brittle and prone to injury.

The **menisci** (singular, **meniscus**), two crescents of **fibroelastic cartilage** (Ch. 7) which sit on top of the articular plateau of the tibia, have greater resilience than articular cartilage. They stabilize the knee by increasing the surface areas which articulate with the condyles of the femur, and they absorb pressure and distribute load.

Fibrocartilage is found at transition points between one tissue and another, at the insertions of ligaments and tendons into bone.

Injuries to cartilage

The commonest injury to cartilage which is seen in a minor clinic is a tear to the meniscus, usually on the medial side of the knee. This is discussed in Chapter 7.

Injuries to the main body of the meniscus are painless. It has neither nerves nor blood supply. Any pain which is felt in meniscus, and any potential that it may have for healing, is at the edge of the structure where there is some circulation and innervation. It is, therefore, common that symptoms experienced in the knee after a meniscal tear are indirect: the inflammation and swelling in the joint triggered by the injury, and the obstruction of normal movement caused by a displaced fragment of cartilage. The joint may 'lock' and may become prone to 'giving way'.

In children, instability of the knee together with pain and interruptions to smooth movement may be caused by an abnormal **discoid** meniscus.

Cartilage healing and treatment

Cartilage is variously described by different authors as a substance which does not heal or one which heals extremely slowly. The cause of this inability to recover from injury is the lack of a blood supply to facilitate healing.

The meniscal cartilage of the knee is the site of most of the cartilage injuries which are seen in the minor injury clinic. The menisci have a blood supply to their outer rims, and some healing and regeneration of excised tissue are possible at these parts. In more central areas, the tissue does not heal. A pattern of recurring problems, gradually or suddenly getting worse, is a well-known feature of meniscal injury.

Treatment in the minor clinic of a suspected acute meniscus injury is addressed to relief of the immediate symptoms. In the knee, there is often swelling, pain and disability, and these can be dealt with in the ways already described. Crutches may be needed. Early physiotherapy can help with recovery of mobility but cannot cure the underlying problem. This should be addressed according to the severity of the situation. If the knee is locked, and this is not resolving, the patient needs referral to a casualty or orthopaedic doctor, depending on the referrals available to clinic, at once. If the patient's symptoms are less severe, recommend a return to active movement as things settle down. In many cases, the problem will quieten down and will not merit surgery. The patient may need referral to a surgeon if the problem goes on, if it recurs, or if it worsens. In this case, the patient should go to the GP for referral.

Ligament

Ligament is a key element in joint stability. It is a soft connective tissue which fastens bones together at the joints. It contains elastin as well as collagen but resists stretching rather than accommodating it. It is often the tissue which limits the range of a particular movement at a joint. It tends to be taut, pulling the articular surfaces together, at the start and end of the range of movement, and lax in the midrange, allowing the bones to separate. If there is extra fluid in the joint, perhaps caused by an effusion, the surfaces are pushed apart and movement is restricted at both ends of the range. The extent of this restriction depends on the size of the effusion and the particular joint which is affected.

Ligament has a poor blood supply and heals slowly, sometimes with scarring and calcification.

It has sensory nerves and injury is a painful event. Through the nerve supply it also has a role in **proprioception** at the joint, helping to coordinate its movement. This may mean, for example, that an artificial replacement for a cruciate ligament of the knee will result in a loss of stability even if the joint is no longer lax.

Injuries to ligament

People with ligament injuries are a common sight in minor injury clinics. The endless parade, on every day of the year, of patients of all ages hobbling and hopping through the door with sprained ankles is a defining spectacle of that area.

Familiarity should not breed a casual approach. Ligament injuries heal slowly and are prone to heal badly. In particular, they are prone to the complications of scarring, calcification, adhesions and chronic laxity. For the patient, that may translate as recurring episodes of pain, as chronic stiffness or instability and a tendency to further injury. Injury to the cruciate ligaments of the knee often causes permanent instability and may contribute to later osteoarthritis.

Injury is normally caused by direct or indirect violence to a joint, forcing it beyond its normal range of movement or in an unnatural direction, stretching and tearing the ligaments. Tears are usually slight, but on occasion there are large tears and complete ruptures of ligament.

The history of a ligament injury is usually clear. The mechanism described means that there will nearly always be a story of a stress to the injured part (although athletes will not always notice the injury if the blood is up in a game like rugby). Ligaments have a nerve supply, and the pain of injury is severe. Patients often describe a feeling of faintness or nausea. Sometimes there is immediate swelling and bruising; more often it happens later in the day. There will be disability, more visible in injuries to the lower limb where weight bearing is compromised.

The injured ligament will be tender to touch and painful when passively stressed, unless it is completely divided, when laxity will be the main sign. If it is possible that the patient has suffered a severe tear (based on exceptional swelling, pain and disability or laxity of the joint), the NP should refer to a doctor. Techniques such as examination under local anaesthetic and stress X-ray are available, and the joint may need immobilization in plaster or even, on some occasions, surgical repair.

An assessment is commenced by excluding fracture. The mechanism which produces a ligament rupture may also cause an avulsion at the bony insertion of the ligament. When this is done, the degree of damage to the ligaments should be established. Sometimes, if the injury is fresh and painful or if instability is severe, there may be muscle spasm, which prevents a true assessment of mobility at the joint. Gross swelling may also prevent an immediate full examination of the injury. The issue of deferred examination is discussed on page 67.

On occasion, commonly at the knee, it is difficult to decide whether an injury is to muscle or ligament. The techniques for testing muscle and joint tissues are described later in this chapter and at the appropriate places for each joint.

Ligament healing and treatment

Soft tissue healing was discussed earlier in this chapter. Ligaments heal slowly, taking more than a year to complete the process. It is common for the patient to experience symptoms for 6 weeks after an ankle sprain. Injured ligaments in the fingers can take months to become painless. Especially in injuries of the lower limb, patients are prone to the complications of adhesions, when the moist, injured tissue bonds to bone, and of contractures and calcification.

The aim of treatment of minor and moderate tears is to steer the difficult middle course between the complications caused by immobility and the complications caused by overuse in order to arrive at a strong, mobile scar of minimum size, with no long-term damage to the proprioceptive functions of the tissue.

In the inflammatory stage of injury, the swelling and bruising around a torn ligament can be massive (especially at knee or ankle), and it is vital to rest the injury. However, total immobility may lead to adhesions, and gentle passive movement and massage are among the techniques which a physiotherapist might employ. A prompt referral for severe cases will be helpful if the NP has that access. The PRICE regimen described earlier in this chapter, is designed to reduce the swelling and allow the healing phase to begin.

Gentle, static muscle exercises involve tightening the muscles around the injury for a few seconds at a time, with very little change in the muscle length so that the joint is not disturbed. These will help to delay muscle wasting and maintain circulation.

Crutches may be necessary at this stage.

In the proliferative phase, the patient will begin a graduated increase in isometric and active exercise. In the case of a lower limb injury, the patient will begin to walk, possibly with the help of a stick. The aim is to walk normally, without limping but to stop if it is becoming painful. Strapping, which holds the injured ligament in a shortened position to protect it from stress (e.g. with the foot in slight eversion for an inversion injury of the ankle), may be applied by a physiotherapist.

The patient will also continue to use ice, compression and elevation to minimize inflammation and swelling.

This is the time when it is most difficult to balance the need of the frail, healing tissue for protection with its need to develop in the presence of movement. Any increase in pain or swelling should warn the patient to ease off.

In the remodelling stage, the patient should gradually increase activity back to normal levels, working to restore normal movement at the joint and good power in the surrounding muscle. This may take several weeks and the pace should not be forced.

Coordination around the injured joint, damaged by loss of proprioception as well as inactivity, may require specific exercises if the injury has been severe or the patient has a high level of physical activity in sport or work. Referral to a physiotherapist may be appropriate.

Synovium

Synovium is a membrane made of loose connective tissue. It is rich in blood vessels but has a poor supply of nerves. It lines the interior of synovial joints, except the cartilage surfaces (Fig. 5.4). It forms the inner layer of bursae and tendon sheaths.

Synovium secretes **synovial fluid** into these spaces to lubricate them. The fluid contains phagocytes to clear debris and fight infection, and it carries nutrients to cartilage.

Injuries to synovium

Synovium is prone to inflammation in the presence of infection, chemical irritation, trauma and certain diseases such as rheumatoid arthritis. This causes increase in the output of synovial fluid, producing an effusion into the joint. This condition is called **synovitis**.

Treatment of synovitis

Treatment of synovitis depends upon the cause. It is an inflammatory condition, and the affected area should be rested at first. Normally, in the case of a small to moderate effusion caused by an injury, the injury is treated on its merits, which will include measures to reduce swelling and to keep an eye on the effusion.

A very large effusion at the knee should be referred to a doctor at once. Apart from the fact that it may indicate a more severe underlying problem, the swelling may require aspiration. In cases where a patient presents with an effusion and no history of trauma, always check the temperature and pulse and consider whether any other signs of infection, such as malaise or raised lymph nodes, are present. Look at the skin around the swelling for any recent break which may have admitted infection. If there is any doubt, and there is a possibility of joint infection, the patient should be referred to a doctor at once. If there are no signs of infection and the patient is sent home, the NP should tell the patient to go to a doctor at once if the injury worsens and should consult a GP at the next available opportunity.

Bursa

A bursa (plural **bursae**) is a sac lined with synovium and filled with synovial fluid. Bursae tend to be found between two musculoskeletal structures which move upon each other, and they reduce the friction between them. Common sites for bursae include knee, elbow and heel. Tendon sheaths are sometimes described as modified bursae. A great many bursae are common to us all, but it appears that they will also develop in other parts of the body in response to repeated stresses caused by particular activities.

Injuries to bursa

Pressure, friction or direct impact may cause traumatic inflammation of a bursa, with redness, heat and tenderness, and a soft swelling. This problem is called **bursitis**. Infection can also cause a **septic bursitis**. The infection may be blood borne or enter through a break in the skin (sometimes caused by previous aspiration of a non-infected bursa).

There are several common sites for this condition. At the front of the patella, **prepatellar** bursitis is also called **housemaid's knee** because the problem affects people whose jobs involve kneeling. Nowadays, roofers and carpet layers are more likely candidates. **Infrapatellar** bursitis occurs at the bursa which lies in front of the patellar ligament, and this is also known as **clergyman's knee. Olecranon** bursitis occurs at the point of the elbow and is often caused by leaning on the elbow.

Treatment of bursal injury

A non-infected bursitis will usually settle with rest and the use of a non-steroidal anti-inflammatory medicine such as ibuprofen (if the patient can tolerate it). A doctor may wish to drain a particularly large bursa, but this action has to be weighed against the risk of introducing infection.

Follow the same advice as for synovitis in dealing with the question of infection.

Fascia

Fascia is a multilayered tissue. The **deep layer** is of particular concern in the study of trauma, especially to the forearm or lower leg (see also the anatomy of muscle fibres (p. 54) and compartment syndrome (p. 57)).

The deep fascia is a tough, inelastic, collagenous membrane which wraps related groups of muscles into parcels (Fig. 5.6). It is a continuous tissue and can transmit muscle tension to its distant attachments. It is also possible for movement at those distant structures to stress the fascia at its connection to bone and cause inflammation (**fasciitis**).

Injuries to fascia

The inelastic nature of fascia is one of the main factors in compartment syndrome (p. 57).

Fasciitis is inflammation at the insertion of fascia into bone. **Plantar fasciitis** is a common cause of heel pain, especially in middle age and later life, and patients often present in minor injury clinics with this complaint. The plantar fascia inserts into the heel on the medial side of the sole, at the **medial tubercle** of the calcaneum, and passes distally to the toes. It helps to support the arch of the foot, and it becomes tighter when the toes are extended. Tension at the insertion of the fascia into bone, with small tears, scarring and inflammation, may cause the irritation. Sometimes a bony spur is present at the painful site, but such spurs are often asymptomatic, and pain may be present without a spur. The patient complains of pain when walking, which has a gradual onset, is worse in the morning and gets easier if the activity continues. It returns whenever walking is resumed after a rest. Tenderness at the medial tubercle of the calcaneum, which is worsened by extending the big toe, is found on examination.

Treatment

Plantar fasciitis is a condition which does not settle easily. The patient should be referred to the GP, who may explore such options as a referral to the chiropodist, steroid injection or referral for ultrasound.

Joints

A joint is the place where two bones meet. The body has three types of joint, immoveable (the skull sutures), slightly moveable (the sacroiliac joint) and, the type which this text will focus upon, the mobile, **synovial** joint (Fig. 5.4).

Synovial joints share certain features. A **synovial membrane** forms the inner of two layers of the **joint capsule**. It secretes **synovial fluid**, a lubricant, into the **joint space**. The outer fibrous layer of the joint capsule, flexible but very strong, links the two bones. The **articular surfaces** of the bones are covered with smooth **cartilage** to absorb pressure and reduce friction when the bones move upon each other.

Synovial joints vary in design, each according to its role, to reconcile opposing demands for stability and free movement. Generally, the joints in the arm are mobile to liberate the hand, while the joints in the leg are restricted to support the weight of the body.

There are six main types of synovial joint (see also Fig. 5.7).

Ball and socket The hip and shoulder joints have a spherical head that fits into a hollow socket; movement can occur in all planes, including rotation about the long axis of the bone. The deep ball and socket of the hip allows a smaller range of movement but more stability than the shallow ball and socket at the shoulder.

Condyloid The metacarpophalangeal joints of the hand (except the thumb) have an oval joint surface that fits a concave depression. It allows flexion, extension and deviation to both sides, movements which combine as circumduction.

Saddle The trapezium–metacarpal joint of the thumb is a joint which is even more mobile than the condyloid. One articular surface is concave and convex in different directions, like a saddle, and fits the matching contours of the other surface.

Plane The intercarpal joints have flat articular surfaces that glide against each other.

Pivot The proximal radioulnar joint pivots as the shaft of one bone (radius) is held parallel to another bone (ulna) by a loop; the first bone can rotate about its own long axis inside the loop. The proximal radius moves in this way to allow pronation and supination of the forearm.

Hinge The elbow has the rounded end of one bone sitting in a notch on the other, like a hinge, allowing only flexion and extension.

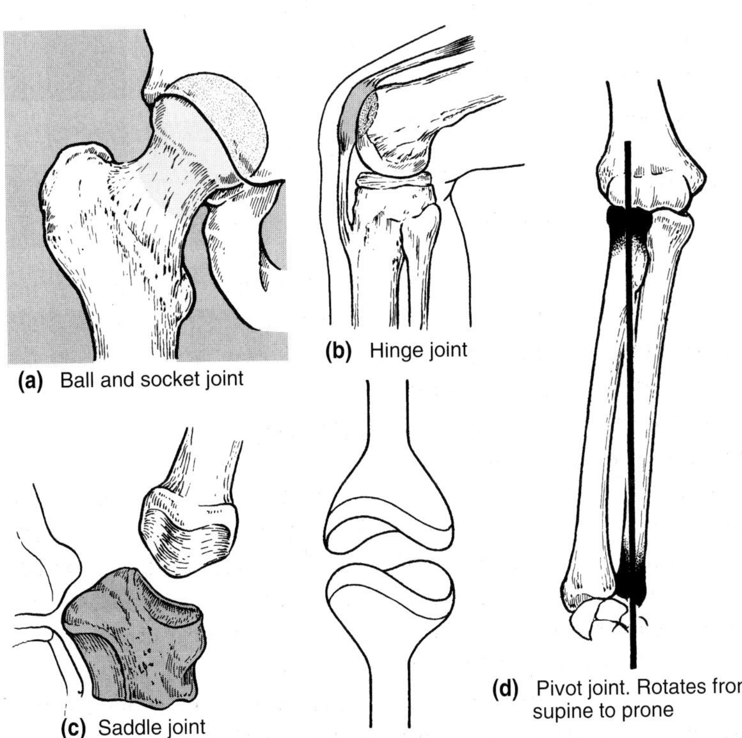

Figure 5.7 Types of synovial joint. (Adapted with kind permission from Dandy and Edwards, 1998.)

Injuries to joints

It is easy to underestimate joint injuries in a minor clinic. Very often, the swelling and pain of a fresh injury make full examination impossible, and a second, later assessment is necessary. In many cases, joints are destabilized by soft tissue injuries which are not apparent on an ordinary X-ray film, and too much comfort is taken from a negative radiograph. Muscle spasm may guard an unstable joint, and laxity of the ligaments is not revealed on examination.

Dislocation is an abnormal separation of the joint surfaces. A lesser injury, where the displacement is only partial, is called **subluxation**. Dislocation may be complicated by the presence of a fracture, for which the term **fracture dislocation** is used.

The articular surfaces of the joint are held in position by soft tissues, particularly the capsule and its reinforcing ligaments and the muscles which operate across the joint. Dislocation cannot happen without damage to some of these tissues. The return of stability depends upon their healing.

A dislocation may be a single traumatic event which will not be likely to recur when healing is complete. It may also be that the first injury will not heal well, and there will be a tendency for the problem to recur. This often happens at the shoulder.

The shoulder is a special case in terms of dislocation. The glenoid socket of the scapula, which articulates with the head of the humerus, is very shallow. The joint is largely stabilized by a complex of muscles and ligaments. This allows an exceptional range of movement but leaves the joint vulnerable to dislocation.

It may also be that an individual, usually a growing girl, is predisposed to suffer repeated dislocations of the patellae by peculiarities of anatomy, laxity of ligaments, shortness of muscle or the angle of a bone.

Treatment of joint injuries

Patients who have a dislocation should be referred for medical treatment. Circulation and sensation distal to the injured part should be assessed. Depending on what part is injured, the NP may use a sling or splint to maintain the unreduced injury in a stable, comfortable position if the patient is to be transferred to another site. If the injury is open, the wound should be cleaned as well as possible and a temporary sterile dressing applied.

In some cases, patients attend with a painful joint and the history suggests a partial dislocation which has corrected itself. In other cases, the patient, a first aider or some other person may have reduced a complete dislocation at the time of injury, often to a finger on the sports field, or a recurrence of patella or posterior shoulder dislocation. In either case, the NP should follow local policies for management of the injury. It is necessary to exclude nerve and blood vessel injury, fracture and severe soft tissue damage, and to make the injury safe and comfortable. Orthopaedic follow-up should be arranged by the agreed procedure for the clinic.

Basic Principles of Examination

Musculoskeletal injury is caused by violence or overuse to the skeleton and to the soft tissues which join and move the bones.

Wounds may be present with musculoskeletal injuries, but the methods of examination and diagnosis which are discussed here are for the assessment of closed injuries. This part deals with the following aspects of examination:

1. Examination and the acutely injured patient

2. Fracture
3. Musculoskeletal examination
4. The joint capsule
5. Referred pain
6. Nerve symptoms.

Examination and the Acutely Injured Patient

In theory, clinical examination is an orderly process. It has to be systematic so that nothing is overlooked. Examination of patients with fresh injuries can make this difficult. The patients may be bleeding, vomiting or feeling faint; they may be immobilized by swelling and unable to walk. They are likely to be in pain, anxious and vulnerable, and they are often embarrassed. In spite of this, patients are expected to allow a nurse to ask personal questions, to intrude upon their space, expose and handle their bodies, and provoke their pain.

The examination of the acutely injured patient is based on the priorities at that particular moment much more than, for instance, a physiotherapist's or an orthopaedic surgeon's examination of the same patient 3 days or 6 weeks after injury. Is this an emergency? Is this really an injury or is the patient ill? How bad is the pain? Who will look after the patient tonight?

If the NP can carry out a full examination, arrive at a diagnosis and complete the patient's treatment on the spot, that is ideal and it should be done. If that cannot be done, the NP needs to decide what the situation requires.

The clinical examination must indicate what injuries are possible and the urgency of diagnosis. It may be possible to exclude a fracture in a finger but not to test the soft tissues because of swelling. Is it enough to send the patient away with advice on possible complications? Should the patient be referred to a doctor at once? Would a doctor have access to extra resources (such as anaesthesia, stress X-ray, specialist referral)? Should the NP decide to review the patient and if so when should this be done?

Much depends upon the local situation. A NP who is based in an A&E department will probably refer any doubtful case at once. If the nearest A&E department is miles away, this will influence the management of the patient's injury. The first priority is to make the patient safe. After that, the approach should be sensible.

The minor injury clinic should have a policy for prompt review of patients who are not fully examined on a first visit. Delay will be pointless if patients do not know how to improve the injury, so they should be given written advice. The worst possible diagnosis should be assumed until it is excluded, and the patient must be made safe. Patients should be told where to seek help if things worsen. A couple of days of rest, using crutches or a splint and treating swelling, often makes examination easier and the results more reliable.

There are two other situations where a NP may restrict examination of an acutely injured patient. In the first, the patient has an injury which clearly needs immediate referral. The NP will then assess the severity of the problem and make the patient safe and comfortable. It may be possible to speed things up by arranging, for instance, an X-ray. At that point, there will be no reason to examine the patient further. It will cause pain and the patient may be less cooperative later for further examinations.

The second situation concerns young children. The NP should minimize distress in an injured child. If the child is safe but needs referral, pain relief and reassurance are the priorities. If the child is upset, the next examiner will start at a disadvantage. The NP should anticipate the problem and refer at once.

Fractures

Examination of an injured patient often begins with the question of fracture. Aspects of examination of the patient with a possible fracture are:

1. Fracture first
2. Signs and symptoms
3. Assessment
4. Aspects of examination.

Fracture first

A patient with a violent injury may present with pain, swelling, bruising and disability. Certain signs are more specific. An abnormally angled bone is broken. A fracture may be visible in a wound. In most cases, the signs are less specific. It may not be clear whether the patient has injured bone or a soft tissue. The diagnosis is reached by exclusion, beginning with fracture.

Fracture comes first for several reasons. It is often the easiest injury to exclude, by X-ray. A fracture is painful, and it should be found with a minimum of discomfort to the patient. The examination and treatment of soft tissue injuries is different to that of fractures, and a negative X-ray film may allow the assessment to proceed without confusion.

Signs and symptoms

Many of the appearances of fracture are not specific to fracture alone.

There will normally be a history of injury. Exceptions are stress fracture (with a history of overuse rather than violence) and pathological fractures (with, perhaps, a suggestive medical history such as cancer or osteoporosis). There will be clinical signs of fracture.

In the case of an open fracture, the broken bone may be protuding from, or be visible in, the wound.

The most specific sign in closed fractures is **deformity**. The bone may be shortened or widened by impaction or overlap, it may be lengthened by separation of the broken ends, it may be rotated or angulated. It can be difficult to distinguish between the deformity caused by a dislocation and a displaced fracture, and the two may coexist.

Also specific is **crepitus**, a grating from the movement of broken ends of bone upon each other. This sign may be mentioned by the patient or accidentally elicited, but it should never be directly sought. The pain is too great, and moving broken bone risks making the injury worse.

Abnormal movement may be a definite sign of fracture depending on its site. Dislocation and ligament injury can cause this sign at a joint.

Among the general signs and symptoms of fracture are **pain**, **bruising** and **swelling**, **local tenderness**, **restricted movement** and **disability**, and **guarding** of the injured part. The patient may be shocked because of blood loss and pain.

Assessment

Fracture may involve displacement of bone, with injury to nerve, blood vessel and any organ. Colour and warmth, pulse, capillary refill time and sensation distal to the injury should be assessed, together with the patient's vital signs if that is necessary.

Broken bone bleeds and is painful. The patient may be in shock. Is the patient restless, pale, cold and sweaty? Is the patient breathing rapidly and shallow? Is the patient sluggish? Vital signs should be monitored and the patient may need oxygen, intravenous fluids and analgesia. There should be a pathway for prompt medical assistance.

If a fracture is unstable, the injury may worsen and movement may cause severe pain. Use splinting and examine with caution.

The mechanism which causes injury at one site may tend to cause simultaneous injury at another. The areas affected may be close to each other (e.g. the radius and ulna) or widely separated (e.g. calcaneal fractures caused by landing on the heels from a height correlate with injuries to the spine).

Fracture may coexist with other presentations (e.g. subungual haematoma, Mallet finger and dislocation). Such fractures will usually alter the management of the injury and it is important not to miss them.

Aspects of examination

The process of musculoskeletal examination, which includes fracture, is discussed later in this chapter. A few points are discussed here about fractures in particular.

Fractures are mechanical events caused by violence and the mechanism of injury is of particular importance. The possible injuries are determined by the forces which have been applied to the tissues. Examination of the patient in the light of the mechanism of injury means that the NP excludes any injury, anywhere in the body, which that mechanism can cause, regardless of the patient's actual complaint. It may be enough to watch the patient walk in from the waiting room to settle some concerns. Detailed examination is usually started from the joint above the injury. If a patient has a painful wrist after a fall on the outstretched hand, the NP will ask the patient to expose both arms above the elbows and will examine from elbow to fingertips. Confirmation that the patient is using the shoulder normally can be achieved by asking the patient to raise a hand behind the head and then to put it up the back. Suspicion of undisclosed injury should be greater with elderly patients and children.

The need to X-ray

Tenderness is the usual indication for X-ray. However, tenderness is a non-specific sign. McRae (1994) advises on how to localize it to bone. A broken bone will be tender at the level of the fracture on every aspect of the bone. If tenderness is confined to one surface of the bone, then it is not likely to be caused by a fracture. Guidelines such as the Ottawa ankle rules (Stiell et al., 1993) attempt to identify patterns of tenderness which are associated with fracture. Local policies vary on the indications for X-ray, and a NP will follow the policies for that clinic.

Guidelines on diagnosis of fractures are generalizations, and patients will always be found who do not fit them. Local tenderness is always present with a fracture, but it can be difficult to elicit in some elderly patients with fractures of the distal forearm (while others, with arthritis, have a great deal of tenderness and no fracture). Children with greenstick fractures may have no bruising or swelling. Patients will walk on fractures of foot and fibula, and sometimes come for treatment weeks after the injury. Consider this when deciding whether or not the patient needs an X-ray.

Musculoskeletal Examination

Many practitioners in minor injuries bring a high level of skill in the care of wounds to their new job. Very few are trained in examination. This part of the text provides a base to build these skills:

1. Preliminary observation
2. History
3. Physical examination
4. Complicating factors in examination.

Preliminary observation

Formal examination is a revealing process, but it is least useful for showing the problems which the injury causes the patient in daily life. Take the fleeting chance to see the patient in the waiting room. Assess movement, appearance and conduct as the patient gets up and walks to your room. How easily does the patient move? Where do any restrictions or difficulties arise? Is the patient in pain, pale, cradling an arm or limping? Does the patient use the injured part? Are the patient's social responses comfortable or are they agitated or lethargic?

The patient should be seen in a quiet, private area. The fact that it is a minor problem does not reduce the right to confidentiality. The patient may have to undress. Patients with minor injuries are often treated, more for lack of space than any view that it is desirable, in curtain-divided cubicles where there is no privacy of speech, and where physical modesty is casually affronted. This kind of inadequate provision may be preventing emergency services from hearing, among other things, the disclosure of cases of domestic violence.

History

The taking of a history has been described in Chapter 3 and the importance of a clear history of injury has also been discussed earlier in this chapter.

If the patient has suffered a violent injury, the mechanism should be established and the NP should have a clear mental picture of the whole episode. The patient may not understand the need for, or be able to give, a full history. Ask questions until you know as much as the patient knows about how the injury happened. Every physical factor contributes to the picture: direction, speed and duration of the force, the type of surface, height of fall, position of limbs and the direction in which they moved. Match the story to the clinical appearance. If they are not consistent, go back to the beginning. The patient may be rationalizing a false connection between an incident and the symptoms.

In many cases the patient complains of an onset of pain with no history of injury, which makes assessment harder. It is often possible to relate an overuse injury to a pattern of daily activity which explains the symptoms. However, in other cases, an orthopaedic or rheumatological problem, or a problem from any other specialty, may surface in a minor injury area. The patient complains of pain and may relate it vaguely to injury. The NP has three prime responsibilites: first, to know when a problem may not be an injury; second, to recognize the most serious possibilities so that an emergency will not be mismanaged; and, third, to make accurate referral so that the patient can be properly treated.

Pain is important. How does the patient describe the pain? Was pain immediate or delayed? Is it getting worse? Is it constant or intermittent? Does anything relieve or aggravate it? Is it related to movement and does continuing movement worsen or improve it? Does it disturb sleep? Is it worse at any time of day? Is it travelling to parts which were not injured? Is it associated with numbness or tingling or is there weakness?

Questions can also clarify events around the time of the injury. Did the patient hear or feel cracking or tearing? Was a joint forced into an abnormal position? Was the patient able to walk after the injury and has walking improved or worsened since? Was there **swelling**? Was it instant swelling (of a haemarthrosis) or a slower (inflammatory) effusion? Has it worsened or improved? Does it come and go?

Further questions elicit facts about the injury's continuing symptoms. Has the patient noticed any **stiffness**? Is movement limited? What limits the movement? Is it pain, or the expectation of pain, or is movement blocked? The patient may describe '**locking**'. What is meant by that? Is the joint still locked? If not, what happened to unlock it? The patient may describe a feeling of **instability** in a joint, often in terms of the joint popping out or giving way. Did the joint pop back, did the patient manipulate it? Ask for examples of where and how, how long, how often and during what movements.

How does the problem affect the patient in **daily life**? What can the patient *not* do? The answers are important, not only because they tell more about the injury but also because the replies indicate the attitude to recovery and the level of activity that the patient expects to resume.

Yet more questions on what **treatments** the patient has tried give an indication as to whether it is improving. Has the patient used ice or taken painkillers? Did any of these help? Has the patient been resting or active since the injury? A large swelling may be quite differently interpreted if the patient has been playing football on a freshly injured ankle.

Physical examination

The patient should undress to show both the area to be examined, and the opposite healthy area. Examination will normally be from the joint above the injury. The patient's modesty should be preserved and there may be a need for a chaperone.

Make the patient comfortable in a position which allows effective examination. This may be sitting at a small table for hand examination, standing for shoulder comparison or lying on a couch with an injured knee. The injured part should be supported so the patient can relax. This may involve the use of pillows and cushions.

A good, even light is necessary for comparison of the injured area with the healthy. Examination of acute musculoskeletal problems is structured around the orthopaedic approach: **look**, **feel**, **move**. Examination always begins by looking. The order of the other parts of the process varies.

If the probable injury is a fracture, palpation or 'feeling', followed by X-ray will be the likely approach. Movement may not be assessed at that stage. The order of examination may also depend upon which part is injured. If the patient is lying down for examination of a painful knee, it may be better to perform the whole face-down part of the examination at one time so that the patient is not constantly struggling from one position to another. In some cases, the diagnosis is clear from the start and the examination is tailored to the variations of that problem. Injuries such as dislocation and Mallet finger are often in that category. In other instances, it may become clear that a certain diagnosis is not possible and examination can be confined to what is relevant.

If the injury seems to be one of soft tissue, movement may become more significant in the assessment, and palpation for tenderness may even be misleading. The diagnosis of possible fracture can be based upon local tenderness because bone pain does not refer to other parts of the body. Pain from injury to soft tissue or to nerves may be felt a long way from the damaged part. The methods of discovering which tissue is injured are based, first, on knowledge of how pain **refers** (p. 76), and, second, on tests of the function of those tissues which may be injured (p. 72). These are tests of movement.

A physiotherapist often begins examination of a patient with a musculoskeletal problem by testing movement and may only use palpation to confirm the findings. A rheumatologist, confronted by a patient with a history of joint pain, may give palpation a larger place in the examination. In the minor injury clinic, there should be a routine of examination, but skills should be applied in a discriminating and appropriate way.

Look

'Look' does not mean 'glance' or 'what you do with your eyes while you reach out to prod that interesting lump'. Looking is a separate, reflective process carried out over a period of time in a structured way. It involves notions like compare, measure and describe.

Looking starts with general observations, of the patient's wellness, alertness, posture, gait and symmetry, and colour and breathing.

Look at the area to be examined and the surrounding area, either by walking around the patient, or by asking the patient to turn. If the patient is lying down, ask the patient to turn over at some point in the process. Compare injured with uninjured side. Note any bruise, redness, rash, wound or scar. Is the skin dry, clammy, flushed, blue, pale? Is there swelling or wasting? Is the swelling localized or widespread? Is there deformity? Is the deformity bilateral? Does it arise from joint or bone; is it traumatic, degenerative or congenital? What is the posture of the joint? Is there rotation or shortening?

It is surprising how long you may look at an injury before seeing a feature such as swelling or redness, which then seems obvious.

Feel

Looking at the patient does not inflict pain, and the patient is in control and can limit discomfort during active and resisted movement. It is harder for a patient to submit to palpation and passive movement. NPs must show, by words, by arrangements for the patient's comfort, and by the care, confidence, restraint and skill of their handling, that they can be trusted with these tasks. Otherwise, the patient will not relax and any reactions will be distorted by anxiety.

Palpation is a systematic assessment by touch of all the structures related to the injury. This will generally include the area from the joint proximal to the injury and the circulation and neurological function of the area distal to it. The back of the hand is more sensitive to temperature variations than the palm. The exploration will be more informative if it is performed gently. Compare with the unaffected side.

Some structures, such as the articular surfaces of the knee, can only be felt with the limb in certain positions. Other structures are exposed by palpation during passive movement. The scaphoid will bulge under the finger if you press into the anatomical snuffbox while passively moving the patient's hand into ulnar deviation. **Crepitus**, **clicking** and other interruptions to normal movement in a joint or tendon sheath will only be felt by moving the part. Elicit these signs gently. Do not look for crepitus from broken bone.

Explore the anatomical landmarks in an orderly sequence. The finger pads are more sensitive, and gentler, than the tips. Feel for each layer of tissue from skin down to bone. The rubbery texture of a thickened synovium at the knee can be felt by lifting the skin and gently rolling it between the fingers.

A tender area should not be directly prodded. It is helpful, with an injured muscle, to begin palpation proximal to the tender spot and move distally until the patient feels the beginning of pain. Draw a line there. Repeat this procedure from the other three directions so that a rectangle of tenderness is outlined without causing more than mild discomfort.

Note the qualities of any **swelling**. Is it general or very localized with clearly defined boundaries? Is it hard or soft, tense or fluctuant, mobile or fixed? Is it anchored to a particular tissue?

A loss of **continuity** may be felt in a tissue, at the displaced end of a fracture or a gap in a muscle or tendon.

The area may feel **hot** or **cold** compared with the normal part.

Note any **tenderness**, but its significance should not be assumed (see movement). Some tissues are normally tender to palpate, so they should be compared with the uninjured part.

Pulses and **sensation** should be checked in the injured area and distal to the injury. Light touch is usually tested for a quick assessment of sensation.

Move

Joint movement is measured precisely with a goniometer, but this level of accuracy is not needed in a minor injury area. Nevertheless, the NP will have to estimate the movement that the patient has lost, and be able to describe the deficit consistently, so that any other person who examines the patient will have a baseline measurement.

Joint movement is measured in degrees, from the anatomical position as zero. There are textbook normal ranges for each joint, and the patient's uninjured side shows what is normal for that individual. Apley and Solomon (1997) advocate a simple system for describing the range of movement, the consistent recording of the range in degrees and whether or not a goniometer is used. Movement in a knee which has lost five degrees of extension, and about half of its range of flexion, is recorded as 'knee – flexion – 5–70 degrees' (a normal range is recorded as 'knee – flexion – 0–140 degrees').

Movement is tested in a very structured way. Each movement has to be performed accurately so that there is no doubt as to which part is being tested. Patients will unknowingly find different ways of carrying out restricted or painful movements. A patient who cannot initiate abduction at the shoulder will tilt the trunk to the side so that the arm falls away from the body by gravity. A patient who cannot flex the shoulder will allow the arm to drift sideways into abduction. Some forms of this **substitution** of one movement for another are subtle. In patients with chronic problems, there may be long established mechanisms of this kind.

Testing of movement is carried out in stages, each with distinct techniques and objectives:

1. Active movement
2. Passive movement
3. Resisted movement
4. Stress testing and accessory movement.

Active movement

Patient performs **active** movements unassisted, using their own muscle power. Difficulty with active movement can arise from disease and from injury to bone, nerve, muscle or joint capsule. A sequence of movements, different at each joint to show its full range of movement, is measured to test the muscles which move the joint, and the joint itself. Any limitations should be noted and the patient asked to describe what is preventing movement: pain, weakness, 'tightness' or 'locking'. In some cases, for example where an 'arc of pain' at the shoulder is suspected, the NP may encourage the patient to push on through the pain to find out if movement becomes painless again in the upper part of the range.

If the range of movement is complete and comfortable, the NP may want to **overpress** the movement. This is when the examiner continues the movement passively from the point where the patient has reached the end of the active range. This stretches the inert joint tissues to the limit and allows the joint to be **cleared** for that movement.

Passive and resisted movement

Injuries to soft tissue and nerve can refer pain to areas where no injury exists, usually distal to the actual lesion. Injured tissues which lie deep, and those in or near the trunk, are the most likely to refer pain and the hardest injuries to locate. Referral of pain is discussed below. At this point, the key fact is that palpation is not a reliable way to locate such injuries. First, because tenderness, caused by the injury, may be localized by the patient to a place which is not injured. Second, a lesion which lies deep may not be palpable. Finally, the lesion which refers pain may not be tender when palpated but may only be painful when it is stretched or pinched during movement (Cyriax & Cyriax, 1993).

Active movements can reveal that an injury is present, but they may not distinguish between damage to joint or to muscle. Passive movements test the inert tissues at the joint. The patient does not use muscles during the movement and, because they are relaxed, they do not cause pain. Resisted movement tests the muscle. The joint is not allowed to move during the test, which eliminates the inert tissues, so that symptoms are likely to be caused by muscle.

The key idea behind this activity is that musculoskeletal tissue is made for movement, and injury (or disease) in any part of the musculoskeletal system will always show itself when that part moves. It may show as pain, weakness, instability, blocked movement or laxity. There will be some evidence of the damage which the tissue has suffered, and this finding, rather than palpation, is the reliable pointer to the part which is injured.

Passive movement

Passive movement aims to eliminate the muscle, tendon and the tenoperiostial junction from the test and to stress inert tissues such as ligament and cartilage. The examiner lifts the injured part and takes the joint through the same movements that have already been tested actively. The patient relaxes muscles so that they are not leading the movement.

If the patient's range of movement is no better than on active testing, and other symptoms remain, then an inert tissue such as ligament or cartilage is the likely cause of the problem. If the range of movement is increased, and the symptoms are less, then it is more likely that the trouble arises from muscle.

Make the patient comfortable as it is difficult for patients to relax to the extent which is necessary. The patient may not be in the same position as when the active range is performed. For example, active shoulder movements may be tested when the patient is standing and passive movements tested with the patient lying down. Lying down enables the patient to relax more and the arm can be handled in elevated positions. Patients need a clear explanation of the purpose of this procedure, and reassurance that it will be performed gently, and that their responses will guide the extent of movement.

Passive movement does stretch muscle at the end of the normal range of movement, and this may cause pain in an injured muscle. In that case the injury to the muscle should also show when it is tested against resistance.

At the point where the passive movement ends, the **end feel** should be assessed. This sensation is experienced through the examiner's hands from the patient's joint and varies according to the cause of the stoppage.

A **hard** end feel is caused by bone meeting bone (e.g. elbow extension). This can be an abnormal finding if the movement is restricted or if that end feel is not normal at the joint being tested. It suggests the presence of some extra growth of bone.

A **capsular** end feel is firm with a hint of stretch, indicating that the movement has been ended by the resistance of the ligaments (e.g. shoulder rotation). This end feel is abnormal if the movement is restricted. Such restriction may indicate arthritis, chronic effusion or contracture of the capsule.

The meeting of the posterior thigh with the calf when the knee is flexed stops that movement with an end feel which Cyriax & Cyriax (1993) call **tissue approximation**.

A hard **twanging** end feel is caused by muscle spasm. This is abnormal and may be triggered by the presence of arthritis or a severe ligament tear.

A **springy block**, preventing completion of the normal range of movement with a rebound, may be caused by a protruding meniscus tear at the knee, or a loose body in the joint.

An **empty** end feel means that the patient stops the movement because of pain, or the expectation of pain. This suggests an acute lesion which is severe and may be serious.

Resisted movement

Injury to muscle or tendon can be detected by passive stretching of the muscle; however, passive movement will also elicit symptoms from the inert tissues of the joint. Only **resisted** testing, with no movement at the joint, isolates the contractile tissue.

On occasion, problems other than muscle injury may cause pain with resisted testing (e.g. fracture, tumour, infection, or an inflamed bursa compressed by the muscle). In some of these cases, there are other indicators which help with the diagnosis. These may be found in the history or in appearances such as fever, redness and heat, tenderness, and pain on passive movement. In other cases, the pain does not restrict itself to the action of one muscle. In practice, these complaints often announce themselves by other signs and symptoms.

Each joint has a **loose-packed** or **resting** position, where the joint capsule is at its most lax. This position, or something near it, is recommended by Cyriax & Cyriax (1993) (see Meadows (1999)) for discussion of different positions during testing) for resisted testing because the inert tissues will not be stressed. Conversely, the **close-packed** position, when the joint surfaces are close together and the ligaments are tense, is less suitable. As a generalization, joint tissues are lax in the mid position of the joint and tense at the extremes of their range.

One hand is used to stabilize the patient. The other offers resistance in the opposite direction to the movement which the patient will attempt. The patient begins an isometric contraction of the muscle against your increasing resistance and increases it until full force is exerted. The patient then gradually relaxes as the examiner reduces resistance.

There are recommended positions for tests of every joint and muscle. The position of the resisting hand should be fairly close to the joint. If it is placed on the far side of a second joint (e.g. resisting shoulder movement by pressure at the wrist) then the test will include muscles at both joints. It may not be clear where symptoms are coming from, and if the elbow is weaker than the shoulder in that movement, the shoulder will not be fully tested. It is sometimes useful to place the resisting hand a long way from the test joint, if the patient has great power at that joint and some mechanical advantage is needed to offer enough resistance. If the examiner is not strong enough to overpower the patient at that joint, the joint will move and the test will be invalidated. There can be problems when a small examiner is testing a large athlete.

There are two abnormal findings, weakness and pain. Cyriax & Cyriax (1993) interpret the combinations as follows:

- a **strong, pain-free** muscle is normal
- a **strong, painful** muscle has a partial injury which hurts but does not reduce function
- a **weak, painless** muscle may have a complete tear of the belly or tendon, or there may a nerve lesion
- a **weak, painful** muscle suggests a major problem, fracture or metastasis.

Accessory movement and stress testing

Accessory movement and stress testing refer to passive tests at the joint of movements which the patient cannot perform voluntarily because they are not under the control of the muscles.

Accessory movements are slight movements which the joint allows, sometimes called **joint-play**, as a result of normal laxity in the capsule. They are tested in the loose-packed position. They are an important aspect of normal movement. A hypermobile joint lacks stability. A hypomobile joint is restricted at the extremes of its range of movement.

Stress testing is the passive stretching of ligaments to detect injury. An acute minor tear will be painful when the ligament is stressed. A complete tear may be shown by pain-free laxity.

Accessory movement is tested when active and passive movements are limited but resisted tests are normal. The patient is shown the loose-packed position for the joint and the examiner uses two hands, placed close to each other on either side of the joint. One of the bones is stabilized with one hand, and the other hand applies traction to open the joint and separate its surfaces. Rotation, rocking and gliding movements may also be used. Accessory movements are often tiny and hard to assess. The patient's range on the normal joint is the best guide. The end feel will usually be capsular, whether the joint is normal or not.

Stress testing is done in the position which best isolates the individual ligament. The result will not be reliable if the patient has muscle spasm around the joint because of pain or instability. The end feel may be capsular with a normal ligament; empty with pain, if it is sprained; empty without pain, if gross laxity is present after a complete tear; and hard, or 'twanging', if muscle spasm stops the movement.

Complicating Factors In Examination

The method of examination which has been described above may produce confusion if other considerations are not weighed in the assessment of the findings:

1. The capsular and non-capsular pattern of pain
2. Referred pain
3. Nerve symptoms.

(The material in this part is largely based upon Cyriax & Cyriax (1993).)

The capsular and non-capsular pattern of pain

Cyriax & Cyriax (1993) describes a pattern of restricted movement in synovial joints which he calls the **capsular pattern**. The pattern is different for each joint but is the same for that joint in different people. When movement is reduced in the capsular pattern, the entire joint capsule is inflamed. Arthritis, haemarthrosis and frozen shoulder are among the complaints which can cause this restriction.

The capsular pattern is seen to the same extent in active and passive movements. The restriction is in certain movements only, and the particular movements affected vary from one joint to another. Most importantly, these movements are restricted in a **fixed proportion** (not in a fixed amount). For example, the capsular pattern for the shoulder is a large restriction of lateral rotation, moderate restriction of abduction and a slight loss of medial rotation. A capsular problem which is not severe at the shoulder may only have a slight effect on lateral rotation to begin with, but as the disability develops the other movements will be affected in turn, abduction first and then medial rotation.

Restriction of passive movement in a non-capsular pattern suggests a lesion which does not involve the whole capsule, such as a ligament injury, a loose body or a lesion which lies outside the joint.

It is important to recognize the capsular pattern when it is present so that restrictions in movement are properly interpreted. Without knowledge of the capsular pattern, it would be difficult to make any sense of certain examination findings. Capsular restriction is not a diagnosis in itself, but it narrows the field of investigation.

The capsular patterns for the main joints are given at the relevant place in Part 2.

Referred pain

Referred pain is pain which is felt in the wrong place. The fact that the brain can misinterpret the source of a pain adds complication for patient and examiner. Pain can be referred to less vital areas from major organs, and life-threatening events can announce themselves with symptoms that can be mistaken for minor musculoskeletal ailments.

Pain referral is not random. The brain receives impressions of pain on a regional basis, and it seems that, on some occasions, it has difficulty distinguishing between the different parts of the region which contains the injury or illness. The part of the body in which the brain perceives pain is determined by which segment of the spine supplies the injured part with sensory fibres, and where the **dermatome** for that segment lies. A dermatome is an area of skin which receives sensory fibres from one segment of the spine, from one posterior spinal root. The same segment also supplies sensory fibres to muscle in a defined area (which may not follow the outline of that segment's dermatome), the **myotome**, and to bone, the **sclerotome** (sclerotomes are less important in this discussion because pain from bone does not tend to refer). The organs, or viscera, are also supplied with some sensory fibres, and **visceral** pain can refer in the same pattern to the dermatome for the segment which supplies the organ.

The apparent randomness of some of these segmental relationships is explained by the fact that they derive from the embryo, and subsequent growth has separated neighbouring tissues. The dermatomes of the limbs are dispersed in a puzzling manner (Figs 5.8 and 5.9), whereas those on the trunk are closely related to their vertebral segment. In the embryo, the limbs are no more than little buds at the top and bottom of the spine. The dermatomes are 'stretched' by the subsequent growth of the limbs, but their original layers can still be detected.

The given explanation (Cyriax & Cyriax, 1993) for the referral of pain is that the brain is organized to receive sensory stimuli from the skin to a much greater extent than from the deeper tissues, and it mistakenly attributes sensations to the skin that in fact come from the myotomes or viscera in a particular segment. Although the brain sometimes fails to indicate the source of deep tissue pain, it can tell which segment the pain comes from and 'refers' it to the dermatome for that segment. Therefore, even if it is not clear where the pain is coming from, the structures that are possible sources is known from which tissues share that segment and that dermatome.

The dermatome for a given spinal segment can be a long way from organs and muscles supplied by the same segment. The heart derives in part from T1 and T2 and so cardiac pain may be felt in the arm. The diaphragm originates from C3 and C4, with dermatomes at the neck and shoulder.

The interpretation of referred pain arising from an organ may be made easier by the fact

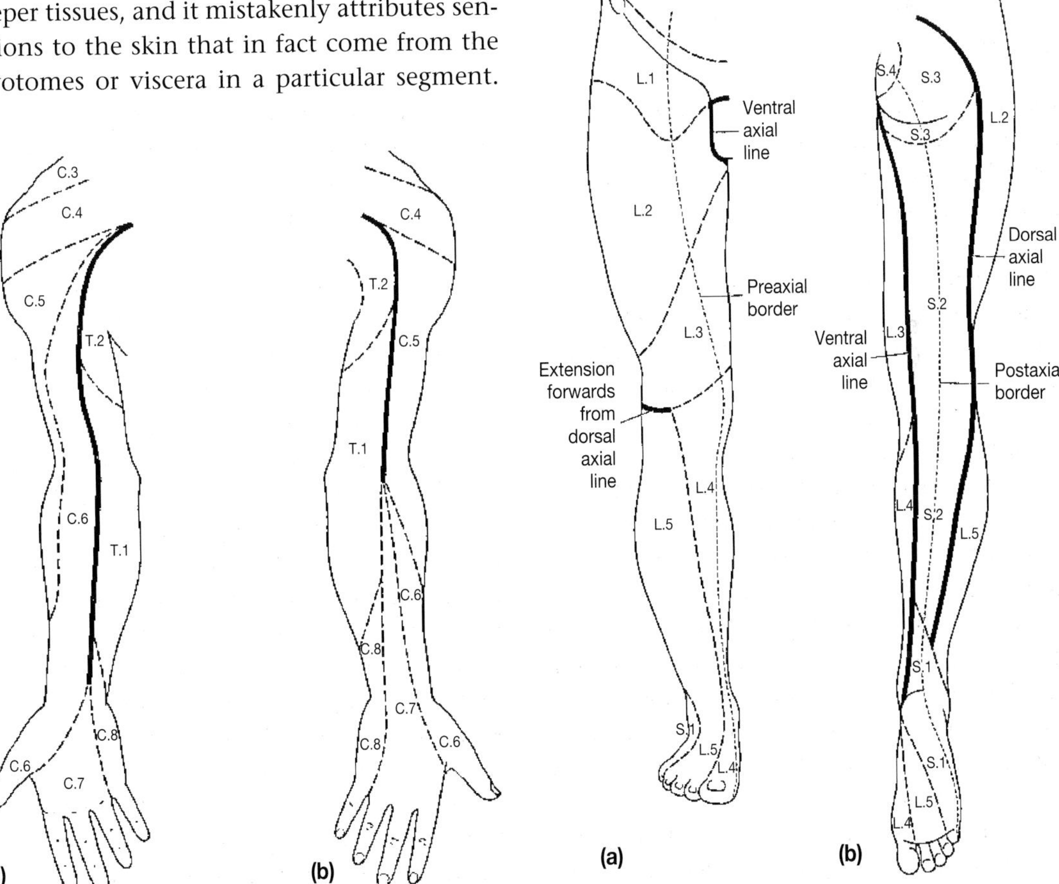

Figure 5.8 Dermatomes of the upper limb. (Adapted with kind permission from Williams, 1995.)

Figure 5.9 Dermatomes of the lower limb. (Adapted with kind permission from Williams, 1995.)

that organ disease of any kind usually produces other signs and symptoms, as well as pain, which will clarify the issue. It may also be that the minor injury clinic will have some means of detecting these changes. There may be features in the history or the patient's general appearance which suggest illness. The NP may examine the area and assess perfusion and nerve supply. Any applicable and available standard tools of assessment can be used: the vital signs, and perhaps urinalysis, blood analysis or electrocardiography. The failure to find a musculoskeletal injury at the painful place warrants a medical review of the patient. A referral to a doctor will be more or less urgent depending on the patient's condition and the differential diagnosis.

The interpretation of pain referred from a nerve lesion is discussed below. The interpretation of pain referred by a musculoskeletal injury or disease is based upon the testing of the tissues which may be involved: those belonging to the myotome which shares a segment with the dermatome where the pain is felt. This is discussed above. The relevant sections in Part 2 contain the information on particular structures.

Referred pain has certain characteristics:

- referral to a great distance from the site of the lesion can occur in the limbs because the dermatomes are long
- even when pain refers a long way, it will remain in the same dermatome
- although the pattern of referral is decided by the position of the dermatome, the patient can tell that the problem is not in the skin as the pain feels 'deep'
- the more severe the pain, the greater the distance it refers
- in most cases, pain refers distally to the lesion
- referred pain does not cross the midline of the body.
- the more proximal the lesion (i.e. the closer to the trunk), and the deeper the source of pain, the more likely it is to refer: patients will localize injuries in the hand very well, whereas they are often vague about the source of shoulder pain

When pain is referred from an injury to muscle or joint, the quality of the pain does not vary according to the tissue which is injured; the injured part is found by testing the function of the possible culprits in that segment.

In cases where it is not clear whether a pain is referred the tissues are tested at the painful site. If the pain is not increased, and function is normal during testing, then it is possible that the pain is referred. The tissues are then tested within the segment where the pain is felt. If that does not reveal the source, referral from a central organ is considered. The neurological and vascular condition of the affected part must always be assessed.

Referral of pain from the dura mater does not follow the segmental pattern.

Nerve symptoms

Pain can be referred from a nerve lesion in such a way that it is not immediately clear whether the problem is musculoskeletal or neurological. Patients also present to minor injury clinics with definite neurological symptoms. Head injuries are discussed in Chapter 9.

The urgency of such problems varies. Some patients will have a long history and be well known to the GP. Other patients may present with new, severe symptoms.

Patients with neurological symptoms should be seen by a doctor. However, that does not settle the matter. The NP needs to have criteria by which to decide whether or not patients have neurological complaints and must examine them sufficiently to assess the urgency of the problem.

It is, therefore, important to discuss some of the neurological symptoms which patients commonly mention in minor injury clinics. The intentions are threefold: first, to be aware when a patient has a neurological problem; second, to have a broad idea of its extent and implications, so that a referral will be appropriate and timely; third, to know when problems are *not* neurological.

Musculoskeletal injury may cause pain and weakness, together or separately. It does not cause tingling or numbness. It will cause some loss of function in the tissue which is injured, and this should be revealed by stressing that tissue. Several situations suggest a possible nerve problem: where spinal movement aggravates peripheral symptoms, where stretching of a nerve (e.g. by straight leg raising) increases the symptoms, where weakness is not accompanied by a history or signs of trauma to musculoskeletal tissue, where the loss of function follows a nerve pathway and involves more than one muscle, or where paraesthesia plays a part in the complaint.

Compression of the central spinal cord and dura mater may cause bilateral symptoms of paraesthesia, weakness and pain, not conforming to a dermatome. This will not be mistaken for a musculoskeletal problem.

Compression of a nerve root's dural sheath at its emergence from the spine causes so-called **radicular** pain. This pain is referred to the dermatome for that vertebral segment. Root compression in the neck may cause pain in the arm; compression in the lumbar and sacral region can refer to the leg. If the nerve fibre inside the sheath is also affected by the compression, there may be dermatomal tingling or numbness, and weakness in the muscles served by the motor fibres of the nerve (which would be shown by resisted testing). Resisted muscle testing may show a loss of power when the nerve root is compressed, but this can be distinguished from a local muscle lesion in most cases. The history may clarify the issue. Aggravation of symptoms by spinal movement suggests compression. Passive stretching of the nerve root and dural sheath causes pain in the appropriate dermatome (some of these tests are shown at the relevant section in Part 2). Weakness without pain distributed through the various muscles served by one nerve suggests a nerve problem. The pain caused by dural compression should not be increased by testing of the local tissues as long as the tests do not move the spine or stretch the dura mater.

Compression or other injury to the sensory distribution of peripheral nerves causes reduced sensation, experienced as tingling or numbness. Injury to the motor distribution of peripheral nerves causes palsy, with eventual wasting of the affected muscles. The symptoms will be experienced in the pathway of the nerve which is affected, unlike the dermatomal distribution of nerve root symptoms. Symptoms will be distal to the lesion. There are many common peripheral neural compression syndromes.

It has been mentioned, in the section on referred pain, that injuries in distal areas such as hand and foot are easier to localize than in central areas like neck and shoulder. It may be difficult to be sure, when dealing with neck, shoulder or back pain, whether or not the symptoms are referred from a nerve. It is also important to exclude an organic disease. Diagnosis of these problems is difficult for specialists and the patient often needs repeated examination and investigations. It is more important for a NP to know the range of possibilities, assess the urgency of the patient's condition, treat the acute symptoms and refer appropriately than to find a label for the problem.

2

Part 2
MUSCULOSKELETAL INJURIES

6 THE NECK AND UPPER LIMBS

CONTENTS

In this chapter, the anatomy, methods of examination and some of the common injuries of the arm, wrist and hand will be discussed.

It is true that the neck is a different issue to the arm, in terms of anatomy and pathology, and in terms of the dangers which injury may bring. However, the neck is often the source of pain in the arm, and it is also the source of many of the structures which cause symptoms in the arm, and it seems sensible to discuss it here.

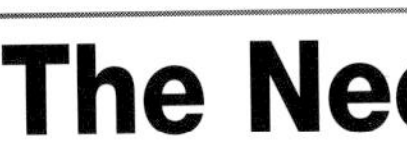

The Neck

Concern about musculoskeletal injury to the neck centres on the cervical spine. Displacement of a part of that structure may damage, or threaten to damage, the function of the spinal cord. Such injuries can easily be lethal or paralyse the patient for life. Dangerous injuries may also appear to be harmless in the first instance, a fact which must weigh heavily with the NP, especially in a stand-alone clinic.

Many of the injuries which people suffer to the neck may be classed as 'minor'. This label does not, however, help the NP confronted by a patient with a problem in that region. There are four difficulties.

1. A neck problem may be minor in the sense that it is not threatening to life or limb, in the sense that no vital structure has been damaged, or in the sense that there is no advanced treatment to offer the patient. However, the problem may not be easy to diagnose or treat, and the patient may suffer from recurrence or prolonged pain and disability.
2. Many patients who present to the NP as 'injured', with pain in the neck, have no history of injury. The nurse has the task of deciding whether the pain has a musculoskeletal source, or whether the patient is ill and needs referral to a doctor. Is the pain referred from a vital organ, or is some other disease process, such as neoplasm or infection, causing the symptoms? This is a heavy responsibility. A medical opinion must be sought in any case which is not clear.

3. It can be difficult, when examining patients with pain in the neck and surrounding areas (including the head, the upper back and the arms), to distinguish between well-localized pain and tenderness at the site of a muscle injury and pain which is referred to those areas from the spine and the spinal nerves. The rules for assessment of those problems are the same as for the limbs, but the task of examination is more demanding, in terms of the time, complexity and knowledge required to reach a diagnosis and exclude dangerous possibilities. In cases where there is a question of this kind, a patient is referred to a doctor.
4. The difficulty of interpretation of radiographs and the range of non-trauma conditions which may be revealed (as well as the questionable value of many radiographs of painful necks) means that it is unlikely for a NP to be allowed to request them. The assessment of the patient by a NP will be restricted to a clinical examination. The patient will need to be referred to a doctor if the patient's problem is one for which an X-ray, or some other form of investigation, is a part of the accepted standard of management.

The NP who works in an A&E department may not have to treat patients with injuries to the neck, but the NP who works in a stand-alone unit, in community or hospital, may have to make at least an initial assessment of every patient who presents. The NP will have to deal with the initial situation and make a correct, and safe, referral. However, it is likely that the protocols or guidelines for the NP clinic will permit a further stage: the treatment and discharge of patients whose problem can be assessed as minor.

In this section, some basic anatomy is given to assist in understanding problems in the neck, and to relate to later information on the arm. The standards by which injuries to the neck may be judged to be minor, or not, will be described. The information which is offered is general. Each practice must be directed by its own protocols or guidelines.

Anatomy

The discussion of neck injuries will begin with a review of those elements of the anatomy of the cervical spine which cast light on recognized patterns of injury.

The cervical section of the spine comprises the upper seven vertebrae and their ligaments and cartilage-covered intervertebral discs. It is a structure which, perhaps more than any other in the body, copes with conflicting demands. It is stable enough to support the weight of the head, yet it is the most flexible part of the spine to permit the mobility which the head requires. At the same time, it provides the armour which protects the spinal cord from damage. It also allows passage for the fibres of the cord, through a multitude of outlets, to the tissues which it supplies. The vertebral artery passes along the cervical spine to the brain.

Bone supplies the rigid elements in the spine. The vertebrae are a vertical stack of irregular bones separated in their frontal sections by pads of fibrocartilage filled with a semi-liquid substance called the **nucleus pulposus** and linked in their rear sections by a succession of pairs of synovial facet joints. The pads, called **intervertebral discs**, allow flexibility between the bony parts of the spine, and they also function as shock absorbers. The spine is arranged in a straight line when seen from the front or back, but in a series of alternating curves when seen from the side. The cervical section has a concave curve on its posterior aspect. The thoracic spine (the 12 vertebrae which articulate with the ribs) is convex. The lumbar (five vertebrae which lie in the lower back and link the whole structure through the sacrum, to the pelvic girdle and the lower limbs) is concave. The sacrum, the section of five, fused vertebrae which articulates with the two wings of the pelvis at the back, is convex. The erect posture of the human is the result of a succession of resilient, variable, dynamic compensations rather than simple straightness, and problems with the alignment of the spine, and the balance of the structures which support it, may be a cause of chronic pain and recurring injury. **Scoliosis** is a term which means that the spine has an abnormal curve to the side. **Kyphosis** means an increase in the normal convexity of the thoracic spine, seen from the side, and **lordosis** refers to the opposite phenomenon in the lumbar area, an accentuation of the curve of the lower back.

The vertebrae are similar in shape and structure along the whole length of the spine. They become larger as they descend to the pelvis. However, the first and second cervical vertebrae (Figs 6.1 and 6.2), sometimes called the upper cervical spine, are specially adapted and rather different from the other vertebrae. They perform the particular task of uniting the spine to the skull and permitting the head to flex, extend and rotate.

The vertebrae of the lower cervical spine (Fig. 6.3), C3 to C7, consist of an anterior part, which is a disc of bone, the **body**, and a posterior part, the **vertebral arch**. The arch is made up of small bony processes united to form an enclosed space. Two small rods project backwards, one on each side, from the vertebral body. These are called the **pedicles**. On each side, the bony projections which begin as the pedicles continue at a new angle, still backwards but turning towards each other so that they meet in the midline, where they fuse. These projections now look flattened rather than rounded and are called **laminae**. The space which is enclosed by the posterior border of the body, the pedicles and the laminae is called the **vertebral foramen**.

Continuing backwards from the point of fusion of the laminae there is, in the cervical region, a **bifid** (meaning, in two parts) bony projection, the **spinous process** of the vertebra. The spinous processes collectively are the most accessible parts of the spine for the examiner. They form the series of bony projections which can be felt in the midline of the back from the top of the neck to the top of the cleft of the buttocks.

Each vertebra also has two **transverse processes**, one projecting from each side of the vertebral body and both pointing in a lateral direction. The transverse processes of the cervical spine are unusual in having a smaller version of the vertebral foramen, a small opening called the **transverse foramen**, enclosed within each process. The vertebral artery passes up through the channel created by these openings to make its way to the cranium.

The three processes, the two transverse and the spinous, are used as attachment points for ligaments and muscles. (In the thoracic area, the transverse processes are part of the articulation with the ribs at the back.)

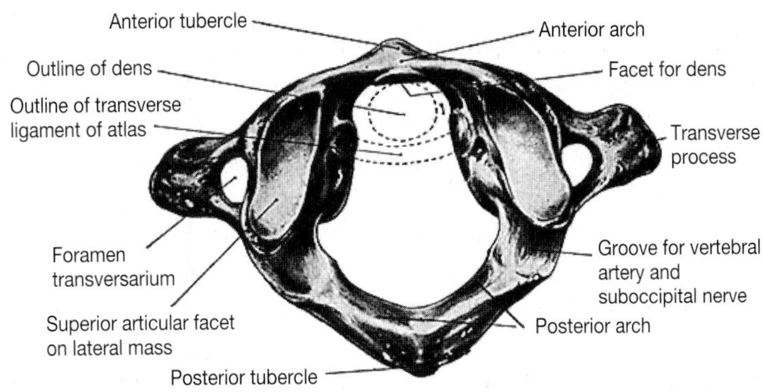

Figure 6.1 The first cervical vertebra (atlas), superior aspect. (Adapted with kind permission from Williams, 1995.)

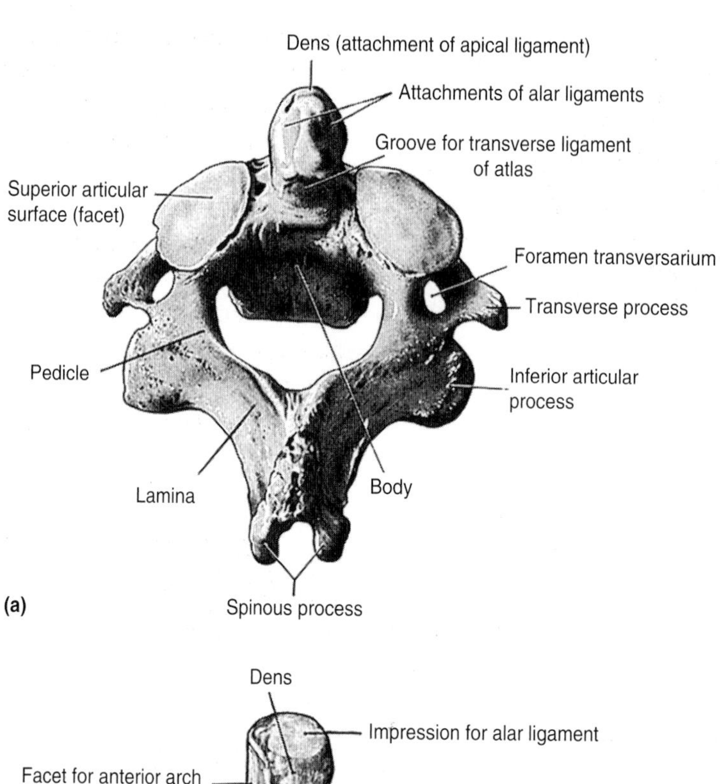

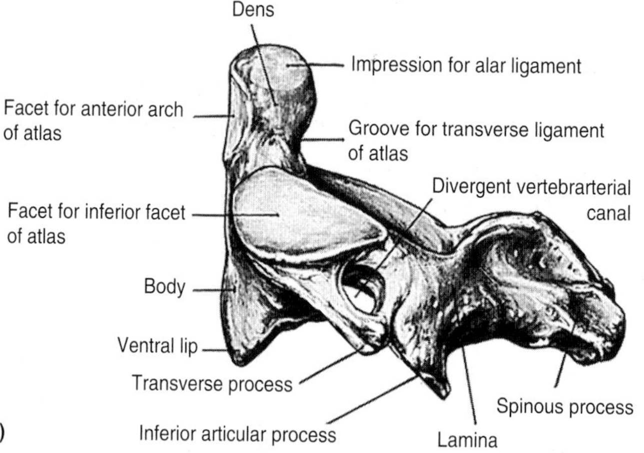

Figure 6.2 The second cervical vertebra (axis): (a) Posterosuperior aspect; (b) left lateral aspect. (Adapted with kind permission from Williams, 1995.)

On the superior and inferior aspects of the arch, at the points where the pedicles meet the laminae, there are articular projections called the **zygapophyses**. The zygapophyses on the upper surfaces of the arch articulate with those on the underside of the vertebral arch above, and so on throughout the spine. The **zygapophyseal joints** are synovial and allow a limited amount of movement, variable from one to another. The surfaces of these articular processes, which are covered with hyaline cartilage, are called **facets**.

There are six intervertebral discs in the cervical area. These are made of a combination of three substances. There is a coating of hyaline cartilage on the opposing surfaces of the two vertebral bodies, which are linked by the disc. These are called the **cartilage end plates**. The disc proper is connected to these. The disc itself has a soft centre, a thick, jelly substance called the nucleus pulposus, which gives the disc its resilience but which can herniate if its retaining outer layer is ruptured (the event known as a slipped disc). The outer layer of the

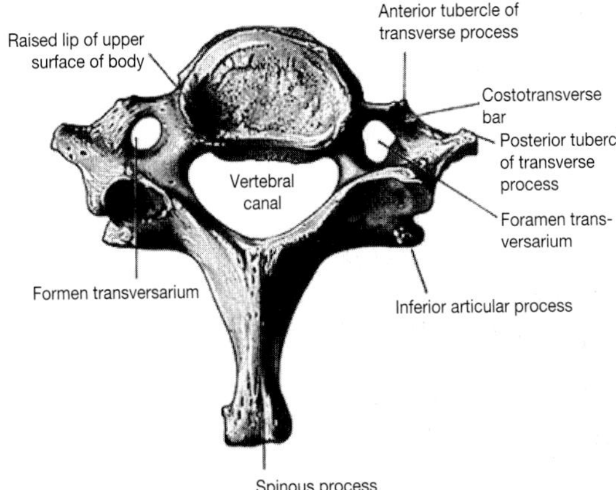

Figure 6.3 The vertebrae of the lower cervical spine: the seventh superior aspect. (Adapted with kind permission from Williams, 1995.)

disc is an arrangement of multiple bands of fibrocartilage, the **annulus fibrosus**, which contains the nuclei.

There is space between the pedicles of neighbouring vertebrae for the passage of spinal nerves into and out of the spine. These gaps between the pedicles are called the **intervertebral foramina** (meaning, openings between vertebrae).

The chain of vertebral foramina which is formed by the arches of the spine is called, in combination, the **vertebral canal**, and it is through this structure that the spinal cord passes from head to pelvis.

The **spinal cord** runs through the vertebral canal. It forms a part of the **central nervous system**. It is described as being divided into a series of **segments**; each segment has a pair of **spinal nerves**, and these nerves pass out into the body through the intervertebral foramina of the spine, where they form part of the **peripheral nervous system**. The parts of the spinal nerve which joins the spinal cord are called the **roots**. Each nerve has two roots, a **ventral** (front) and a **dorsal** root. The ventral root carries **efferent** (from the Latin, to carry out of) motor fibres from the cord to the spinal nerve. These nerves ultimately pass to muscles and stimulate them to contract. The dorsal root delivers **afferent** (from the Latin, to carry to) sensory fibres from the spinal nerve to the cord. The cervical segments are numbered from one to eight. C1 to C7 nerve roots emerge from above the vertebra for which they are numbered, and C8 emerges from between C7 and T1.

The **brachial plexus** (see also **lumbar plexus** (Ch. 7)) is a combination into a network of the ventral nerves from C5 to T1, with exchanges of fibres between the different segmental nerves. It occurs after the nerve has emerged from the spine but before it reaches its peripheral distribution. The brachial plexus supplies the shoulder and arm with motor and sensory fibres (Fig. 6.4).

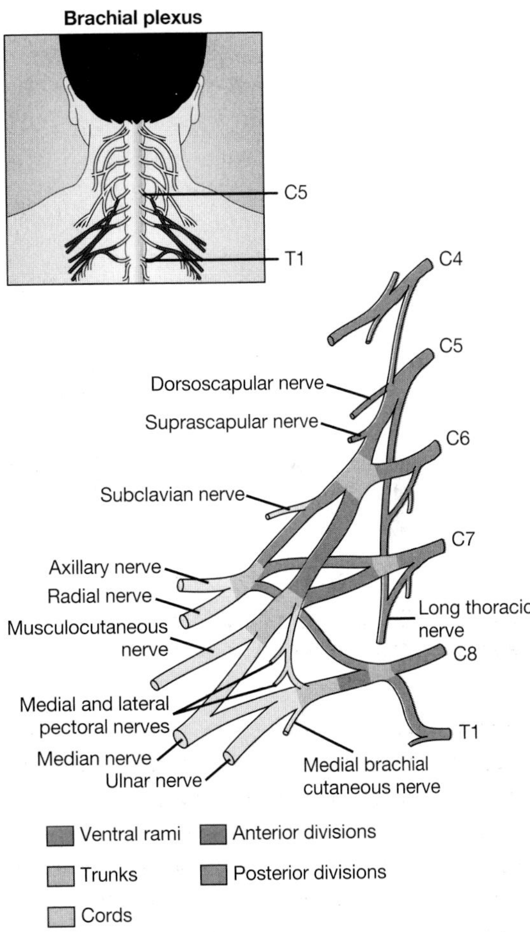

Figure 6.4 Brachial plexus. Three trunks form from the five rami (C5 to T1) and then subdivide into divisions then cords. The cords give rise to the individual nerves leaving the plexus. (Reproduced with kind permission from Thibodeau and Patton, 1999.)

The intervertebral discs which lie between each vertebral body are also, on their posterior aspects, in close contact with the spinal cord, and any injury which causes a herniation of the disc in a backward direction may interfere with the function of the cord. Cyriax & Cyriax (1993) point out that the anterior dura mater covering the spinal cord where it meets the vertebral bodies and discs, and the dura mater, which covers nerve roots as they pass out from the spine, are innervated, and pain will be felt if either is overstretched or compressed. There are two possibilities.

1. A backward herniation of the disc will impinge first on the dura mater where it covers the central cord and cause extrasegmentally referred pain, usually on one side only (see pain referral, Ch. 5). In the cervical area, this pain may be felt in the neck, over to the forehead, or, most commonly, in the scapular and shoulder area.
2. A herniation which is backwards but to one side or other, rather than central, will impinge upon the nerve root on that side, which is also covered at that point in a sleeve of dura mater. This will only cause pain if the pressure is slight but will cause signs of nerve compression (weakness, paraesthesia and reflex suppression) if the pressure is deep enough to reach the nerve within the sheath. These symptoms will refer to the dermatome for that nerve root.

Three of the cervical vertebrae have special features which require further description. C7 (Fig. 6.3) has a larger body than the other cervical vertebrae and a longer, non-bifid, spinous process. It offers a conspicuous landmark at the base of the back of the neck, at the point of transition between the cervical and the thoracic spine. T1 is also seen, even more prominent than C7, and just below it.

In the upper cervical spine, C1, also called the **atlas**, (Fig. 6.1) after the mythic Titan who carried the weight of the heavens upon his shoulders, bears the weight of the skull. It has two articular facets on its upper surface, and the **occipital bone** lies upon them at the **atlanto-occipital joints**. These joints permit some degree of flexion and extension of the head. The undersurfaces of the atlanto-occipital joints are also adapted for articulation with the upper surfaces of C2, at the **atlanto-axial joints**. The atlas has no vertebral body or intervertebral disc. It is simply a bony ring made up of a front and rear arch, linked at the sides by its articular masses. The atlas has a transverse process on each side, which can be felt just under the mastoid processes (the prominences behind the ears) of the skull. Unlike the other vertebrae it does not have a projecting spinous process at the rear. There is only a **posterior tubercle**, a little button of bone which is difficult to palpate.

C2 (Fig. 6.2) is also called the **axis**. It does possess a vertebral body but has a unique feature: a peg-like bony projection rises from its superior surface like a tooth (hence, its names, the **dens**, or the **odontoid process**, both derive from terms for teeth). This peg projects upwards through the arch of the atlas. It is stabilized there by ligaments, inside the **foramen magnum** (meaning, large opening) of the skull, which gives access to the cranium on the underside of the occipital bone. The **transverse ligament** crosses behind the dens and the **alar ligaments** pass from the dens to the occipital bone on each side. The atlas, and with it the skull, rotate about the fixed point of the axis. Half of the neck's range of rotation occurs at this joint. The alar ligaments are placed to prevent excessive rotation on the side opposite to each ligament (i.e. the alar ligament on the left tightens as the head rotates to the right). The alar ligament also prevents separation of the axis from the atlas. It becomes tighter as the neck is flexed. Injury which involves forced flexion and rotation of the head may rupture the ligament, allowing excessive rotation on the side which is opposite to the tear. Patients will sometimes demonstrate the frightening sense of instability which this type of injury inspires by holding onto their heads as if to prevent them from falling off.

Other ligaments stabilize the spinal column as a whole. The **anterior longitudinal ligament** is strong and passes down the front of the spine, attaching to vertebrae and to discs. It limits the range of extension of the spine. The **posterior longitudinal ligament** passes up the back of the spine, attaching to the intervertebral discs. This limits the range of spinal flexion. **Ligamenta flava**, a series of individual ligaments rather than a continuous band, reinforce the rear of the spine, linking neighbouring laminae and forming a part of the vertebral canal. In the cervical area the **ligamentum nuchae** also passes from the occipital area to the spinous process of C7.

Movement in the cervical spine is allowed and limited by the same forces, the action of the various ligaments, the disposition of the zagapophyseal joints and the mobility of the intervertebral discs, which have a capacity for compression, rotation and for stretching. In the cervical area, the discs are relatively thick, and this adds to the range of movement. The muscles of the neck offer a dynamic force for stability and mobility, and they exert a powerful protective influence when injury occurs by going into spasm to immobilize the injured area. This is one of the factors which can, initially, conceal the extent of the instability caused by an injury. Box 6.1 gives the normal cervical spine ranges of movement.

The cervical spine houses the **vertebral artery**. This is a branch of the subclavian artery. It joins the cervical spine at the transverse processes on each side of the C6 vertebra. It then passes up to enter the skull through the spine's point of access to the cranial cavity, the foramen magnum, at the back and underside of the skull in the occipital region. The two branches of the artery unite at this level to form the **basilar artery** within the cranium. This artery, along with the internal carotid artery, carries the brain's blood supply. The vertebral–basilar contribution is about one fifth of the total. Interruption of its function may be caused, among other things, by degeneration or subluxation of the cervical spine, which may stretch or compress the vessels and will affect cerebral activity. Excessive movements of extension and rotation of the neck, common in so-called **whiplash injuries**, may compromise the artery in the region of the foramen magnum. The pathological process will be of ischaemia in the areas supplied. A NP should be aware of suggestive elements in a patient's history. Patients who suffer from cervical spondylosis or rheumatoid arthritis may be affected. A common first complaint, which should alert to the possibility of vertebral artery insufficiency in a patient with neck pain or injury, is of dizziness, and there may be light headedness and nystagmus. These symptoms are not specific to vertebral artery insufficiency alone.

Box 6.1 Cervical Spine Statistics

The ranges of movement quoted here are the composite ranges, made up of smaller movements in different parts of the spine.

Capsular pattern a greater limitation of side-flexion and rotation, a lesser limitation of extension.

Joint positions close packed is extension; loose packed is a small degree of extension.

Flexion approximately to 90°; end feel is firm.

Extension approximately to 70°; end feel firm.

Rotation occurs to each side to approximately 80°; end feel firm.

Side-flexion occurs to each side up to approximately 45° (there is a wide variation between individuals); end feel firm.

Circumduction rotation of the head achieved by combining a fluent sequence of the above movements.

Examination

The patient's history should include any diseases which affect the spine or spinal cord, and any long-standing symptoms which might confuse examination.

A patient with a stiff neck will rotate the whole trunk in order to turn the head. The patient may have a torticollis, usually a combination of rotation and side-flexion of the head. This is usually caused by muscle spasm; however, on occasion, more serious rotational deformities at the facets of the spine may occur. An acute, stiff neck can be very painful. Examination should be sensitive.

Where is the pain? Does it radiate to the shoulder? Does it pass down the arm? How far does it radiate, and in to which part of the arm? Is there a headache? Is there pain in the lower back? Is the patient able to walk?

A posterior disc herniation will refer pain in a non-segmental way, as will injuries to facets and ligaments in the neck. Such pain may cause headache or scapular pain. Posterior/lateral herniations, compressing nerve roots, will cause dermatomal referral (see Ch. 5).

Palpation of the cervical spine

Palpation of the cervical spine is most easily accomplished if the patient lies face down on a trolley with the chin pulled in. Some examination trolleys have a space cut in the head rest to allow more flexion of the neck. At the top of the neck, in the midline, it is easy to feel the spinous process of C2. Below that, the next clearly prominent landmarks are the large processes of C7 and T1. The intervening processes of the cervical spine can be felt, with more or less difficulty, depending on the patient, in the central hollow of the neck. Establish that each process is present, with no gaps or deviations. The transverse processes of the atlas are large and placed just below the mastoid processes of the skull. The others are felt by placing the fingers lateral to the central columns of muscle in the middle of the neck. Once again, the processes of C7 are particularly large.

Palpation of the muscles of the neck and shoulder may reveal tenderness and spasm.

Examination of the range of movement

Movement has to be assessed with particular care when the neck has been injured (Fig. 6.5). In all cases of neck pain and injury, the patient should first demonstrate the active range of movement which feels safe and comfortable. The rationale for this is that a patient will avoid movements which make an instability worse. Any passive testing should be very gentle, and nothing resembling manipulation should occur. In cases where there has been an injury, and its nature and severity are not yet known, passive movement should be avoided completely. Be very careful not to exacerbate the patient's symptoms or worsen the problem.

Nerve tests in the arms

The NP should exclude a loss of sensation or power to the arms in any patient who has suffered a neck injury. Awareness, with the eyes closed, of light touch, comparing one side with the other, is usually an adequate assessment of sensation in a minor injury area. If any defect is found, further investigation is required. The area of any deficit should be mapped with its depth and nature to allow a distinction between problems at the root and the peripheral system.

Power in the myotomes supplied by segments C5 to T1 can be assessed by resisted tests of the following movements:

C5: shoulder abduction (deltoid)
C6: elbow flexion (biceps)
C7: elbow extension (triceps)
C8: thumb extension (extensor pollicis longus)
T1: finger adduction (intrinsics).

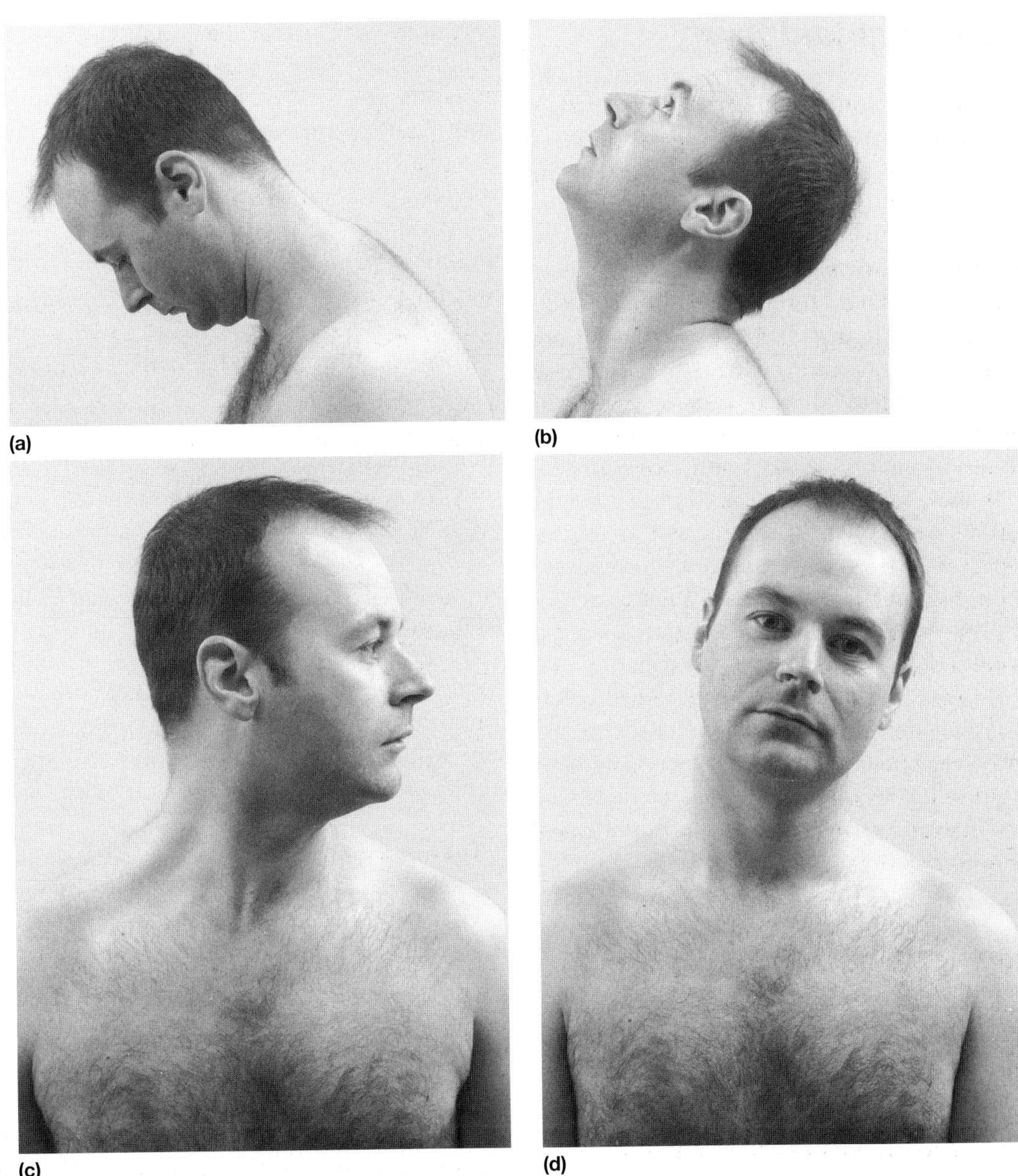

Figure 6-5 Active Neck Movements. (a) Flexion; (b) Extension; (c) Rotation (right and left) and (d) Side flexion (right and left).

These tests are all illustrated later in this chapter.

Once again, any weakness will require further investigation, and a distinction must be made between a root lesion and a peripheral nerve problem. This can be done by testing other muscles which are supplied by the same nerve root and comparing the result with tests of muscles which have the same peripheral supply but a different nerve root.

A patient who has a very painful, acute injury, such as a whiplash or an onset of severe neck pain, may not be able to comply with resisted tests, and any weakness or pain may be misleading. Such a patient will probably need medical referral.

Neck Pain and Injury

In the stand-alone minor injury clinic, there should not be many self-evidently serious neck injuries. These patients will usually be taken by ambulance to more appropriate centres. However, any medical service will occasionally be used as the nearest port in a storm by people who panic and bundle an injured person into a car. There must be plans for that contingency.

Patients should be assumed to have a serious neck injury if there is a severe mechanism of injury, such as a fall from above 10 feet (3 metres), a dive onto the head from a height into shallow water or a car crash at greater than 30 miles per hour, and if they have severe signs and symptoms of injury, such as a very painful, rigid or unstable neck, neurological deficits, loss of consciousness or collapse. The neck should be immobilized in a hard collar the spine kept in neutral alignment with the patient lying flat and the head taped and held in position with sandbags. It may be necessary to initiate a resuscitation, and urgent help is certainly needed by the route that is set up for such situations. The neck must be assessed for all patients who present with complaints of head injury or shoulder pain (see Ch. 9 and later in this chapter).

There are two main categories of neck problems: trauma and pain with no history of injury.

Neck trauma: whiplash

The commonest traumatic neck complaint which patients bring to minor injury clinics is so-called whiplash. The term is controversial, but that is only of interest here to the extent that a a standard pattern of injury cannot be assumed because the tale that one patient tells will be very like that of another. The patient has been involved in a car crash and will probably be distressed and unclear about the exact mechanism of injury.

Factors such as the position of the head at the moment of impact are important in assessing the risk of fractures, subluxations and ligament injuries. Other aspects include the exact position of the patient in the car, the direction and speed of both vehicles, the point where the vehicles struck each other and movement of the patient's car afterwards. Was the patient wearing a seatbelt? Was there a headrest? Which way was the patient looking at the collision? Did the patient's head hit anything?

The patient's signs and symptoms should be established from the time of the injury to the time of the examination and when they resolved, if they did. Was the patient knocked out? Is the patient suffering from headache, amnesia, discharge from nose or ears, neck pain, blackouts, visual disturbances, nausea and vomiting, hearing disturbances, dizziness, coordination problems or weakness or loss of sensation in the limbs? Does the patient have any wounds, bruises or swelling? Are there injuries to clavicle or chest caused by the seat belt?

The patient's posture and demeanour should be observed. Patients who have just emerged from a car crash may look pale and sweaty or they may be distressed and tearful, because they are reacting to the incident rather than because of injury. Give them some time to settle.

A common account is of a patient stopping the car for a traffic light, or making an emergency stop, and a vehicle behind driving into the rear. The patient's head is thrown about, and neck pain follows some minutes or hours later.

Corrigan and Maitland describe (1998) the mechanism:

1. The impact drives the patient's body forward, throwing the head back and hyperextending the neck
2. The muscles at the front of the neck reflexively contract, and the neck is flexed
3. The head and neck decelerate.

The most traumatic aspect of this event is the hyperextension, because the chin will hit the chest before any significant hyperflexion of the neck can occur. Hyperextension can damage muscles, ligaments (especially the anterior longitudinal ligament), the discs (by compression at the back of the disc, overstretching at the front, or tearing of the whole disc from the endplate) and the zygapophyseal joints, which may suffer fractures.

The degree of severity of presentation varies widely. The Quebec classification of severity of whiplash-associated disorders is shown in Table 6.1.

Patients who present in a minor injury clinic will most commonly have injuries at grades 1 or 2. Management of such patients in a minor injury clinic is problematic. NPs are not likely to be able to request neck X-rays. In fact, X-rays are not likely to demonstrate many of the problems which the patient may have, especially in the initial period after injury. However, it is widely accepted that, as a part of correct management of whiplash injuries, the patient should have an X-ray to exclude fracture. The Royal College of Radiologists (1998) recommends X-ray of the cervical spine for patients who have a history of a neck injury and have neck pain. Wardrope and English (1998) say that X-ray examination is not necessary for the patient who has suffered a low-speed impact (less than 10 miles per hour), who is alert and who has a full range of movement and no local tenderness. On this basis, patients with grade 1 injury or worse should have X-ray examination. Local guidelines or protocols will give specific routes to follow with patients who have whiplash injuries.

Examination

Examination of the patient should include:

- palpation of the neck and surrounding structures to assess tenderness and spasm
- assessment of active range of movement only (avoiding any manipulation, including passive movement)
- a neurological assessment.

A neurological assessment should test power and sensation in the arms. A patient who is walking and shows normal coordination and agility in leg movements does not require a full examination of the lower limb. Wardrope and English (1998) recommend that legs can be functionally assessed by asking the patient to stand on one leg, and then the other, with the eyes closed.

Treatment

If the minor injury clinic has access to a physiotherapist, guidelines should be established for the treatment of patients with this type of injury, and appropriate referrals. It is likely that the physiotherapist will favour early and active intervention. This situation will obviously be related to the guidelines for medical referral and X-ray examination.

Table 6.1 The Quebec Scale for severity of whiplash-associated injuries

Grade	*Presentation*
0	No neck pain, no physical signs
1	Neck pain, stiffness and tenderness, no physical signs
2	Neck complaint and musculoskeletal signs
3	Neck complaint and neurological signs
4	Neck complaint and fracture or dislocation

From Corrigan and Maitland (1998) based on Spitzer et al. (1995).

The guidelines for the treatment of soft tissue injuries should be followed (Ch. 5). A soft collar may make the patient more comfortable if movement is restricted and painful. It can relieve the patient of the need to guard against painful movements. However, it will increase stiffness and should not be worn constantly; it is not worn when eating, drinking or sleeping. Gentle movements in the same pattern as for neck examination, within the limits of pain, will help to prevent unnecessary stiffness. There is no evidence that a soft collar shortens the time for recovery. It should be fitted properly. The patient should be able to fit two fingers between collar and neck. It should not force the head into a painful position. If it does not help, or if it makes pain worse, the patient should stop using it.

Ice should be used on the first 1 to 2 days (see Ch. 5), and heat applications should be avoided. Muscle spasm may become a problem, and gentle use of heat in later days, and lying or reclining in positions which support the head and neck, may help.

In bed, supporting the head and neck in a neutral position, using rolled up towels or the like to support the hollow in the back of the neck when lying flat, and higher pillows when lying on the side, will maintain comfort.

The pain may worsen over the first few days. Ibuprofen, for patients who can tolerate it, combines analgesic and anti-inflammatory benefits. Advise the patient to see a GP if pain relief is a problem.

Neck pain with no history of injury

There are many degenerative, inflammatory and mechanical causes of neck pain and restriction, and other illnesses may refer pain to the neck. Patients with such problems require a general assessment, and, perhaps, the exclusion of serious infections such as meningitis and events such as myocardial infarction. Treatment of such patients is outside the framework of the minor injury clinic, and an appropriate referral should be made, often to the patient's GP.

Torticollis or wry neck

Torticollis is a description of a clinical appearance rather than a diagnosis, and it should be treated with caution. The cervical spine is twisted, muscle spasm is present and the patient cannot straighten the head. This may be a non-specific response to something wrong in the neighbourhood of the spasm. In the absence of a clear history of injury, keep an open mind about what that might be. Infection and neoplasm are among the possible causes. The problem is commonest in young adult women, and the usual history is of waking with a sudden pain in the neck. The neck is usually twisted away from the painful side (this is more marked in some cases than others), and attempts to move it back will hurt and feel impeded. There are usually no neurological deficits. Corrigan and Maitland (1998) ascribe the cause, tentatively, to a zygapophyseal joint derangement. They think that the youth of the typical patients makes a degenerative disc problem unlikely. They recommend physiotherapy to treat it.

The Shoulder

ANATOMY

The dynamic relationship of the arm to the trunk is established by a bony girdle the main feature of which is mobility rather than stability. Such stability as the shoulder has is maintained by soft tissues, muscles, ligaments and capsular tissues.

The bones of the shoulder girdle are the **scapula**, the **clavicle** and the **humerus**. The scapula articulates with the chest wall (the **scapulothoracic** joint), the clavicle (the **acromioclavicular joint**) and the humerus (the **glenohumeral joint**) (Fig. 6.6). In addition, the clavicle articulates at its medial end with the sternum (the **sternoclavicular joint**).

The Scapula

The scapula is a triangular plate of cupped bone, with its concavity lying on the wall of the posterior thorax between the second and seventh ribs (Fig. 6.7). It is attached to the trunk by muscles only. The apex of the triangle points downwards. A prominent bony ridge, called the **spine of the scapula** (a visible and palpable landmark on the upper back), crosses the dorsal surface of the scapula from high on its medial border to the superior, lateral corner of the bone, where it expands to become the **acromion process** (process means bony projection). This process articulates with the lateral end of the clavicle at the synovial acromioclavicular joint.

The dorsal surface of the scapula is divided by the spine into a small **supraspinous fossa** (meaning, the hollow above the spine), and a larger **infraspinous fossa**. The front surface of the scapula forms a single hollow called the **subscapular fossa**. Many of the muscles of the shoulder girdle are attached to these

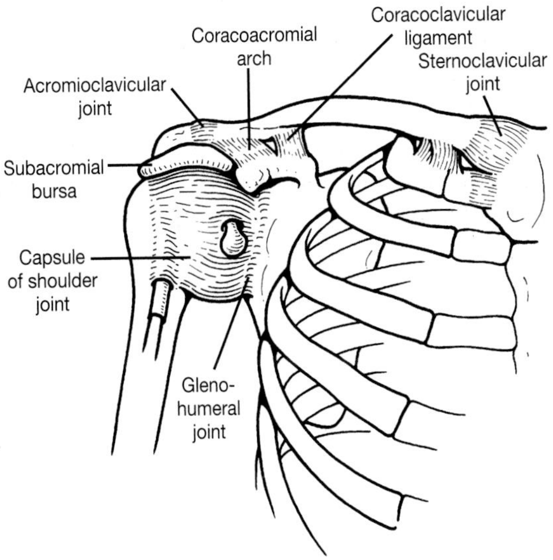

Figure 6.6 The joints of the shoulder region. (Adapted with kind permission from Dean and Pegington, 1996.)

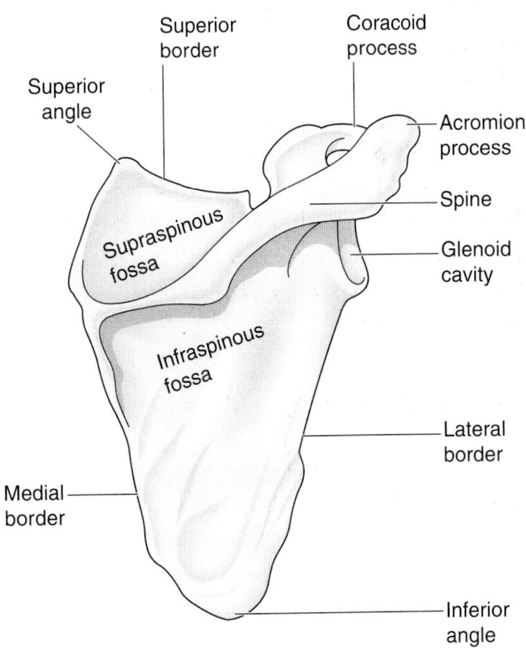

Figure 6.7 Posterior view of the right scapula. (Reproduced with kind permission from Waugh and Grant, 2001.)

surfaces. At the **acromial angle** of the scapula, slightly inferior to the bony arch, two important structures are found. The **glenoid fossa** is the shallow socket which articulates with the head of the humerus to form the shoulder joint. The **coracoid process** is a bony hook which points forwards and offers attachment for muscles and ligaments. It lies above the glenoid fossa, in the shelter of the acromion process. The bony arch over the shoulder is reinforced by the **coracoacromial ligament**, which crosses from the acromion to the coracoid process.

The scapula has a large repertoire of movements and contributes much to the mobility of the shoulder. It can be moved straight up and down, it can be adducted and abducted and it can rotate so that the glenoid fossa faces up or down.

The acromioclavicular joint

The acromioclavicular joint forms the bony arch which covers the shoulder joint proper. The joint has, in addition to its own capsule, the reinforcement of the **coracoclavicular ligament**, a two-part ligament made up of the **conoid** and **trapezoid** ligaments, which anchors the clavicle to the coracoid process of the scapula. No muscles cross this joint and its movement is passive only. The joint moves to allow movements of the scapula laterally and medially round the chest wall, up and down, and to allow scapular rotation when the shoulder is flexed.

The clavicle

The clavicle, seen from above, is a bone with curves following a long, flattened S-shape from the sternoclavicular joint, medially, to the acromioclavicular joint at its lateral end. It is superficial and forms a very distinctive dividing line between neck and chest. The clavicle braces the arm at the distance from the trunk which is necessary for it to have freedom of movement.

The sternoclavicular joint

The synovial sternoclavicular joint is the only point where the shoulder girdle is fixed to the trunk. Like the acromioclavicular joint, it has no capacity for active movement because no muscles cross it. It permits the clavicle to angle up and down, and forwards and backwards, and to rotate to a limited extent on its own axis (a movement which is initiated by rotation of the scapula).

The humerus

The humerus is the long bone of the upper arm (Fig. 6.8). At its proximal end its rounded head,

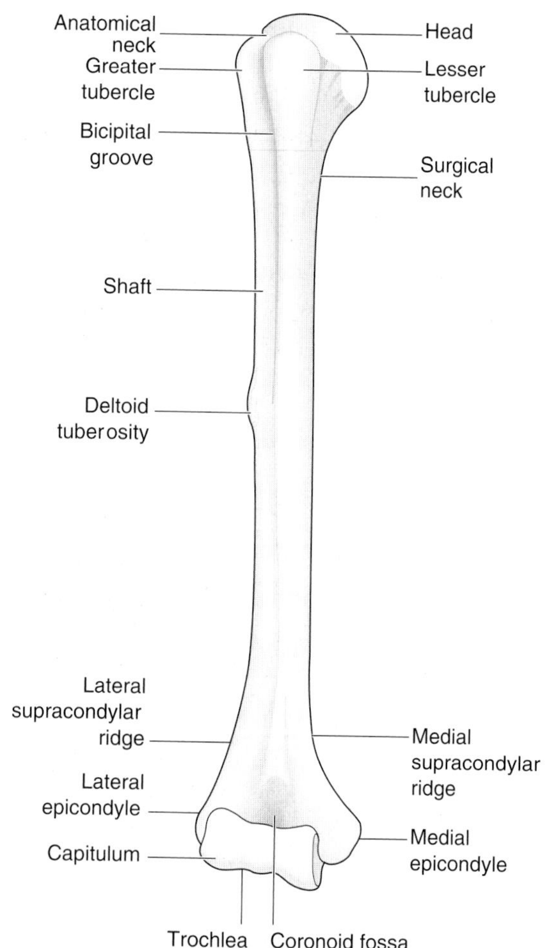

Figure 6.8 Anterior view of the right humerus. (Adapted with kind permission from Waugh and Grant, 2001.)

tilting up and backwards, articulates with the glenoid fossa of the scapula to form the shoulder joint. The head is separated from the tubercles of the humerus by the anatomical neck. There are two **tubercles** (a tubercle is a rounded bony projection for the attachment of muscles), which crown the top of the shaft of the humerus. The **greater tubercle** is just lateral to the head of the humerus. The **lesser tubercle** is on the anterior aspect of the humerus under the anatomical neck. Between the tubercles is the **intertubercular sulcus** (sulcus means groove) also called the **bicipital groove**. The tendon of the long head of the biceps muscle lies in this groove. The humerus narrows below the tubercles, at the **surgical neck**, and continues as the **shaft** of the bone.

The glenohumeral joint

The glenohumeral or shoulder joint is an unstable ball and socket joint. The glenoid fossa is shallow but slightly deepened by a fibrocartilaginous rim, the **glenoid labrum**. The capsule of the joint passes round the anatomical neck of the humerus and is strengthened in front by three ligaments: the **superior**, **middle** and **inferior glenohumeral ligaments**. The capsule is also reinforced by the insertion around it, on the humerus, of the tendons of four scapular muscles, known collectively as the **rotator cuff** (Fig. 6.9). These muscles are **supraspinatus**, which abducts the shoulder, **infraspinatus** and **teres minor**, which are lateral rotators of the shoulder, and **subscapularis**, which medially rotates the shoulder. They can be remembered by the acronym **SITS**.

The tendons of the supraspinatus muscle and the long head of the biceps pass over the humerus and under the bony arch of the girdle. Between the tendons and the bone, lies the **subacromial bursa**, to minimize friction. These soft tissues are vulnerable to various forms of degeneration, inflammation and trauma because they are liable to compression, or **impingement**, between two mobile bony surfaces. This can be aggravated if the subacromial space is narrowed for any reason (such as the formation of osteophytes) or if the soft tissues swell.

Movement at the shoulder

Movement of the shoulder does not occur purely at the glenohumeral joint. During flexion

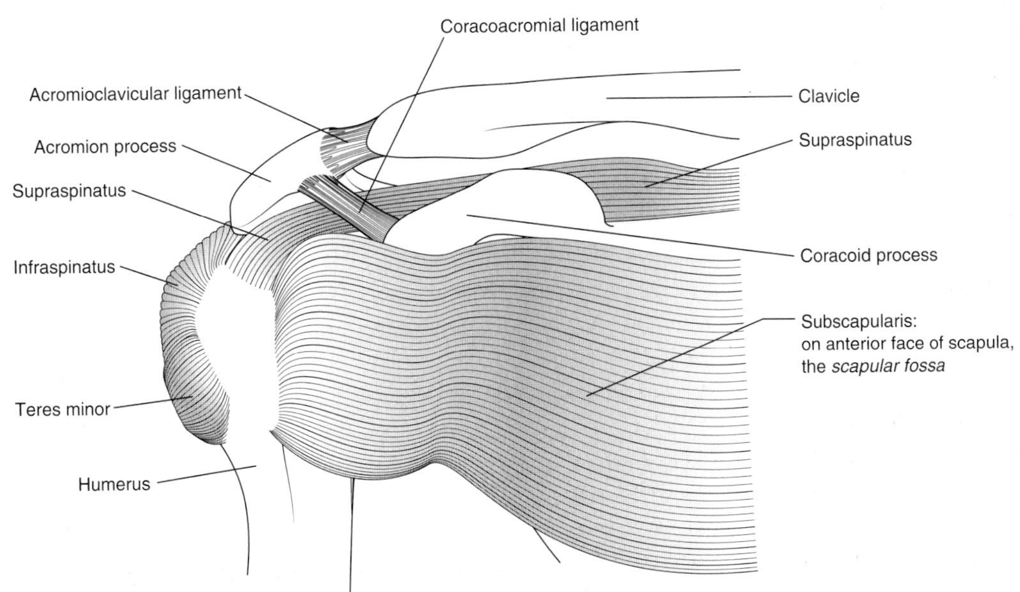

Figure 6.9 The rotator cuff of the glenohumeral joint.

of the shoulder, the early part of the movement (60° approximately) is glenohumeral. The scapula then shares the movement, by rotating upwards, and contributes about one third of the total range. Box 6.2 gives the movement statistics for the shoulder.

Box 6.2 Shoulder Statistics

Capsular pattern restriction in three movements, the largest being lateral rotation, the next abduction, and the least is medial rotation.
Joint positions loose packed is 60° abduction and 30° horizontal adduction; close-packed position is in combined full abduction and external rotation, and in combined full extension and internal rotation.
Flexion 0–180°; end feel firm; capsule stretching.
Extension 0–60°; end feel firm; capsule stretching.
Abduction 0–180°; end feel firm; capsule stretch.
External rotation 0–90°; end feel firm; capsule stretch.
Internal rotation 0–70°; end feel firm; capsule stretch.

Box Shoulder Examination

Ask the patient to expose both shoulders. Assess distal sensation and circulation:

- **LOOK** at the neck.
  Look and compare the shoulders, front, back and sides.
  Is there asymmetry or wasting?
  Is there redness, swelling bruise or deformity?
- **FEEL** the main landmarks.
  Feel the cervical spine.
  Feel the anterior structures, the sternoclavicular joint, clavicle, acromioclavicular joint and the coracoid process.
  Feel the upper humerous, the greater and lesser tuberosities, the bicipital groove and the insertion of the supraspinatus.
  Feel the scapula. Find its borders and the superficial ridge of its spine.
- **MOVE**
- Assess **ACTIVE NECK MOVEMENTS** (see Fig 6.5). Do they cause the patient pain?
  Observe the scapula during shoulder flexion. It contributes 60° of the upper part of the movement by rotating and tilting the glenoid upwards.
  If the patient feels pain at about 70° of abduction, gently encourage him to continue. If pain disappears in the upper half of the movement he may have an arc of pain, caused by supraspinatus impingement.
  It is easiest to assess all active movements together, resisted together and passive together.
- Two **SPECIAL TESTS**
  (1) The **DROP ARM TEST** to show a rotator cuff tear.
  Abduct the shoulder passively at 90°. Ask the patient to slowly lower the arm.
  Pain and/or weakness is positive.
  (2) **HORIZONTAL FLEXION** to elicit pain from an acromio-clavicular sprain. The patient abducts his shoulder to 90° then passes his arm across his chest, putting his hand on the opposite shoulder.

Examination

The basic shoulder examination is illustrated in Figures 6.10–6.13.

Every shoulder examination where there is no history of direct trauma to the shoulder should begin with an assessment of neck movement (see above). If neck movement triggers or worsens the patient's pain, a problem at the neck must be excluded. All joints should be palpated and the insertion point of the supraspinatus muscle on the lateral humerus, and the groove of the biceps on the anterior humerus. The subacromial bursa can be made more accessible by palpating the superior aspect of the humerus with the shoulder in extension.

Shoulder Injuries

The shoulder can be injured by violent trauma, and a variety of bone, joint, ligament and muscle injuries are common. The shoulder is also disposed, by its anatomy, the effects of its large range of movement and the often heavy demands made upon it, to suffer inflammation and degeneration. It is also, like the hip, a common site for referral of nerve pains from the spine and pain from the organs.

Violent trauma most commonly affects the shoulder when there has been a direct blow to the joint, or when force is transmitted by a fall on the hand. The patient will have a clear history of injury. There may be deformity, pain and disability. Vital structures in the arm, and occasionally in the neck, may be compromised.

Sternoclavicular dislocation

Sternoclavicular dislocation results from injury to the ligaments joining the proximal end of the clavicle to the sternum and the first rib, causing displacement of the clavicle. It is usually caused by a direct blow or a fall on the outstretched hand.

There will be asymmetry of the sternoclavicular joints and tenderness at the site.

Dislocation is normally anterior and uncomplicated, but a posterior displacement can threaten the airway and circulation. A fracture should be excluded and the dislocation is treated as a ligament injury.

Fracture of the clavicle

The clavicle can fracture after a direct blow or a fall on the outstretched hand. There will be pain, tenderness and swelling; frequently, there will also be deformity with crepitations and a palpable step or angulation at the site of fracture (usually at the outer third of the bone). Fracture at the distal part of the bone can involve the acromioclavicular joint.

There can be complications, neurovascular injury and pneumothorax. Torticollis can indicate a simultaneous rotational injury to the cervical spine.

The patient should be referred to a fracture clinic. The injury is usually rested in a sling in the early stages of healing.

Acromioclavicular dislocation

A sprain at the acromioclavicular joint is common, but complete dislocation is much less so. Rupture of the acromioclavicular ligament and, in some cases, the trapezoid and conoid ligaments (sometimes accompanied by capsule and muscle tear and fracture), which stabilize the outer end of the shoulder girdle, cause separation of the clavicle and scapula.

A blow to the point of the shoulder or a fall onto the shoulder, the point of the elbow or the outstretched hand are the usual mechanisms of injury.

The patient will have pain and tenderness on top of the shoulder with loss of movement, active and passive. The separated distal end of the clavicle will probably bulge upwards and will not move backwards with the acromion when the scapula is adducted.

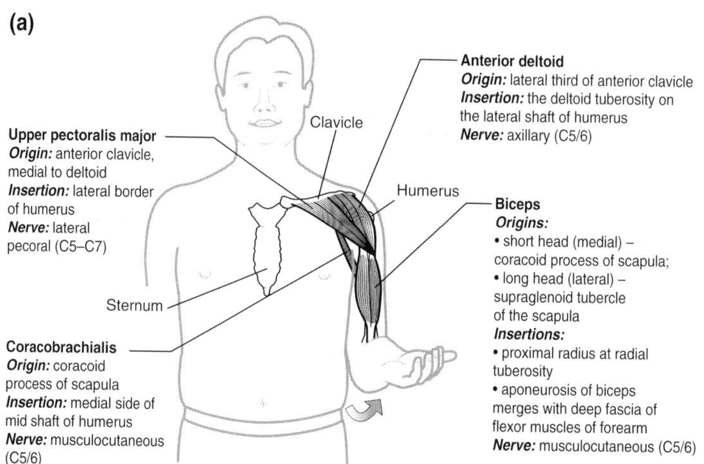

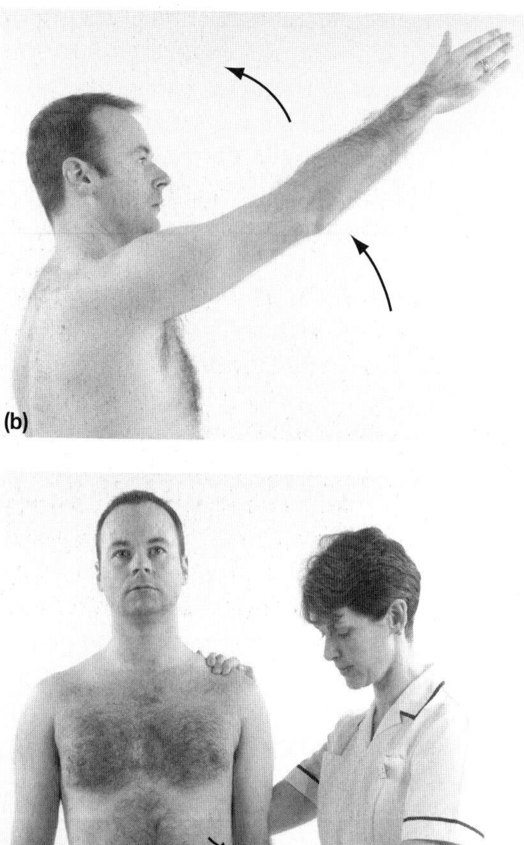

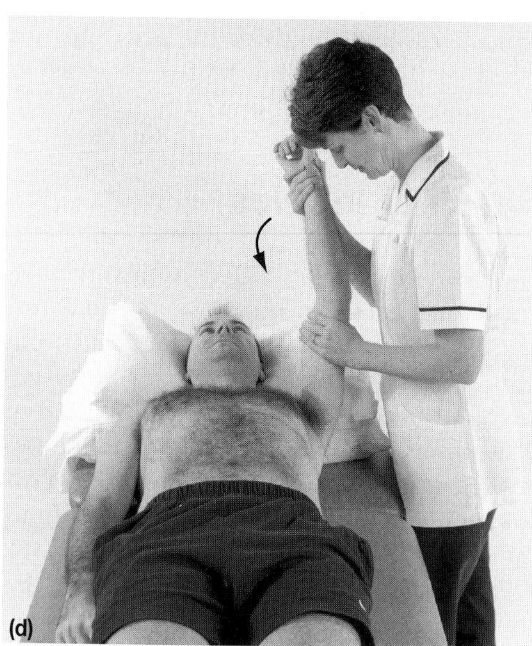

Figure 6.10 **(a) The flexors of the shoulder. (b) Active flexion – observe scapular movement during the upper part of the range. (c) Resisted flexion – test the movement in two parts, offering resistance above the elbow, and then below it to assess the biceps. (d) Passive flexion.**

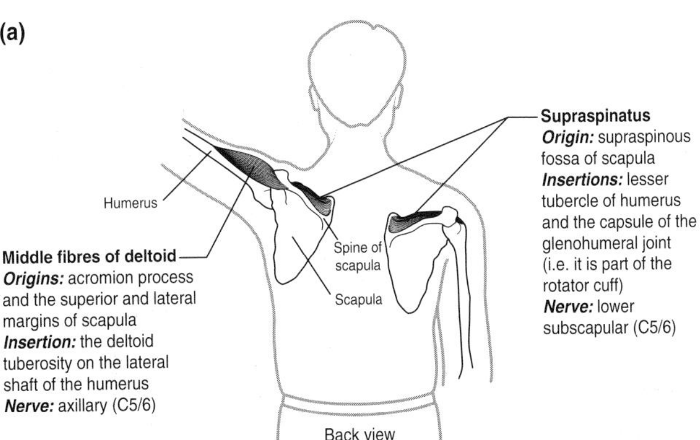

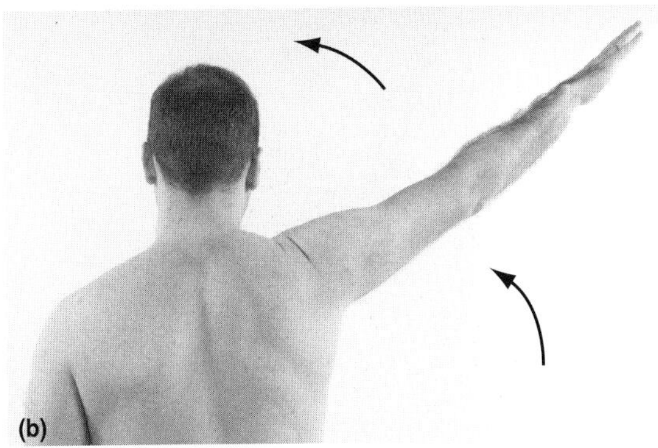

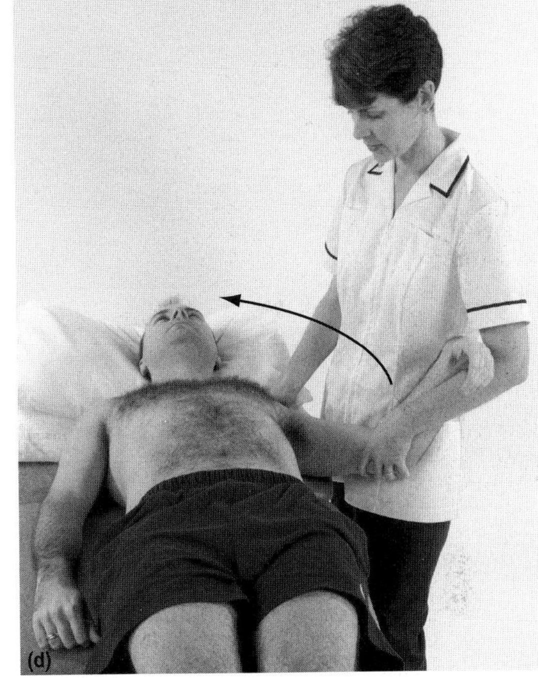

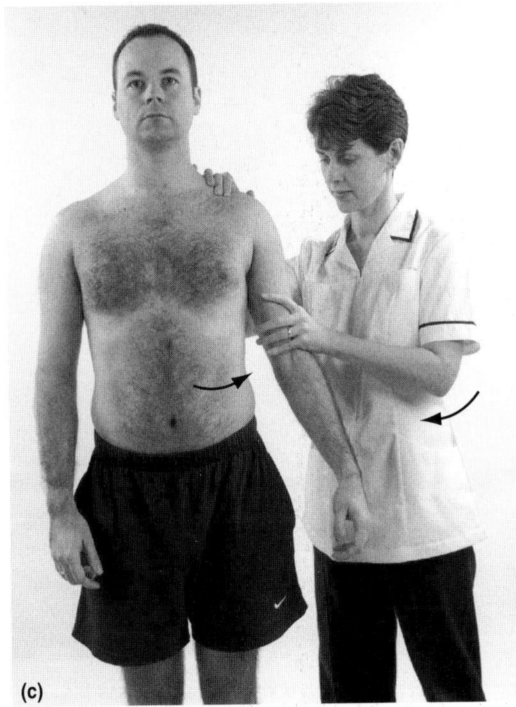

Figure 6.11 **(a) The abductors of the shoulder. (b) Active abduction – observe scapular movement during upper part of the range. Is there an arc of pain? (c) Resisted abduction. (d) Passive abduction.**

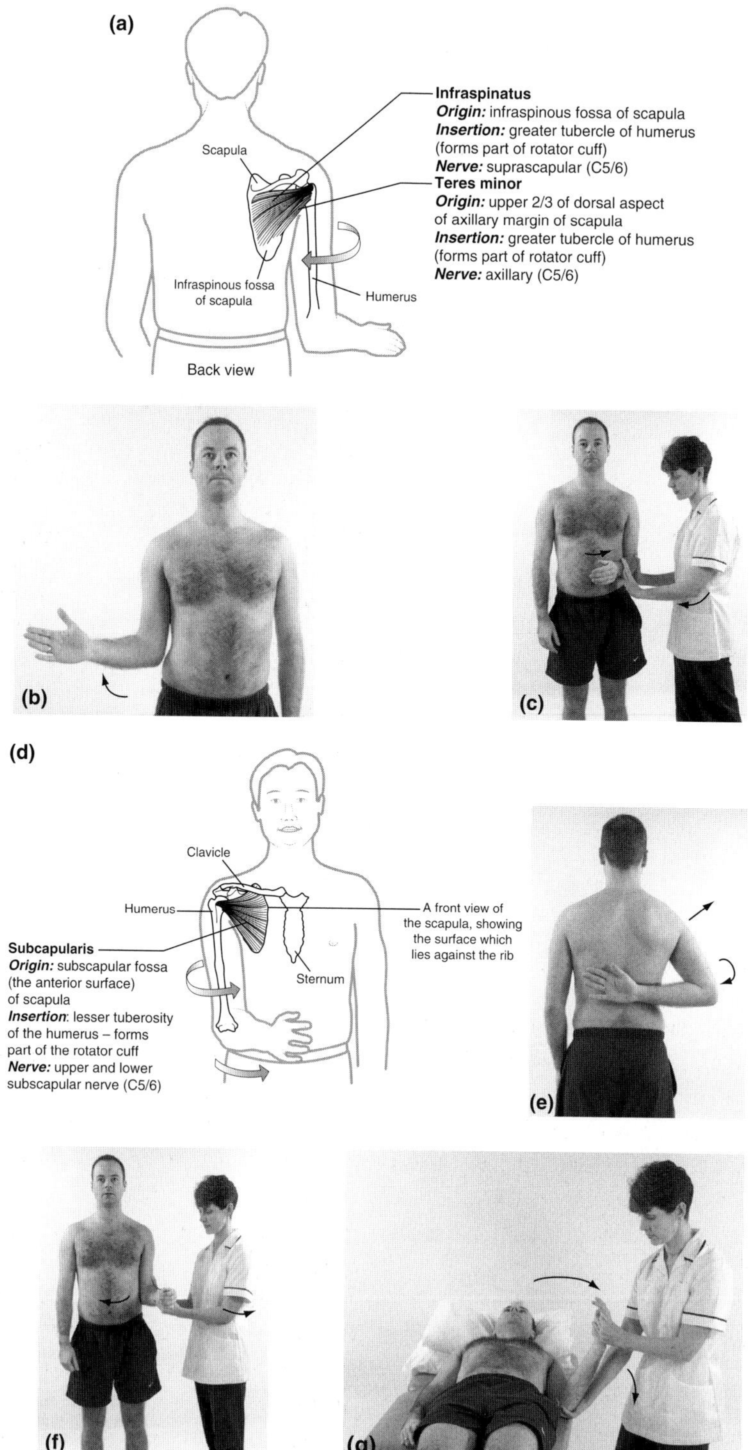

Figure 6.12 (a–c) The lateral rotators of the shoulder. (b) Active lateral rotation – the patient flexes his elbow so that forearm rotation will not complicate the movement. (c) Resisted lateral rotation – keep the patients elbow close to his body so that he does not use abduction instead of rotation. (d–g) The medial rotator of the shoulder. (e) Active medial rotation. (f) Resisted medial rotation. (g) Passive lateral rotation – with the shoulder in 90° abduction, medial rotation can be performed.

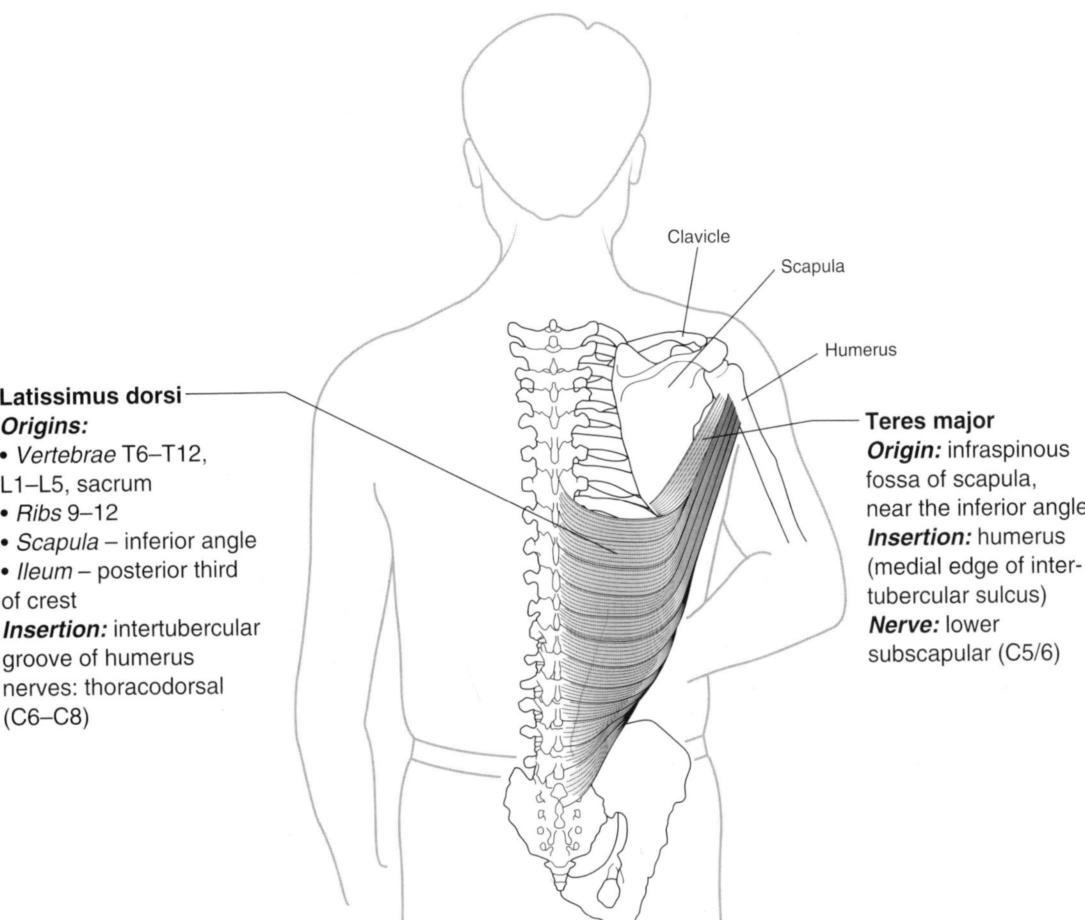

Figure 6.13 The extensors of the shoulder.

X-ray film of the two shoulders with the patient holding weights in the hands will demonstrate the gap caused by the sprain.

Later arthritic degeneration of the shoulder can follow dislocation, and the injury needs orthopaedic assessment. Surgical repair is sometimes needed for severe tears, but mobilization and physiotherapy are the usual treatments.

Anterior shoulder dislocation

Anterior shoulder dislocation is a fairly common injury, with a history of previous episodes also common. Displacement occurs of the head of the humerus, forward and down, from the glenoid cavity of the scapula.

The patient usually falls on the outstretched hand with external rotation of the arm. There may have been a violent pull on the arm, outwards and back, or a blow to the back of the arm which forces the head of the humerus forward. Previous dislocation often predisposes the patient to recurrence with only a slight injury.

The patient presents with an internally rotated arm held against the body by the other hand. There may be a hollow under the acromion and a flat appearance of the outer shoulder when viewed from the front, both caused by the slippage of the head of the humerus.

There is a risk of injury to the axillary nerve and artery. There may be fractures to the humerus or glenoid rim. The injury often recurs.

The patient requires transfer for reduction of the dislocation.

Posterior shoulder dislocation

Posterior shoulder dislocations are less common than anterior dislocations but, in those affected, a history of recurrence is common. There is displacement backwards of the head of the humerus from the glenoid cavity of the scapula.

A fall on outstretched arm is often the cause of the injury, most likely if shoulder is flexed to 90 degrees and the elbow extended. Other mechanisms include a direct frontal blow to an internally rotated arm or a direct blow to a flexed elbow, which drive the humerus back. This injury may be present in patients with shoulder symptoms after electric shock, epileptic fit and with certain neurological conditions (obstetrical and Erb's palsies).

The injury can be missed. General pain, local tenderness and loss of shoulder movement are seen, sometimes with deformity. The displaced head of humerus is seen at the back, below the acromion.

Complications may include neurovascular injury, rotator cuff injury and recurrence.

Fracture of the proximal humerus

The proximal humerus can fracture with a direct blow, a fall on the side of the shoulder or a fall on the outstretched hand.

The presentation includes pain, loss of movement, local tenderness and, often, deformity, swelling and bruising.

Complications may include neurovascular compromise of the arm. Anterior dislocation of the humerus often accompanies severe comminuted fractures and surgery is sometimes needed.

Rupture of the rotator cuff

Two patterns of injury are seen in the rotator cuff, the first more common.

- an older, manual worker who is predisposed by degeneration of the joint and who suffers an acute, possibly slight, injury
- a violent acute episode, often in a young athlete.

A tear occurs in the tendinous insertion, at the head of the humerus, of one or more of the muscles which support the shoulder joint. Typically, the site of a small tear will be the supraspinatus, with larger tears also including the infraspinatus, teres minor and subscapularis in that order.

The mechanism may be a fall on the outstretched hand or direct violence. Contraction of any muscle of the cuff, against resistance, can tear that muscle.

Presentations are variable. A complete tear may not be painful. There will be disability. There will be a loss of active abduction, especially at the start of range and, perhaps, local tenderness. The patient will fail the 'drop arm' test – lowering the arm from full abduction – losing active control and letting it fall at 90 degrees.

Small tears are treated conservatively, but large ones may require surgical repair. Complications include poor recovery, even with surgery, for larger lesions.

Supraspinatus tendinitis

Supraspinatus tendinitis is an overuse injury of an abductor muscle of the shoulder, which tends to be inflamed by use of the arm with the shoulder abducted above 90 degrees or laterally rotated.

The patient has pain, with tenderness at the insertion of the muscle, and a **painful arc** during abduction (this means that the movement begins and ends without pain but the patient has pain during the movement, usually at about the range of 80 to 120 degrees of abduction). The patient will have pain on resisted, but not passive, abduction.

This injury can be of a chronically inflamed type. The pain may be associated with a tendon tear and may require surgery.

The problem may settle with rest. It often needs physiotherapy and responds well to treatment. The GP may give a steroid injection.

Acute calcific tendinitis

Degeneration of the supraspinatus tendon, especially in those over 30 years of age, can make it prone to inflammation when overused, and this can be followed by the depositing of calcium salts in the tendon.

There is a sudden onset of pain with tenderness in the upper anterior shoulder, sleeplessness, inability to work, guarding the arm and reluctance to have it examined. The calcium deposit will be visible on X-ray film.

Treatments include rest and analgesia, steroid injection, aspiration of the deposit in some cases and physiotherapy for exercise. In cases which do not settle, surgical treatment, curretage of the deposit, may be needed.

Subacromial bursitis

Inflammation of the subacromial bursa can be caused by overuse or impingement, and trauma to the shoulder may cause bleeding in the bursa. Other shoulder problems such as a supraspinatus tear or impingement may also be present.

There is a fairly quick onset, pain that disturbs sleep and prevents lying on the affected side, a sensation of having a 'heavy arm', referral of pain to the humeral deltoid insertion, a painful arc between 80 and 120 degrees of active and **passive** abduction. There may be tenderness and a boggy feeling at the head of the humerus when the shoulder is examined in extension.

Treatment is rest followed by gradual mobilization, which may settle an acute form. The bursa may need aspiration if there has been bleeding. A more difficult chronic form may respond to a steroid injection. Prolonged inflammation caused by adhesions in the bursa may result.

Impingement

Impingement is the pinching or compressing of soft tissues between the hard surfaces of the shoulder joint, caused by swelling of the soft tissues or narrowing of the bony space. It leads to inflammation, thickening, atrophy and sometimes rupture of the tissues. The tendons of the supraspinatus, infraspinatus, teres minor, subscapularis and long head of biceps muscles, and the subacromial bursa and glenoid labrum, can all be affected.

Pain occurs through an arc of abduction, between 80 and 120 degrees approximately, and there will be pain on passive movement. The pain will discourage the patient from lifting the arm over the head. There may be pain at night and difficulty lying on the affected shoulder.

Treatment includes reducing inflammation by rest, and then, possibly, physiotherapy with ultrasound and exercise. Steroid injections are sometimes needed, depending on severity and which tissue is impinged.

Complications include chronic inflammation, intractable restriction, which requires surgery, and damage to the impinged tissues.

Referred Pain to the Shoulder

A patient presenting with a shoulder problem, but no history of injury, will usually complain of pain. Where there is no clear history of injury, an injury cannot be assumed to be present. Three other categories of problem must be eliminated.

1. Disease affecting the joint. Sepsis is the most urgent condition in this category.
2. Illness at another site, referring pain to the shoulder. The list is long and includes life-threatening events. Some of these are:
   - myocardial infarct
   - pneumothorax
   - pneumonia
   - tumour
   - aneurism
   - gallbladder infection
   - ruptured spleen
   - ectopic pregnancy.

3. The cervical spine can refer pain to the shoulder and should always be assessed as part of a basic shoulder examination.

During assessment of a patient, a nurse should be alert, looking for the unwell patient, a high temperature or abnormal vital signs. A careful past medical history should be taken and considered for possible connections to the presenting complaint. The patient's account of the complaint, its onset, duration, pain and so on, should be examined to see if it is consistent with injury. These questions should be asked again if the shoulder examination does not reveal an injury. If no answer is obtained a medical opinion should be sought.

The Elbow

Anatomy

The elbow is a synovial hinge joint. It is placed in the middle of the arm and, like the shoulder, its ultimate purpose is to place the hand wherever in space its owner wishes it to be. It allows the hand to turn back towards the body and this makes it possible for the hand to be brought to the face (Box 6.3). It has many structural similarities to the knee but, perhaps surprisingly in view of the greater mobility of the arm compared with the leg, the elbow joint is simpler.

The elbow lies in close relation to the proximal radioulnar joint. This will be discussed with the wrist and hand. There are three bones at the elbow, the distal **humerus**, the head of the **radius** and the proximal end of the **ulna** (Figs 6.14 and 6.15).

The humerus

The humerus, seen from the front, has a triangular appearance at its distal end as the shaft

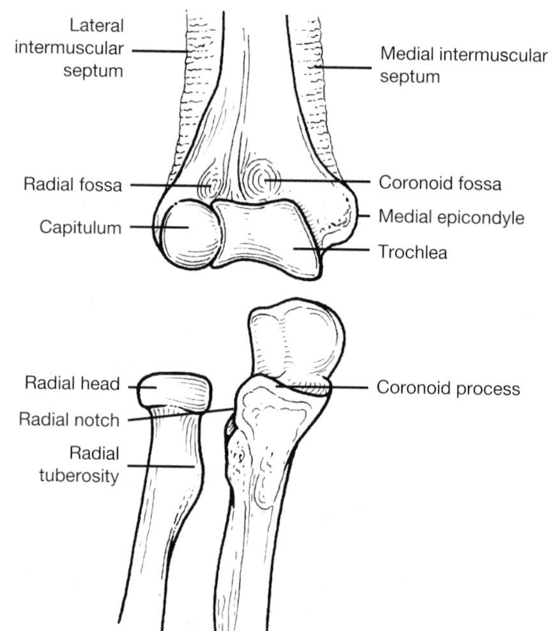

Figure 6.14 Anterior view of the bones at the elbow. (Reproduced with kind permission from Dean and Pegington, 1996.)

Box 6.3 Elbow Statistics

Capsular pattern greater limitation of flexion than extension.

Joint positions loose packed is 70–90° flexion with 10° supination; close packed is full extension with supination.

Flexion 0–150° with tissue approximation end feel as muscle meets muscle. If the patient is thin the end feel may be hard as the coronoid process enters the fossa. Extension has a hard, bony end feel as the olecranon enters its fossa. There can be 10° of hyperextension at the joint.

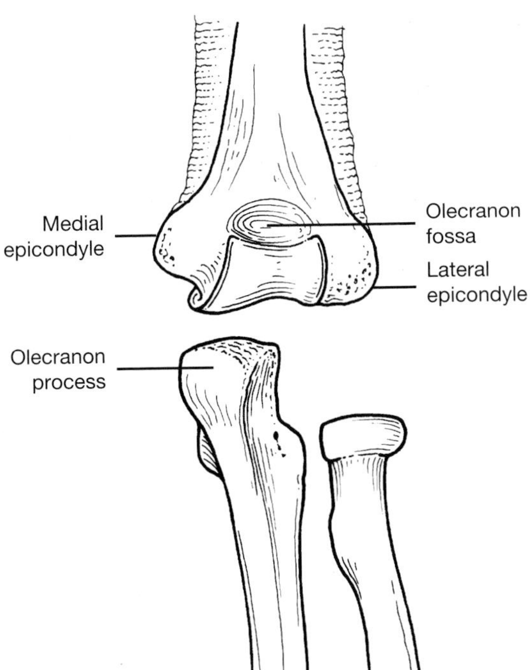

Figure 6.15 Posterior view of the bones at the elbow. (Reproduced with kind permission from Dean and Pegington, 1996.)

broadens and becomes flattened. The medial corner of the triangle is the **medial epicondyle**, and at the lateral side is the smaller **lateral epicondyle**. The borders of the triangle, which pass from the shaft of the humerus to the epicondyles, are called the **medial** and **lateral supracondylar ridges**. Seen from the side, the elbow articulation of the humerus has a bulbous appearance and a forward curve. The rounded appearance is caused by the articular area, which lies between the epicondyles. The lateral part of the articular surface is the **capitulum**, a rounded prominence for articulation with the head of the radius. The medial articulation is the **trochlea**. It has a waist between two prominences, of which the medial is larger. This inequality causes the ulna to sit at a valgus angle of 10–15 degrees, slightly more for women (the **carrying angle**) when the arm is straight. There are two hollows on the front surface of the humerus, just above the two articulations. Above the capitulum is the **radial fossa**, and above the trochlea is the **coronoid fossa**. The head of the radius and the coronoid process of the ulna fit into these hollows when the elbow is fully flexed. On the back of the humerus, at the same level, is a larger single hollow, the **olecranon fossa**, where the olecranon process of the ulna fits when the elbow is fully extended.

The radius

The radius is the lateral of the two long bones of the forearm. Its head, sitting on top of a slender neck, resembles the head of a nail, and it has a concavity on its top surface for articulation with the capitulum. The radius is bound to the ulna proximally by an **annular ligament** (meaning ring), which keeps it close to the ulna while leaving it free to rotate axially.

The ulna

The ulna is the medial long bone of the forearm. At its proximal end, the bone is expanded with an articular surface which is slightly like a cupped hand. There are two processes in this area. The **olecranon process** is like the clawed fingers of the hand. Its rear part forms the point of the elbow and sits in the olecranon fossa when the elbow is extended. Its front part is cupped, the **trochlear notch**, and it articulates with the trochlea. At the base of the trochlear notch, in front, is a projection called the **coronoid process**, which sits in the coronoid fossa when the elbow is flexed. On the lateral aspect of the coronoid process is a small hollow, the **radial notch**, which articulates with the radial head.

The ulnar collateral ligament

The ulnar collateral ligament of the elbow reinforces the joint capsule on the medial side and stabilizes the joint against valgus stress and, with the radial collateral ligament, limits the range of abduction, adduction and rotation (Fig. 6.16). It also helps to stabilize the relationship between humerus and ulna. The ligament spreads out in a triangular shape from the medial epicondyle

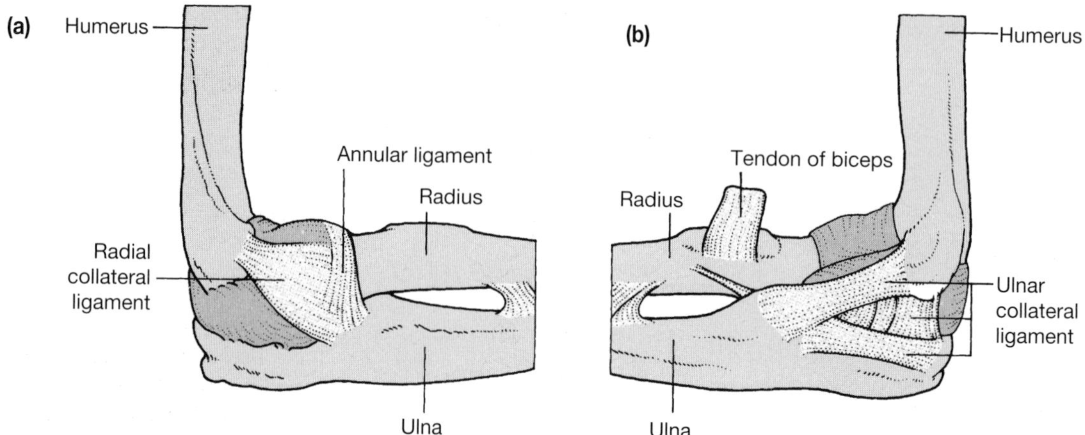

Figure 6.16 The elbow joint and its ligaments. To stress the ligaments of lateral elbow, flex patient's elbow and supinate the hand. Grip the humerus near the elbow and the forearm near the wrist. Move the forearm medially. To stress the medial ligaments, move the forearm laterally. Pain or laxity offer positive tests. (Reproduced with kind permission from Rogers, 1992)

to the coronoid process in front and the olecranon behind. There is also a stabilizing transverse band between the front and back bands.

The radial collateral ligament

The radial collateral ligament (see Fig. 6.16) arises from the lateral epicondyle and joins the annular ligament and the radial notch of the ulna. It limits varus angulation of the joint.

Examination

Palpation should include all the bony landmarks. A patient with olecranon bursitis will have heat and a boggy swelling over the olecranon.

The main muscles groups, and their tests, are described in Figure 6.17 and 6.18. The collateral ligaments can be stressed in a similar manner to those of the knee (Ch. 7), by the application of varus and valgus stresses to the joint with the elbow slightly flexed.

Elbow Injuries

A wide range of bone injuries are possible at the elbow. Three types of fracture will be briefly discussed here: supracondylar, radial head and tip of olecranon. Also discussed is pulled elbow. Fracture/dislocations of the forearm will be discussed with the forearm.

Supracondylar fracture of the humerus

A supracondylar fracture occurs in the distal third of the humerus but proximal to the articular surface of the elbow. It is common in children (Ch. 4). The fracture occurs from a fall on the outstretched hand.

The patient will have a tender distal humerus. A child will guard the arm and be unwilling to be examined. In cases where there is displacement, the distal fragment may be dislodged dorsally, and this may cause occlusion of the brachial artery. Occlusion of the artery can result in a **Volkmann's ischaemic contracture** of the forearm, the result of necrosis of avascular muscle tissue. It is important to check nerve and circulation repeatedly and obtain swift treatment for such injuries.

Radial head fracture

A radial head fracture is caused by direct violence or a fall on the outstretched hand which compresses the radial head against the capitulum.

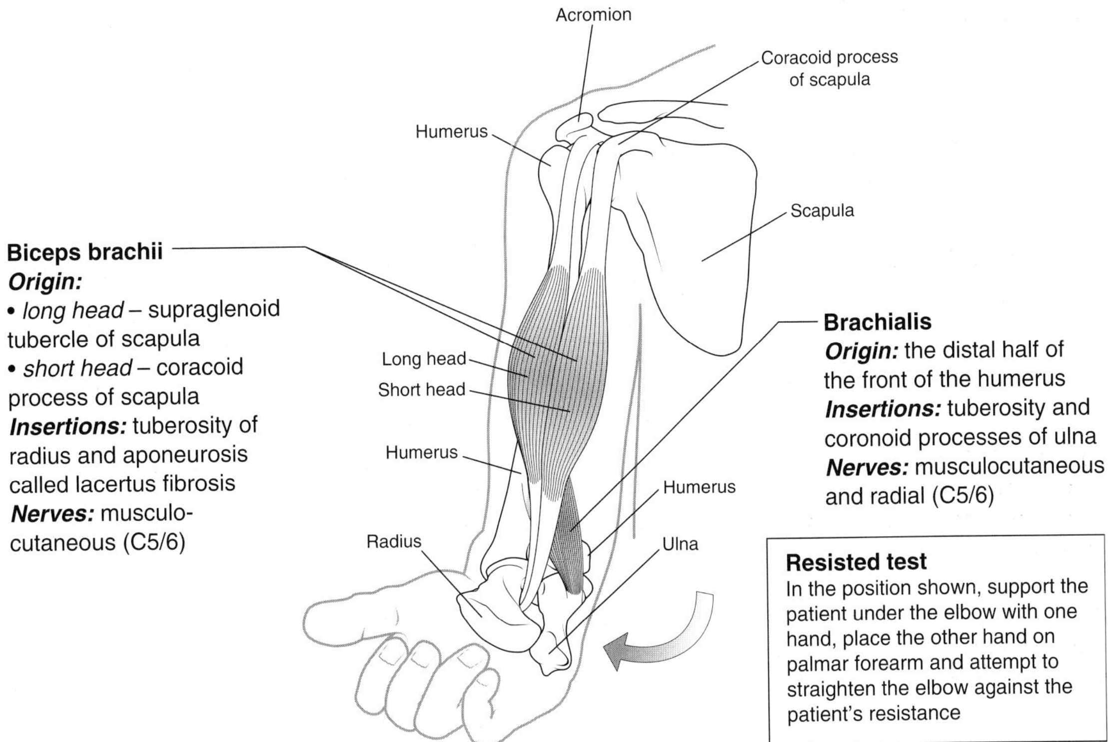

Figure 6.17 The flexors of the elbow.

The patient will hold the elbow flexed at 90 degrees. There may be swelling caused by haemarthrosis. The radial head will be tender; it should be palpated through the range of pronation and supination. Forearm movement may be present, but the patient will not wish to extend the elbow.

Severe fractures may require excision of the radial head and this can cause the radius to rise in relation to the ulna, with problems at the wrist joint. Recovery of forearm movement may not occur in conservatively treated fractures, and these sometimes need surgery later.

Olecranon fracture

The usual mechanism for an olecranon fracture is a fall onto the point of the elbow, which breaks the end of the olecranon. The triceps muscles are attached to this fragment and may displace it by pulling it away from the rest of the bone.

There will be tenderness and swelling and the patient will not be able to straighten the elbow.

Displaced fractures will need surgery, either for screws/wiring of the displaced fragment or, in some cases, excision of the piece and repair of the muscle.

Radial head dislocation

Radial head dislocation (pulled elbow) occurs in children under 6 years of age when the radial head slips from its annular ligament. It is usually caused by an adult pulling on the arm, as in swinging the child in play or restraining the child while holding the hand.

The child will not use the arm and will be distressed by any attempt to examine the elbow, and especially to supinate the forearm. There may be some tenderness and swelling at the radial head.

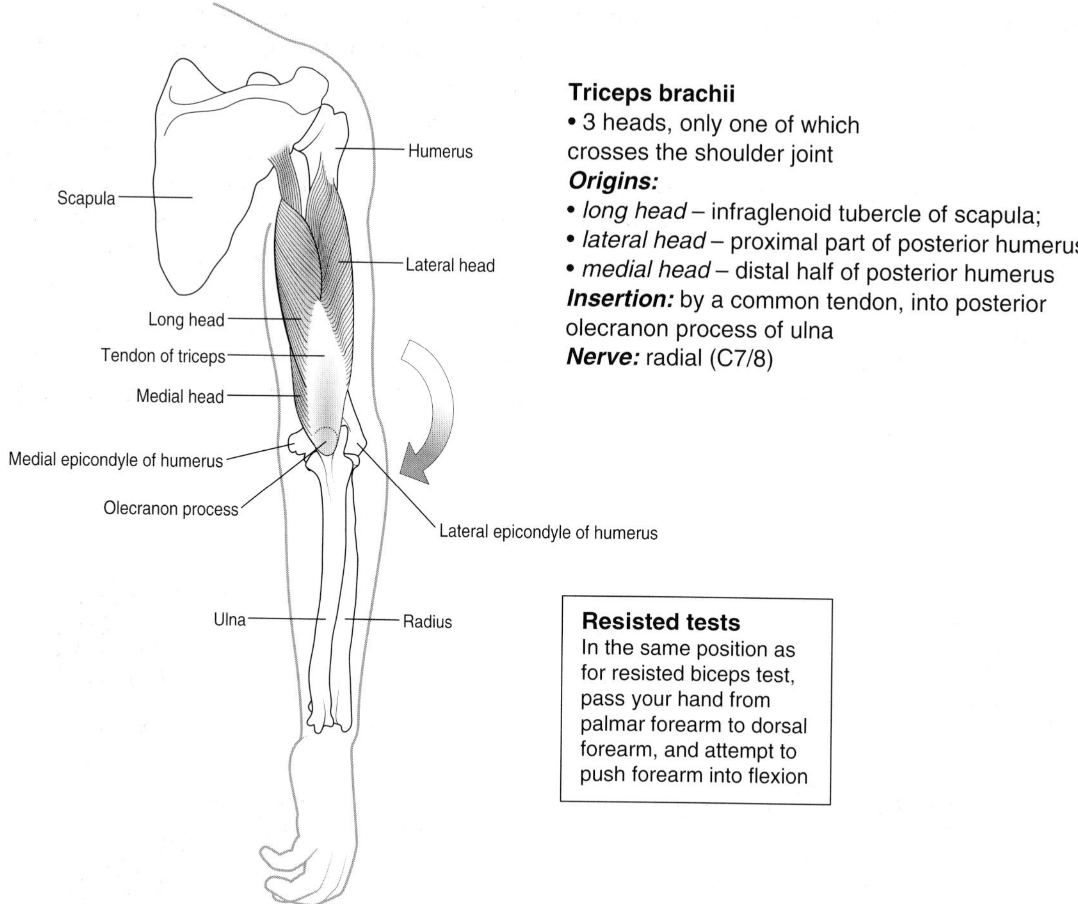

Figure 6.18 The extensors of the elbow.

Give the patient analgesia. Different doctors vary slightly in the method they use to reduce the dislocation. Combined supination of the forearm while flexing the elbow is advocated by Glasgow and Graham (1997), followed by resting the arm in a sling.

The problem may recur while the child is under 6 years of age but it settles after then.

Olecranon bursitis

Pressure or friction can cause inflammation of the olecranon bursa. A blow to the olecranon can cause a bleed into the bursa, which irritates the synovial tissue and causes inflammation. Infection can also cause a septic bursitis.

There is a prominent, round, red, soft, hot and tender swelling over the olecranon process and pain and restricted flexion of the elbow. If bleeding has occurred, there should be a history of trauma, and bruising may be visible. If there is infection, other signs may be present, such as malaise and pyrexia, and there may be broken skin in the vicinity of the swelling.

A simple bursitis should settle with rest. A bleed into the bursa may require aspiration. Infection may require aspiration and antibiotics will be given. An infection in the joint would be excluded.

Epicondylitis

Epicondylitis is an overuse strain on the common tendinous insertions of the extrinsic extensor and flexor muscles of the wrist and hand at the lateral and medial epicondyles of the humerus, respectively (Fig. 6.19). It can give rise to inflammation at their tenoperiosteal junctions. These problems are called lateral epicondylitis or **tennis elbow** and medial epicondylitis or **golfer's elbow**. Tennis elbow is commoner and tends to be more troublesome.

There is a history of pain at the appropriate side of the elbow, which can radiate up and down, with pain and loss of function in wrist and hand movements. Elbow movements are not affected. The epicondyle is tender.

Both problems do settle but may take a long time to do so. The GP will often give a steroid injection. Physiotherapy manipulations are sometimes tried, as are rest and, occasionally, surgery.

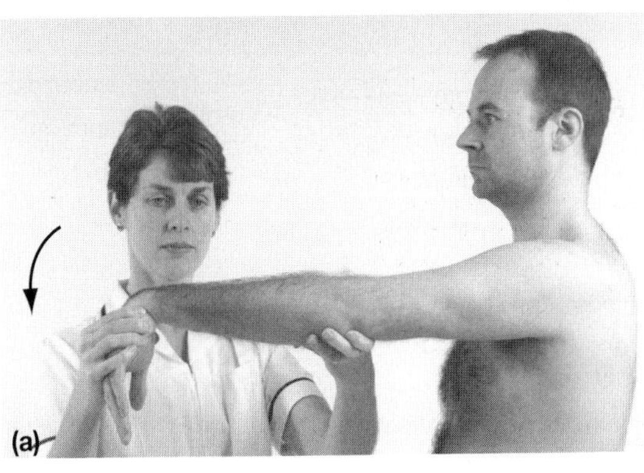

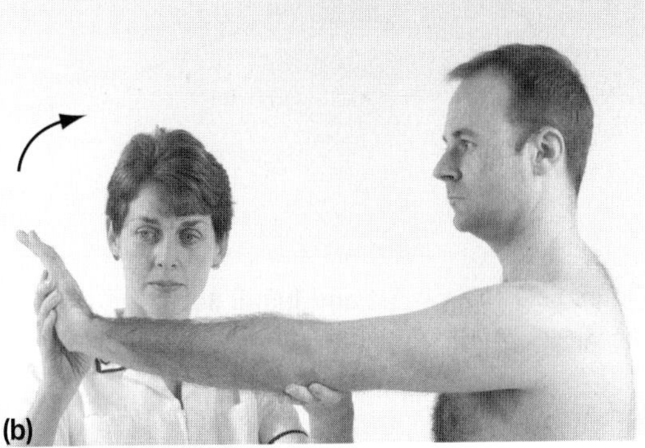

Figure 6.19 Epicondylitis. (a) To test for tennis elbow, passively stress the common extensor tendon by flexing the wrist with the elbow extended. Pain at the lateral epicondyle is positive. (b) To test for golfer's elbow, passively stress the flexors of the wrist by extending the wrist with the elbow extended. Pain at the medial epicondyle is positive.

The Forearm, Wrist and Hand

Anatomy

Terminology

The terminology used to describe structures and positions of the hand are somewhat different to other parts of the body. This is because the positions of other areas are named in relation to a fixed point, the midline of the body. The mobility of the arm in general, and the hand's capacity to be rotated about the axis of the arm, makes a nonsense of fixed points of reference. Instead, its positions are described in terms of fixed internal relationships and descriptive rather than directional names.

Surfaces

The surfaces of the hand (Fig. 6.20) are **palmar** and **dorsal**: its margins are **radial** (thumb side)

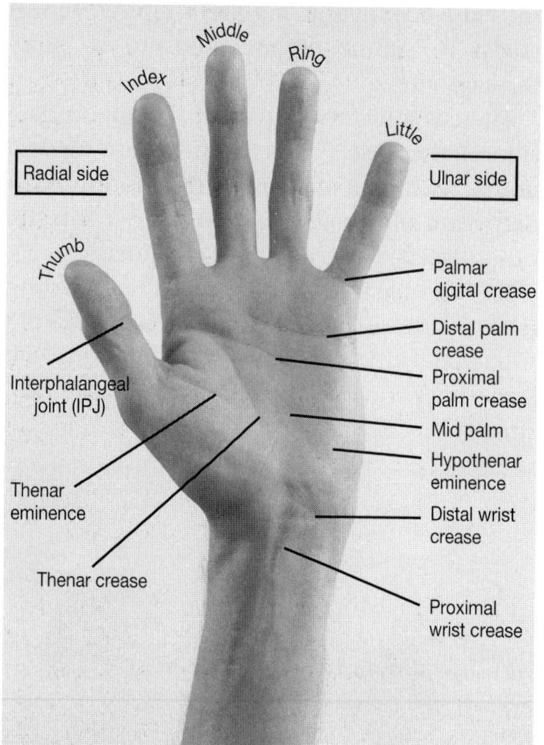

Figure 6.20 The wrist and hand: surface markings and terminology.

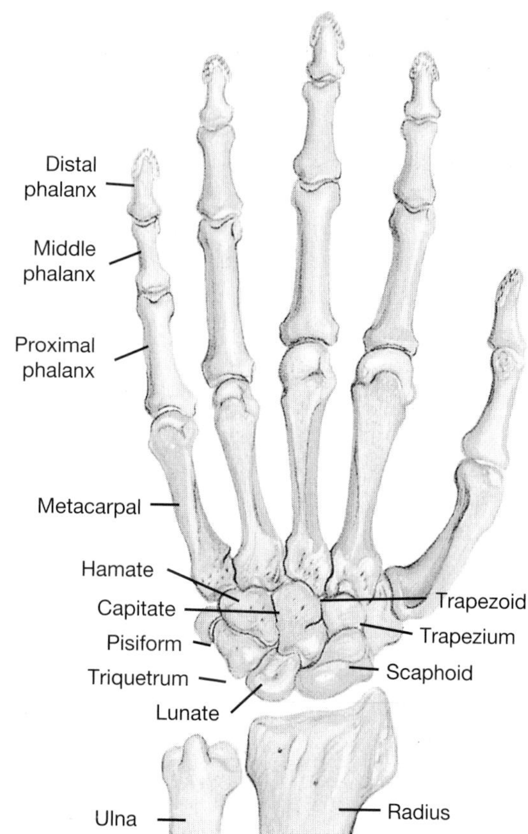

Figure 6.21 Palmar view of the bones of the wrist and hand. (Reproduced with kind permission from Thibodeau and Patton, 1999.)

and **ulnar** (little finger side). The fingers are referred to by name (not by numbers, which can cause confusion), **thumb**, **index**, **middle**, **ring** and **little**. The palm is divided into three zones. The **thenar eminence** is the mound of muscle which covers the metacarpal of the thumb. The **hypothenar** covers the metacarpal of the little finger. Between these lies the **mid-palm**.

Bones

Every bone in the hand and wrist (Fig. 6.21) belongs to one of three groups: the **carpals**, **metacarpals** and **phalanges**.

The eight carpal bones lie in two rows, **proximal** and **distal** and they articulate with each other in a complex manner, side to side and across the rows. The proximal row also articulates with the distal ends of the forearm bones, the **radius** and **ulna**, to form the wrist joint. The distal row articulates with the bases of the five metacarpals and with the proximal row of carpals.

The metacarpal bones provide the main bony structure of the palm. They are numbered one to five from the thumb to little finger. At the distal end, or head, each metacarpal articulates with the proximal phalanx of a finger.

The thumb has two phalanges: proximal and distal. The other fingers have three phalanges: proximal, middle and distal.

Joints

The joint between metacarpal and finger is the **metacarpophalangeal joint** (**MCPJ**). The proximal/middle phalanx joint is the **proximal interphalangeal joint** (**PIPJ**). The middle/distal phalanx joint is the **distal interphalangeal**

joint (**DIPJ**). The articulation between the phalanges of the thumb is the **interphalangeal joint** (**IPJ**).

The forearm

The radius and the ulna are the two bones of the forearm. The wrist joint is formed by the articulation of the distal end of the radius with the proximal carpal row. The ulna does not articulate directly with the carpal bones.

The radius is a long, arched bone. In the neutral position, it lies on the lateral side of the forearm alongside the ulna and articulates with it at two joints, separated by almost the entire length of the bones. In spite of this separation, these two joints are best considered, for understanding of function and the problems caused by trauma, as a single unit of movement. Proximally, the radial head rotates on its own axis. The radial head is in contact with the capitulum of the humerus but has much less to do with the elbow joint than the ulna. It is held against the proximal ulna by a ligamentous loop, the **annular ligament** (Fig. 6.16), which leaves it free to rotate about its own axis. Distally, the radius travels 180 degrees in an arc, passing around the ulna (which functions, at the wrist, as a pivot for the radius), carrying the hand between the palm up (**supine**) and the palm down (**prone**) positions. The relative length of these two bones, and the space between them, must be correctly maintained for proper function of the lower arm's intricate system of bone, ligament, fibrous tissue, muscle and tendon.

Any bony injury which changes the relationship between the radius and ulna (e.g. a fracture of the distal radius) or disrupts an important soft tissue attachment (e.g. a displaced fracture of the ulnar styloid) may be more crippling than simple X-ray appearances would suggest.

The wrist joint (radiocarpal)

The expanded articular surface of the distal radius is a concave triangle with two cartilage-coated sockets for articulation with the **scaphoid** and the **lunate**. The proximal row of carpal bones is more curved in its outline than the distal radius, and moves upon it in a gliding fashion.

The radius and the ulna each have a **styloid process**, a button of bone on their carpal articular surfaces for the attachment of ligaments. The radial styloid is usually distal to the ulnar styloid, and the dorsal margin of the radius, at the wrist, is distal to the palmar margin; this creates a two-way slope and means that the neutral position of the hand tends to be slightly palmar and ulnar.

On the dorsum of the distal radius, in the centre, is a projection called **Lister's tubercle**, best felt with the wrist flexed. It provides a channel for the passage of extensor tendons of the hand. It lies in line with the third finger and the capitate and is a useful landmark for palpation of the midcarpal bones.

The wrist joint allows movements of flexion and extension, **radial deviation** and **ulnar deviation** (Box 6.4). These combine with rotation of the forearm to allow precise placement of the hand in any plane.

The carpal bones

In the proximal row of carpal bones, from radial to ulnar sides, lie the **scaphoid**, **lunate**, **triquetrum** and **pisiform** (Fig. 6.21). The pisiform lies directly in front of the triquetrum, on the palmar aspect, and cannot be palpated on the dorsal wrist. The distal row comprises the **trapezium**, **trapezoid**, **capitate** and **hamate**.

The carpal bones are six sided. They articulate with each other, with the forearm and with the five metacarpals. Their articular surfaces are covered with cartilage and their palmar and dorsal surfaces are rough for the attachment of ligaments.

The carpal bones form an arch from side to side, concave on the palm and convex on the dorsum. Opposition of the thumb depends upon the concavity of the palmar arch. The wrist is more stable in flexion than extension,

Box 6.4 Wrist Statistics: The Radiocarpal Joint

Capsular pattern equal restriction of flexion and extension.
Joint positions loose packed is 10° wrist flexion with slight ulnar deviation (the neutral position of the hand at rest); close packed is full extension with radial deviation.
Flexion 0–80°; end feel firm; capsule and ligament stretch.
Extension 0–70°; end feel firm; capsule and ligament stretch.
Ulnar deviation 0–30°; end feel firm; capsule and ligament stretch.
Radial deviation 0–20°; end feel firm and capsule and ligament stretch or end feel hard and scaphoid meets radial styloid.

partly because of its palmar concavity but also because of the strength of its ligaments. The palmar concavity of the wrist is also important in balancing the action of the extensor muscles of the wrist with the flexors of the fingers. The dorsal curve is longer than the palmar and the individual bones tend to be wider on the dorsal surface. This means that if they dislocate, they will normally do so dorsally. The lunate is an exception and is also the carpal bone most likely to dislocate.

The carpus is a transition from the levers of the forearm to the complex adaptibility of the hand. Each carpal bone has a distinctive shape, an individual role and a range of movement different from its neighbours. They combine to provide the two conflicting needs of the transition: stability and movement.

Most wrist movements occur at the radiocarpal and the midcarpal joints. The proximal row, the key to these movements, is not a simple articular block tilting in two planes. The bones of the proximal row, especially the scaphoid and the lunate, change their positions by mutual displacement (by gliding obliquely, rotating and rocking) so that a convex surface will be presented to the distal radius at all stages of movement, and a concave hollow will receive the distal row.

The distal row, with the capitate at its core, is much less mobile than the proximal. The metacarpals of the index and middle fingers are rigidly joined to it to form the fixed part of the hand. There is more mobility at the articulations of the hamate with the fourth and fifth metacarpals; consequently, the ring and little fingers can move across the palm into opposition. The saddle joint of the trapezium with the base of the metacarpal of the thumb is the most mobile single joint in the hand, permitting a complete range of circumduction at the base of the thumb.

The scaphoid

The scaphoid is the largest bone in the proximal row. The **tubercle** of the scaphoid, a round projection on the distal palmar surface, is an attachment for the **flexor retinaculum**, which forms the fibrous roof of the bony channel called the **carpal tunnel**. The scaphoid articulates with five bones: the radius, lunate, capitate, trapezium and trapezoid. It crosses between the two carpal rows, making it prone to stress in its mid-section (called the **waist**). It is, by far, the most commonly injured carpal bone. A fall on the outstretched hand forces the bone back against the dorsal lip of the radius, causing fracture.

The scaphoid is pierced on its dorsum by nutrient foramina, to allow the passage of blood vessels. In many people these foramina are only found on the distal part of the bone, which means that, for them, the bone is perfused in a distal to proximal direction. A fracture through the waist of the scaphoid can cut the blood supply to the proximal part if the fracture does not unite. This can cause avascular necrosis of the proximal scaphoid and, later, serious disability of the hand.

The scaphoid is both highly mobile and a major source of the stability of the carpus.

The carpal tunnel

The carpal tunnel is a narrow passage running from forearm to palm, with the midcarpal bones of both rows for its floor, the prominences of the carpal bones at both sides for its walls, and a roof of fibrous tissue known as the **flexor retinaculum**. Without its contents, the tunnel is deep enough to receive a fingertip.

On the radial side, the wall of the tunnel is formed, proximally, by the tubercle of the scaphoid (which can be felt at the base of the thenar eminence) and, distally, by the tubercle of the trapezium. On the ulnar side, the pisiform, proximally (which can be felt at the proximal border of the hypothenar eminence), and the hook of the hamate, distally, form the wall.

The flexor tendons of the fingers and the median nerve of the hand pass through this restricted space. Excess fluid in the wrist can cause compression in the tunnel and disability of the hand, with the symptoms of compression of the median nerve.

The bones of the hand

The bones of the hand are a succession of long bones (the metacarpals' digital appearance disguised by the flesh of the palm) designed to perform a huge range of tasks within the area of its palmar scope, requiring varying degrees of power, finesse, complexity and precision. The joints are all simple synovial hinges, except those of the MCPJs of the index to little fingers, which are condyloid and capable of abduction and adduction as well as flexion and extension (Fig. 6.21).

The particular mobility of the thumb, and especially its capacity to oppose the other fingers, is the source of the human hand's dexterity and power. When the thumb is opposed, the palmar surface of its distal phalanx is pressed against the same surface of the opposing finger. This position is quite different to the pinch grip, which can be obtained by flexing the distal phalanges of two fingers and putting the tips together.

Ligaments

The annular ligament of the proximal radioulnar joint has been mentioned. At the wrist the ulna does not articulate with the carpal bones. It is separated from them by a thick pad, the **triangular fibrocartilage** (Fig. 6.22), which also articulates by ligamentous fibres with the distal radius, controlling and permitting the range of pronation and supination at that joint. The ulna is linked to the carpus by the **ulnolunate ligament** and the **ulnar collateral ligament**.

There are a large number of radiocarpal ligaments; these are the main stabilizers of the wrist and are chiefly arranged across the palmar aspect of the carpus. The **space of Poirier** is a thinning of the palmar carpal arrangement in front of the lunate, and it is this small weakness which allows the lunate to dislocate anteriorly with a rupture of the ligament.

The metacarpal bones have a system of interconnected transverse ligaments in the palm, reinforced by the general density of fascia and a large number of tendons.

The digits have two collateral ligaments at each joint, linked on the palmar surface to a **volar plate** (Fig. 6.23), a thick, resistant palmar reinforcement which is inserted into the base of the distal bone at the joint and connected to the proximal bone by the collateral ligaments. These plates limit extension at the joint to varying degrees, most severely at the PIPJ.

The ulnar collateral ligament of the MCPJ of the thumb is often implicated in abduction injury of that digit.

Examination

Palpation of the head of the radius should be performed while the forearm is moving, if that is possible.

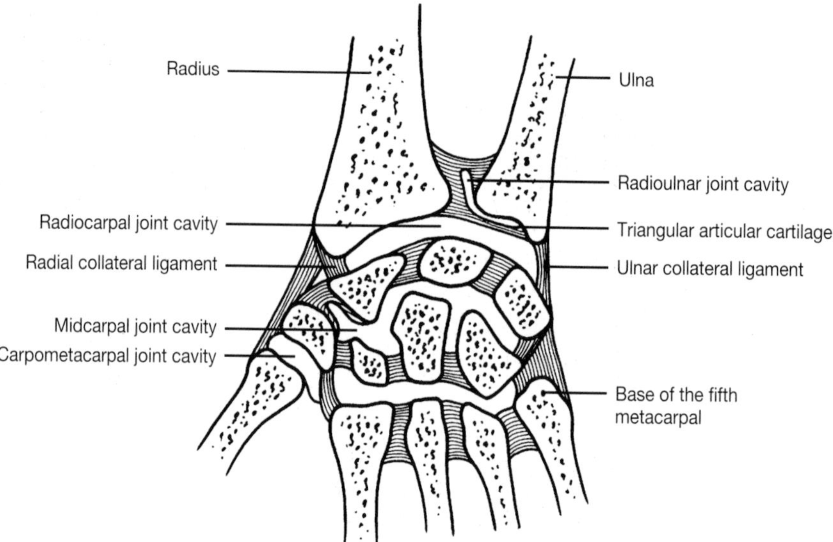

Figure 6.22 The ligaments and joint capsules of the wrist, carpal and carpometacarpal joints. (Reproduced by kind permission from Dean and Pegington (1996); after Ellis (1983).)

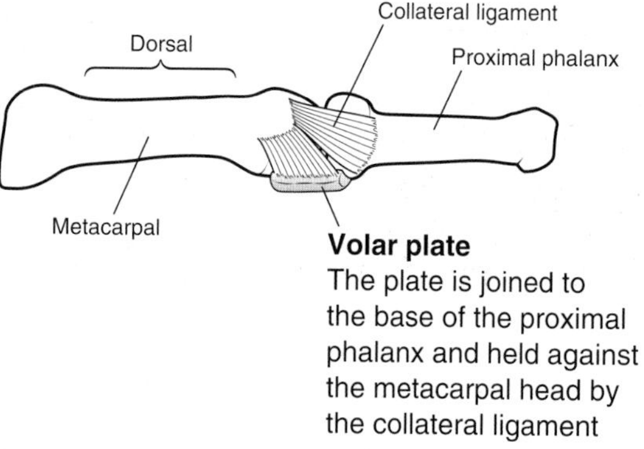

Figure 6.23 The volar plate and collateral ligaments of the hand.

Examination of the carpal bones is summarized in Figures 6.24 and 6.25.

A detailed description of the muscles of forearm, wrist and hand, and a method of resisted examination of each of these, is given in Figures 6.26–6.40. This emphasis on the hand is justified, not only by the numerous and subtle closed injuries which it suffers, but also because such knowledge is essential when assessing wounds to the hand.

The peripheral nerve distribution is shown for sensory nerves in the hand, and for the motor distribution in the forearm, wrist and hand (Figs 6.41–6.46). Resisted tests for the relevant muscles are shown.

Forearm, Wrist and Hand Injuries

The complexity of the hand, its ceaseless and varied activity and the fact that it is raised to defend the body from any expected impact mean that the upper limb is the part of the body which is most often injured. These injuries are too numerous for any inclusive list. A few common presentations are described here.

Hand splinting

If the hand is to be splinted or restrained by a heavy bandage, the NP should be aware that prolonged immobilization can cause joint contractures and is not beneficial for the intrinsic muscles. The collateral ligaments of the MCPJs contract if the joints are kept in full extension. The volar plates of the IPJs contract if those joints are held in flexion.

The so-called **safe** position (also known as the **Edinburgh** position) of the hand requires

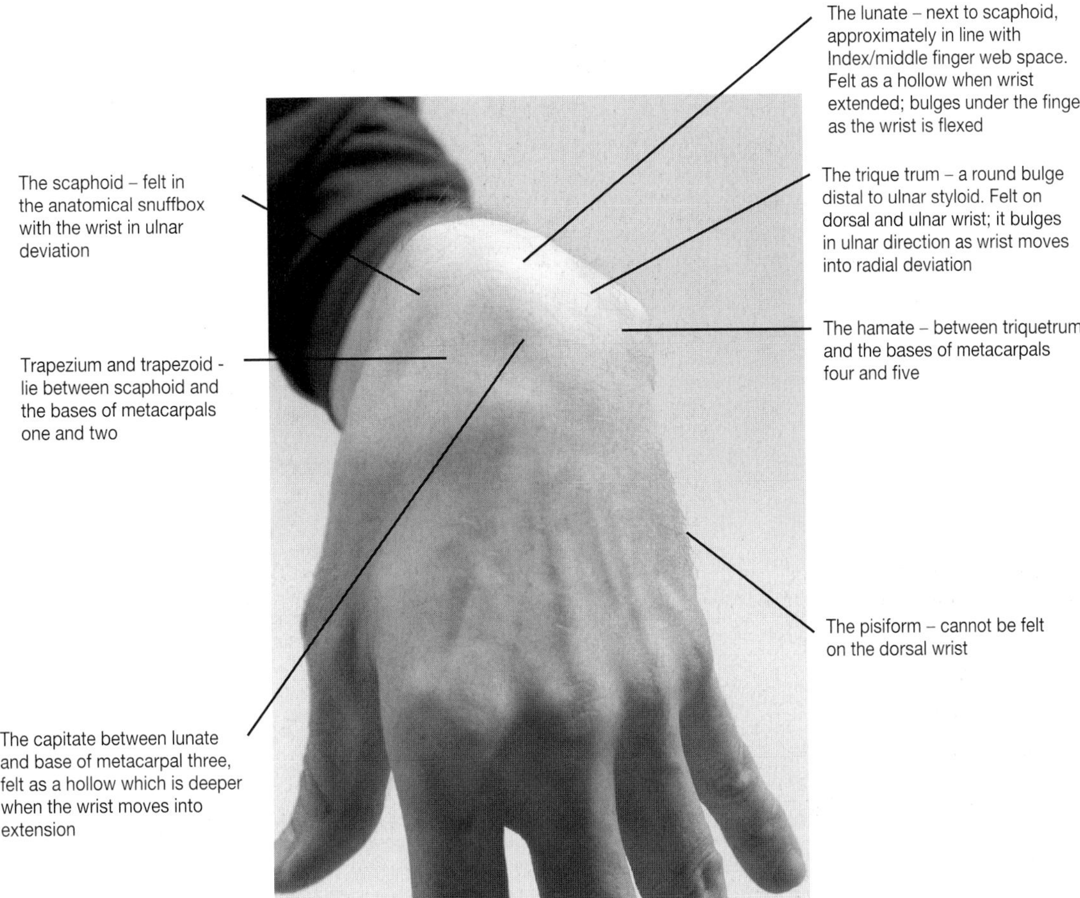

Figure 6.24 Examination of the dorsal carpal bones of the wrist.

that immobilization is carried out with the MCPJ flexed to about 80 degrees and a very slight flexion of the IPJs, for comfort, and the thumb in abduction. Different texts give slightly different details of this position, but the principle is clear.

Fractures

The fall on the outstretched hand

Falling onto the outstretched hand results in a forceful impact through a straight arm with the wrist extended and the forearm pronated. Injuries to ligament (and other soft tissues), bone and joint can occur anywhere in the wrist and arm.

In the forearm, fractures occur in either the radius or ulna, or, commonly, in both. Any severe angulation or displacement of one bone will cause a dislocation between these two bones at the proximal or distal articulation. The **Monteggia** pattern of injury is of a fracture of the ulna with dislocation of the radius at the proximal joint. The injury termed **Galeazzi** is the reverse pattern, with radial fracture and dislocation of the distal ulna.

The older person who falls on the outstretched hand is likely to incur a **Colles fracture**. This has a characteristic 'dinner fork deformity' of the wrist, caused by displacement of the distal radius. The deformity is of dorsal and radial displacement with a dorsal tilt of the radial head and impaction. The ulnar

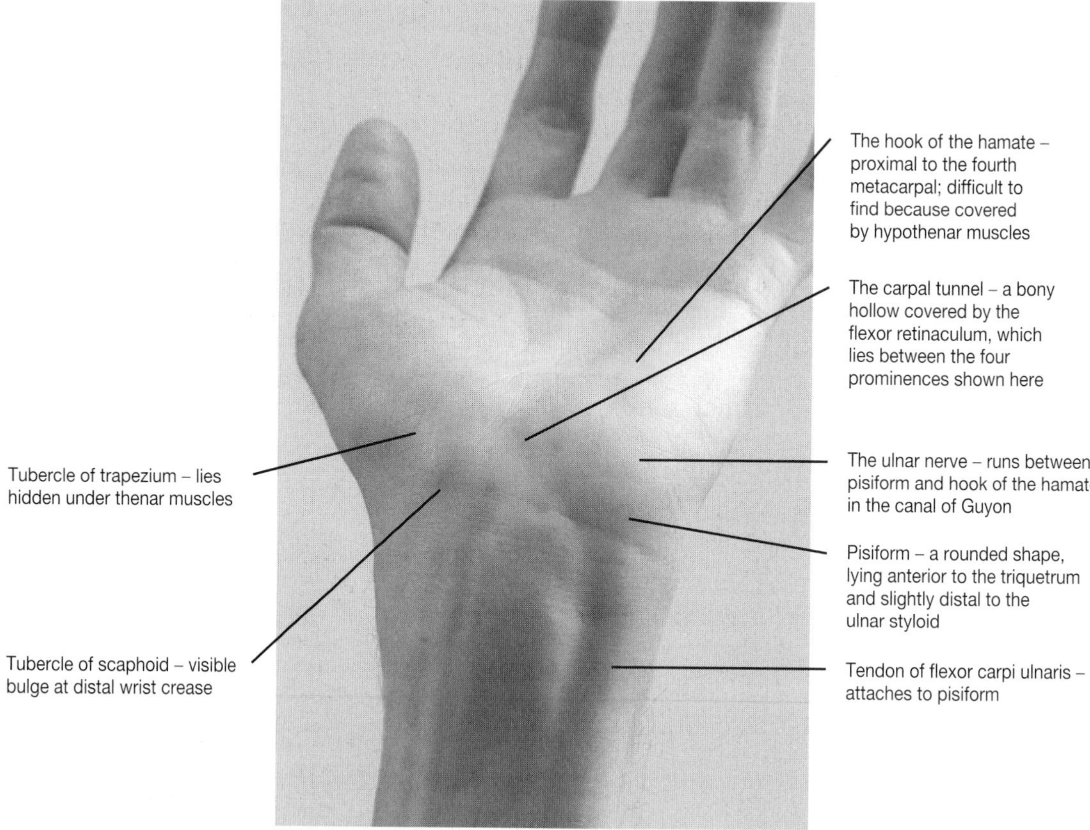

Figure 6.25 Examination of the palmar carpal bones of the wrist.

Box Muscles of forearm, wrist and hand

The muscles of the wrist and hand fall into two large groups, the **EXTRINSICS** and the **INTRINSICS**. The extrinsics originate from outside the wrist and hand, some from above the elbow. The intrinsics both originate and insert within the wrist and hand.

The extrinsics are in two groups:

- The **EXTENSORS** which arise from the lateral elbow and pass along the dorsal forearm to the hand.
- The **FLEXORS** arise from the medial elbow and pass along the palmar forearm.

The intrinsics can be described as being in three groups: the **THENAR**, the **HYPOTHENAR** and the **INTEROSSEUS/LUMBRICALS**.

The thenar muscles supply the thumb, and the hypothenar the little finger. Apart from muscles for flexion, abduction and adduction, they also permit **OPPOSITION**.

Opposition is a vital function of the hand. The first metacarpal can swivel across the palm, bringing the palmar surface of the distal phalanx of the thumb into powerful contact with the palmar surfaces of the other digits.

The interosseus muscles act as abductors and adductors of the fingers. (Movements which occur around the midline of the middle finger). However, with the lumbricals, they also form part of the extensor mechanism of the fingers. They interact with extrinsic muscles to allow the hand to achieve combined flexion in its metacarpal phalangeal joints, with extension of the other finger joints.

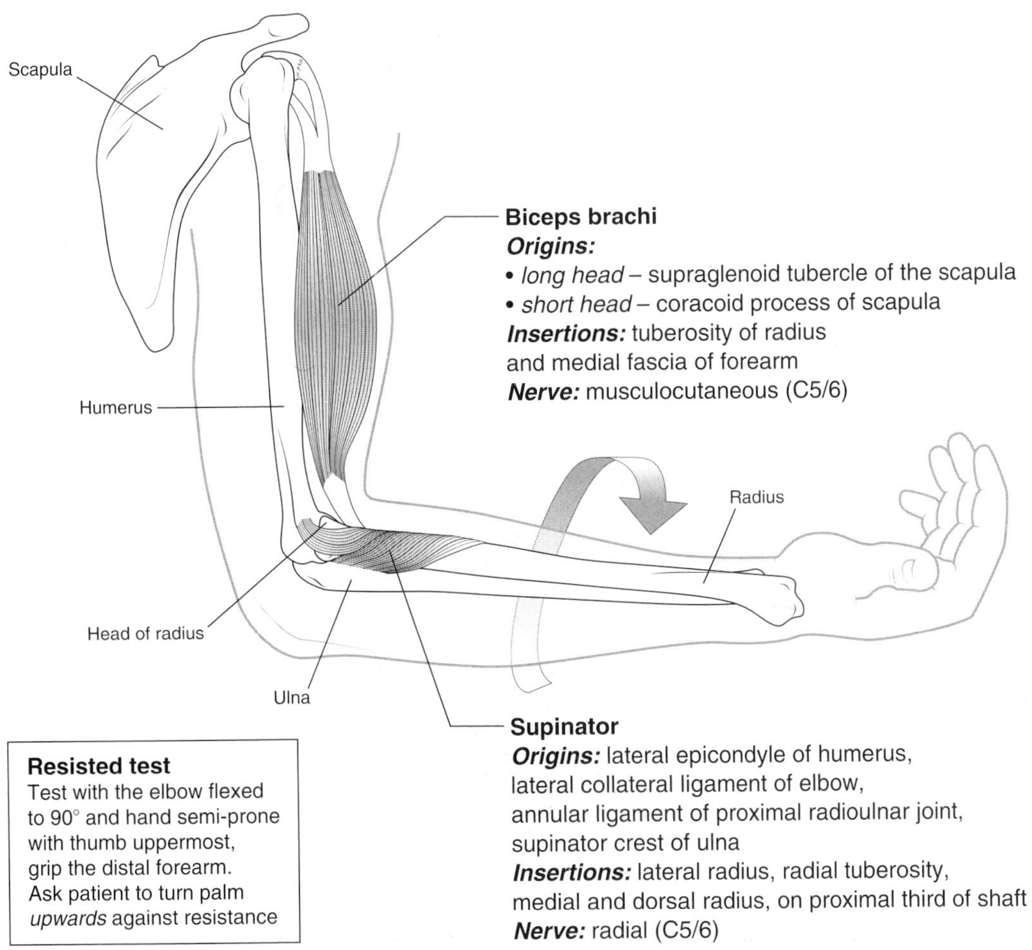

Figure 6.26 Supinators of the forearm.

styloid usually suffers avulsion. There is a specific risk of compression of the carpal tunnel. The neurovascular condition of the hand should be assessed carefully. These patients often require reduction of the deformity under local anaesthetic.

Children can also have severely angulated forearm fractures, which require correction, but greenstick fractures with minimal deformity are more common. There is often very little to see in the way of bruising or swelling with these injuries, but there will be pain, local tenderness, guarding of the limb and a reluctance or inability to use it. As with all forearm fractures, the elbow must be carefully assessed to exclude a double injury. It is common for an adult who falls on the outstretched hand to suffer a fracture of the scaphoid, especially across the narrow waist of the bone, which is forced against the lip of the radius by the hyperextension of the wrist. The hazards which non-union of a scaphoid fracture can cause have been discussed above. Tenderness in the **anatomical snuffbox**, especially if reinforced by tenderness on the palmar and dorsal aspects of the bone, is the chief clinical sign of scaphoid fracture (Fig. 6.34). Swelling over the anatomical snuffbox and inability to oppose the thumb to the little finger because of radial wrist pain are other indicators. The wrist should be X-rayed and either three or four (according to local policy) **scaphoid views** taken. Scaphoid fracture may not be detectable on the first X-ray film, even if it is present, and

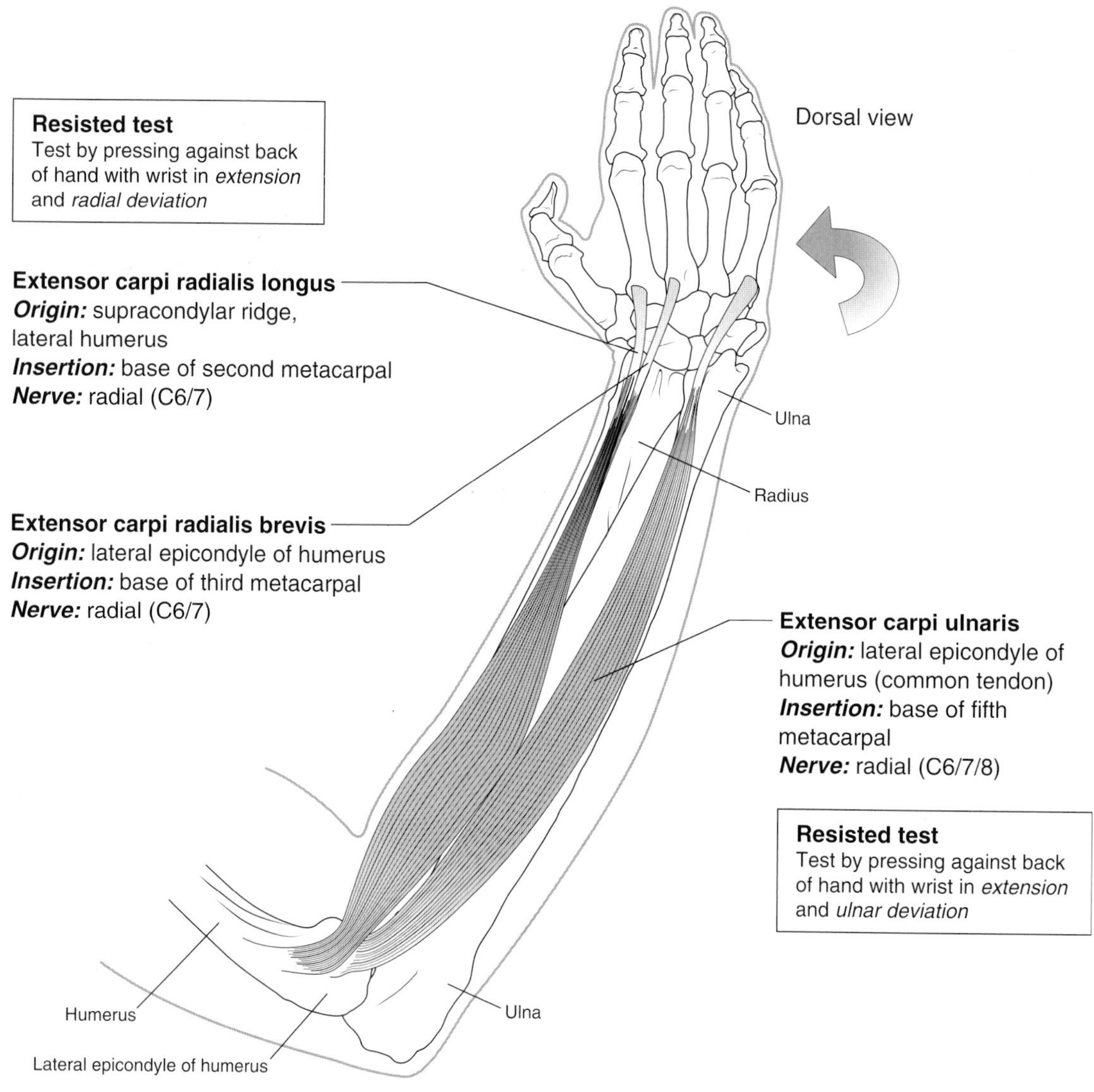

Figure 6.27 Extensors of the wrist.

the fact that the clinical signs are present means that the patient must be assumed to have a fracture. Each clinical area has its own variation on the policy of immobilizing the injury in a scaphoid splint or plaster (with the thumb held in a straight line with the axis of the forearm) and reviewing the patient between 1 and 3 weeks later. A fresh series of X-ray films may then reveal the signs of a healing fracture, and the patient can be reassessed clinically. Any case where doubt remains on clinical grounds should be treated as a fracture.

Hand fractures

The base of the metacarpal of the thumb can be fractured, usually by forced abduction or the impact on the thumb of punching. The thumb looks shortened and is swollen at its base. The **Bennet's fracture** divides the base of the bone, leaving a small medial fragment sitting on the trapezius while the force of the pull of the abductor pollicis tendon dislocates the rest of the bone proximally. This injury needs orthopaedic review and may need surgery.

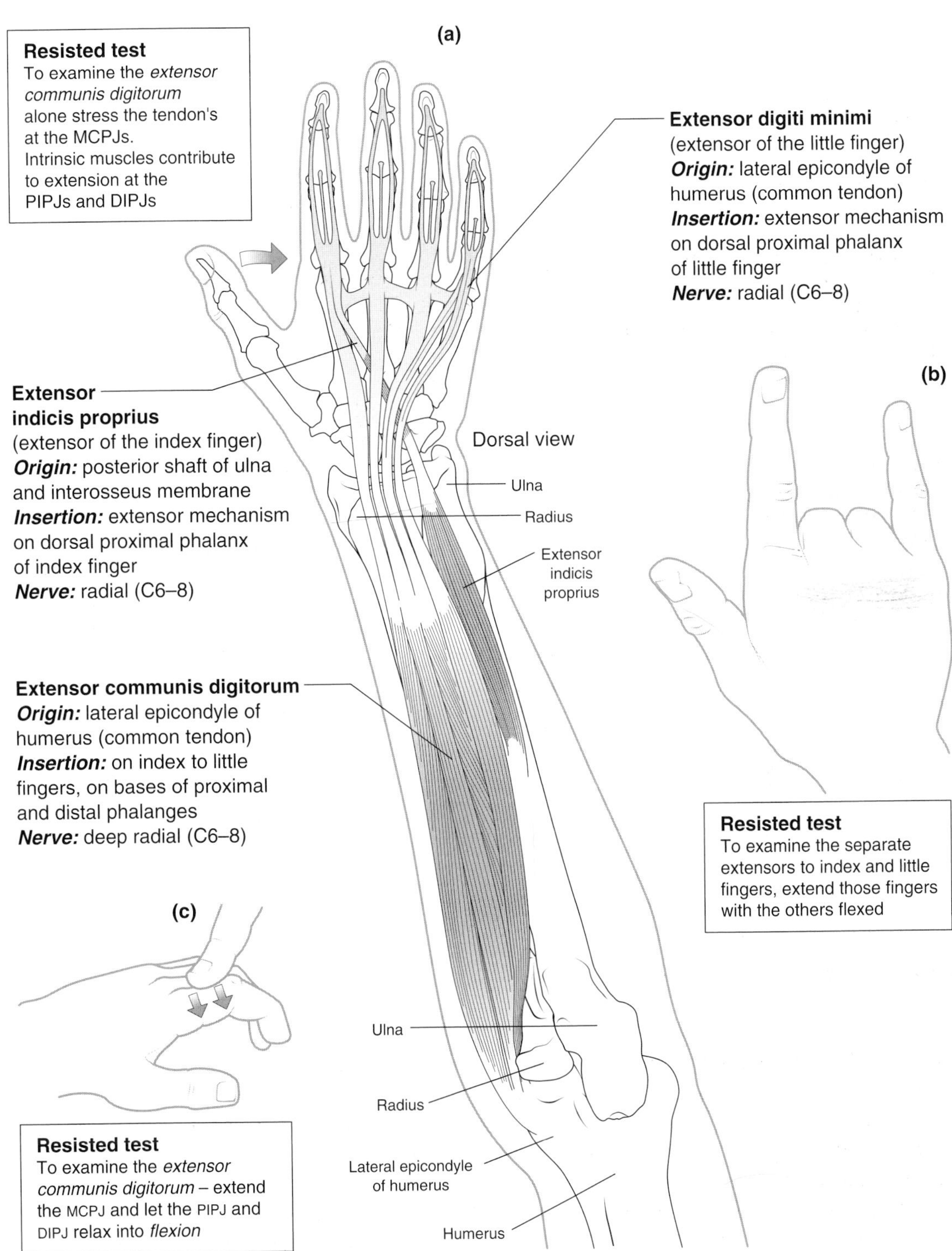

Figure 6.28 Extensors of the fingers.

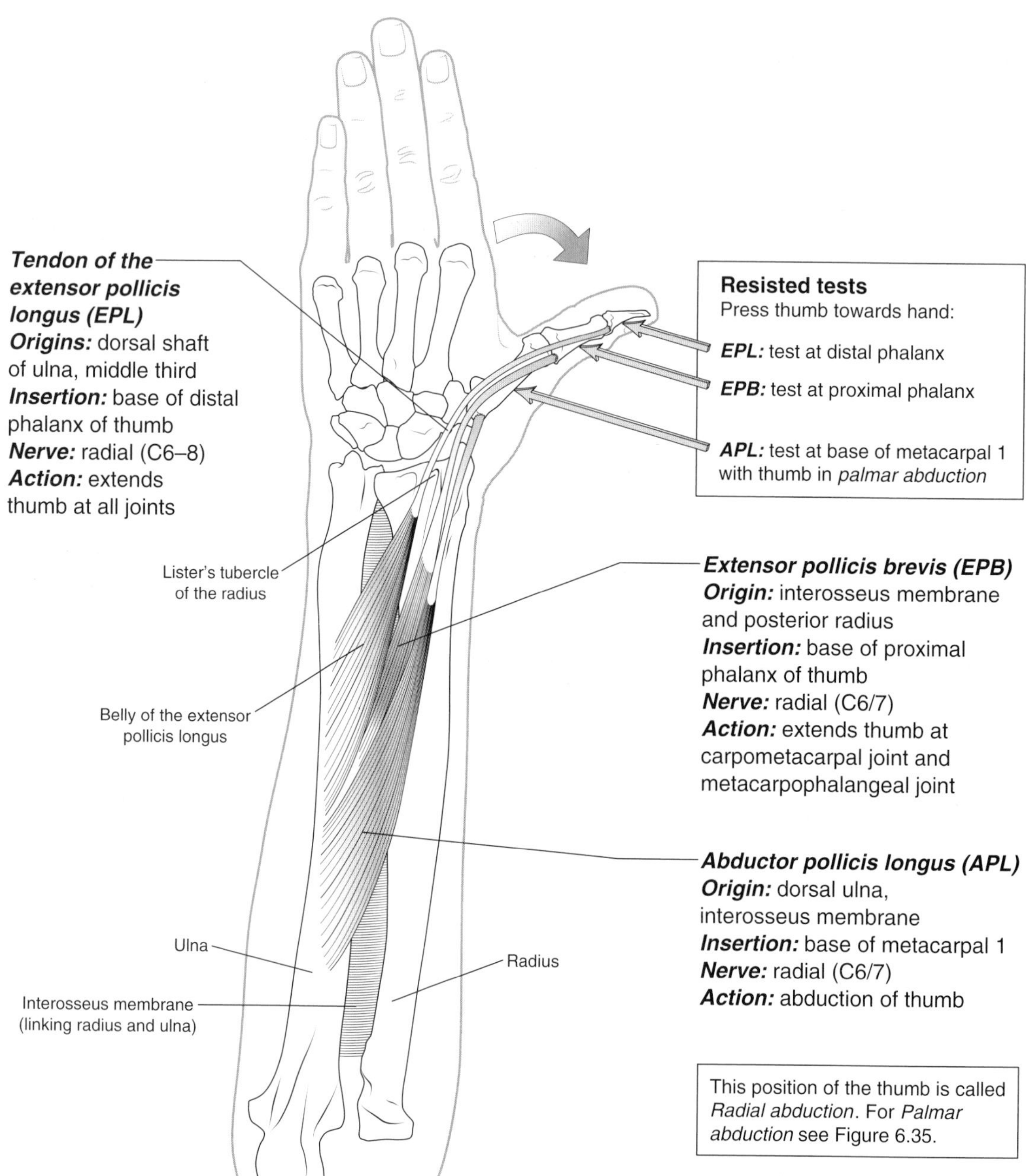

Figure 6.29 Extrinsic abductor and extensors of the thumb.

Another punch injury, called the **boxer's fracture**, is an angulated fracture of the fifth metacarpal. The injury is usually close to the head of the bone. The definition of the knuckle is lost (it is tilted into the palm) and extension of the MCPJ is much reduced. There is usually gross swelling in the ulnar half of the dorsal hand. Any small wounds on the injured knuckle should be closely inspected. Human tooth wounds are a common feature of this injury. Policies vary for management of this fracture, and sometimes the angulation needs correction; however, a combination of buddy strapping and tubigrip is often the only splinting it receives.

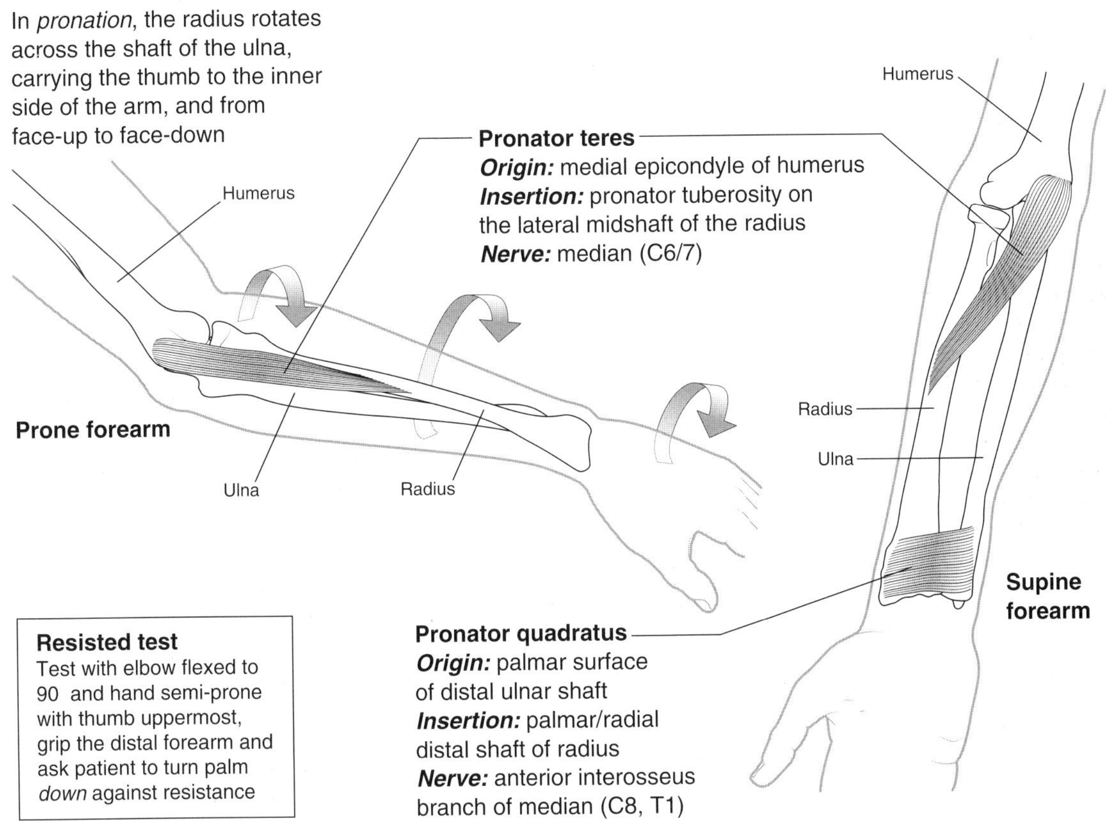

Figure 6.30 Pronators of the forearm.

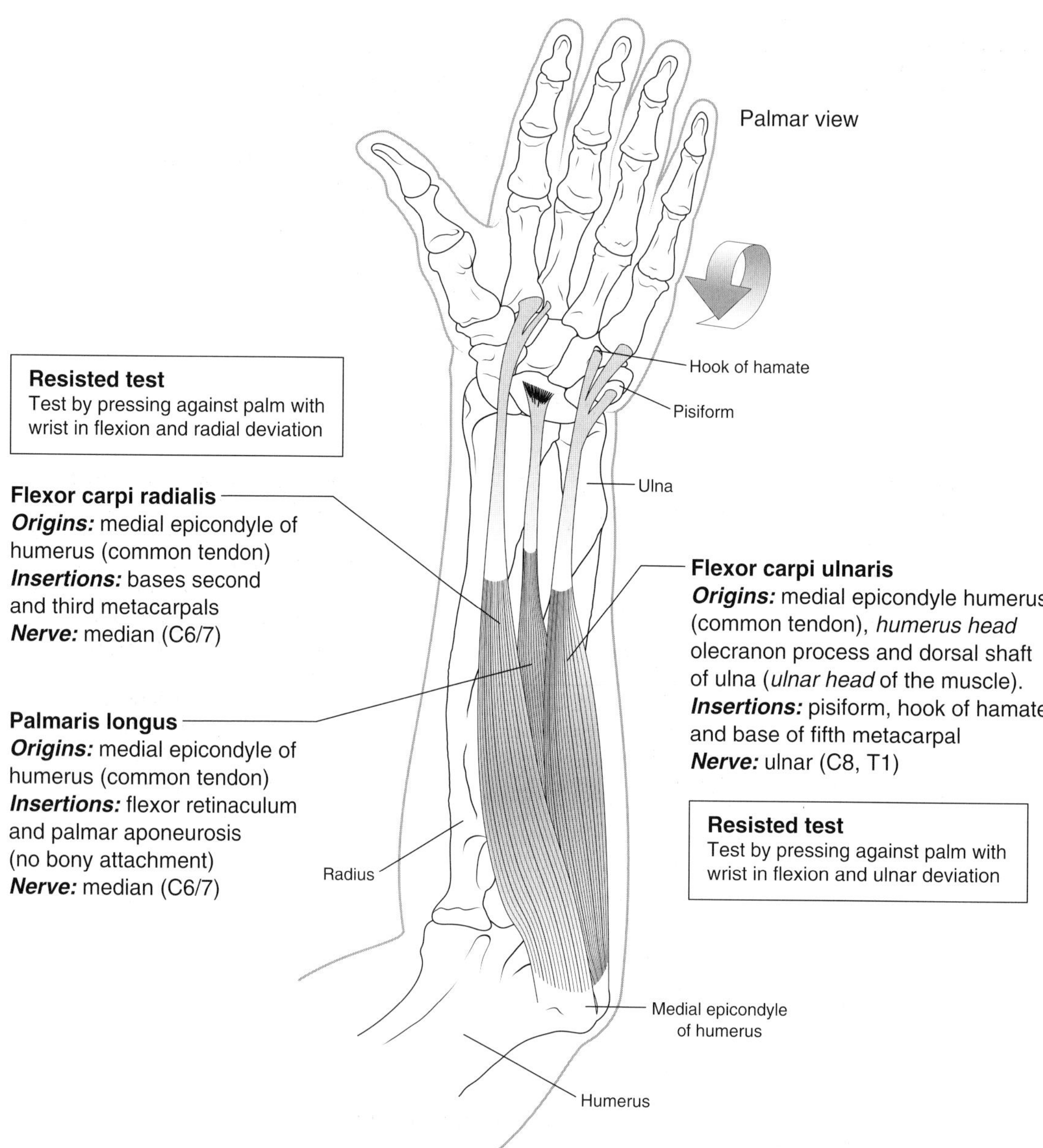

Figure 6.31 The flexors of the wrist.

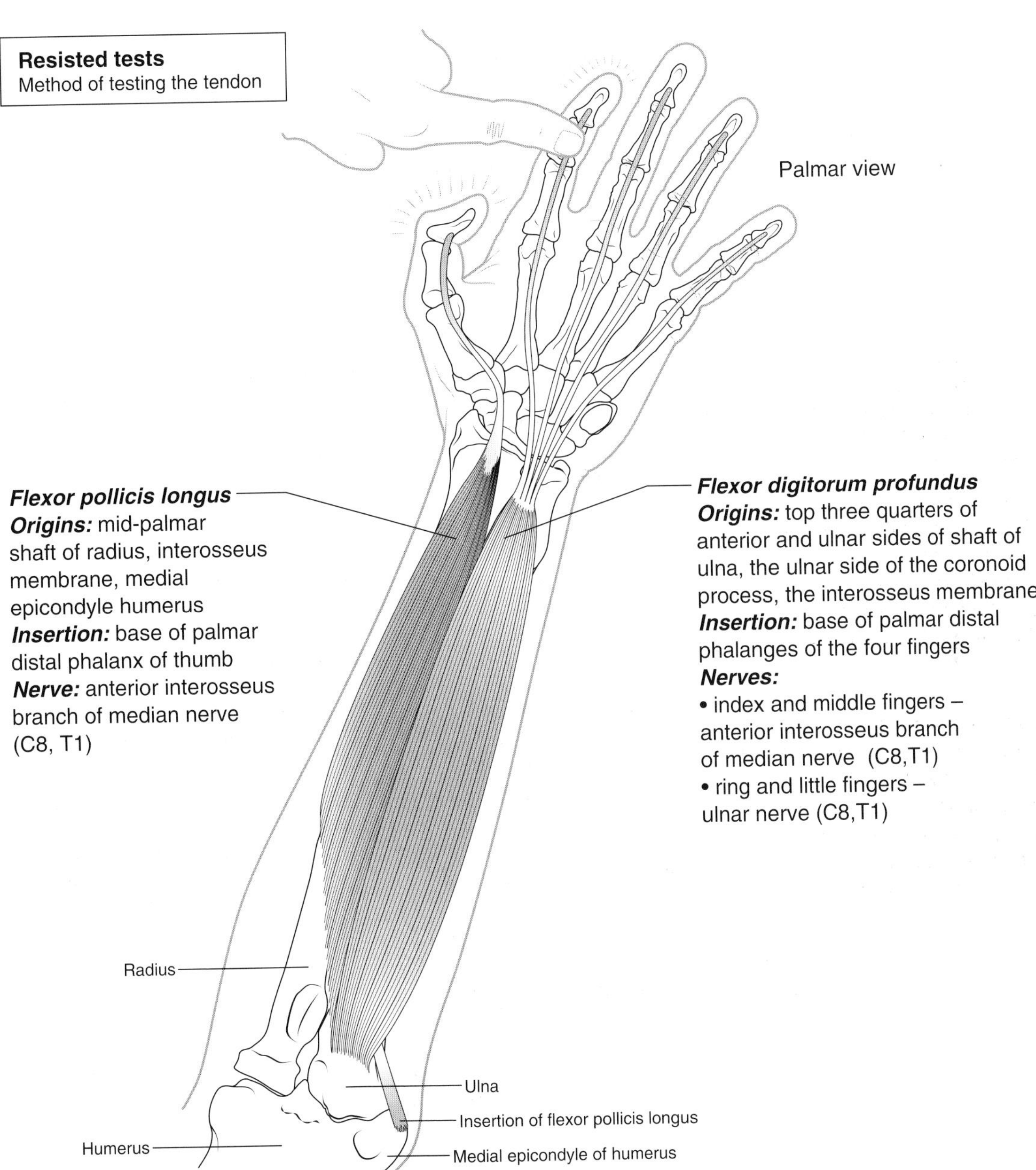

Figure 6.32 Deep flexor of the fingers and long flexor of the thumb.

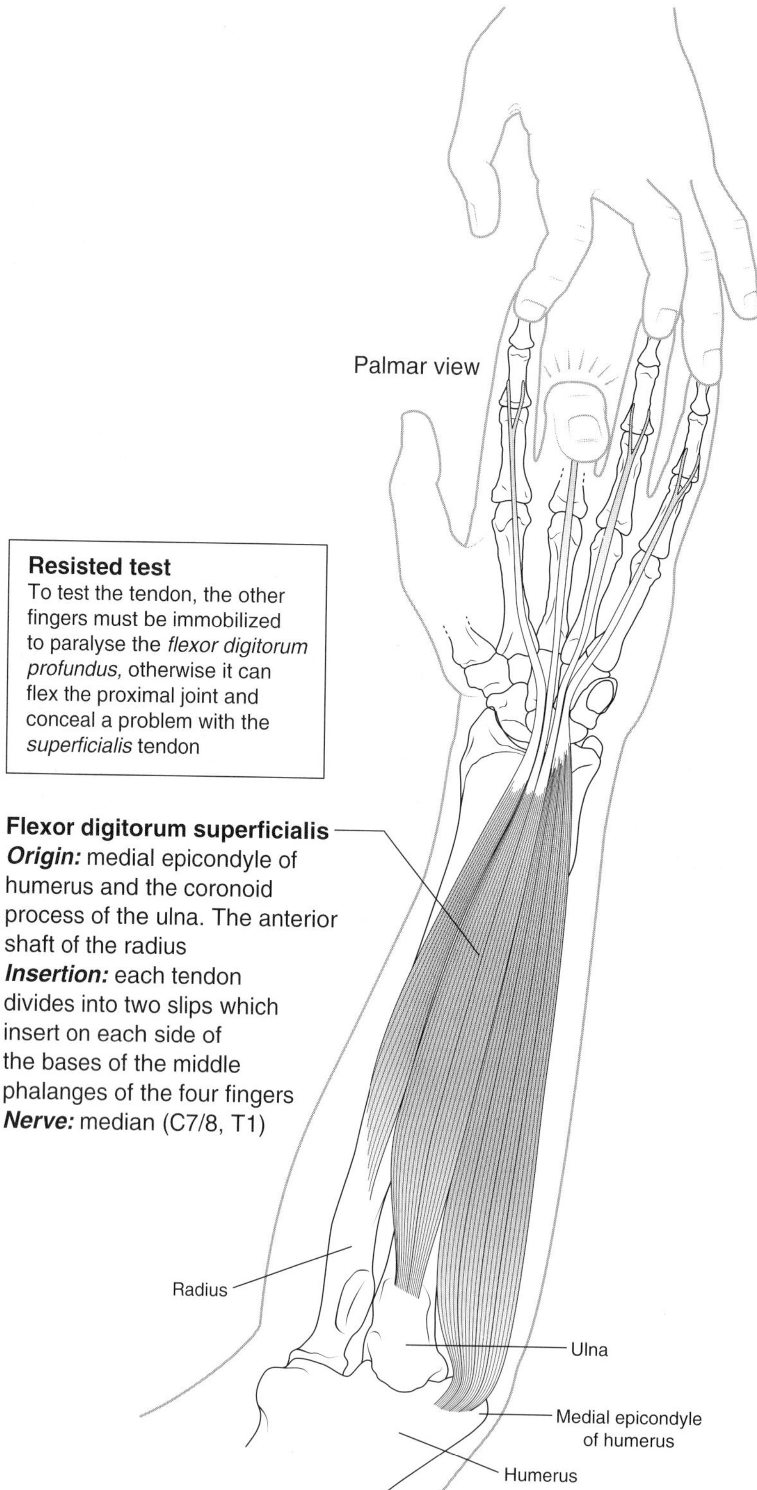

Figure 6.33 Superficial flexor of the fingers.

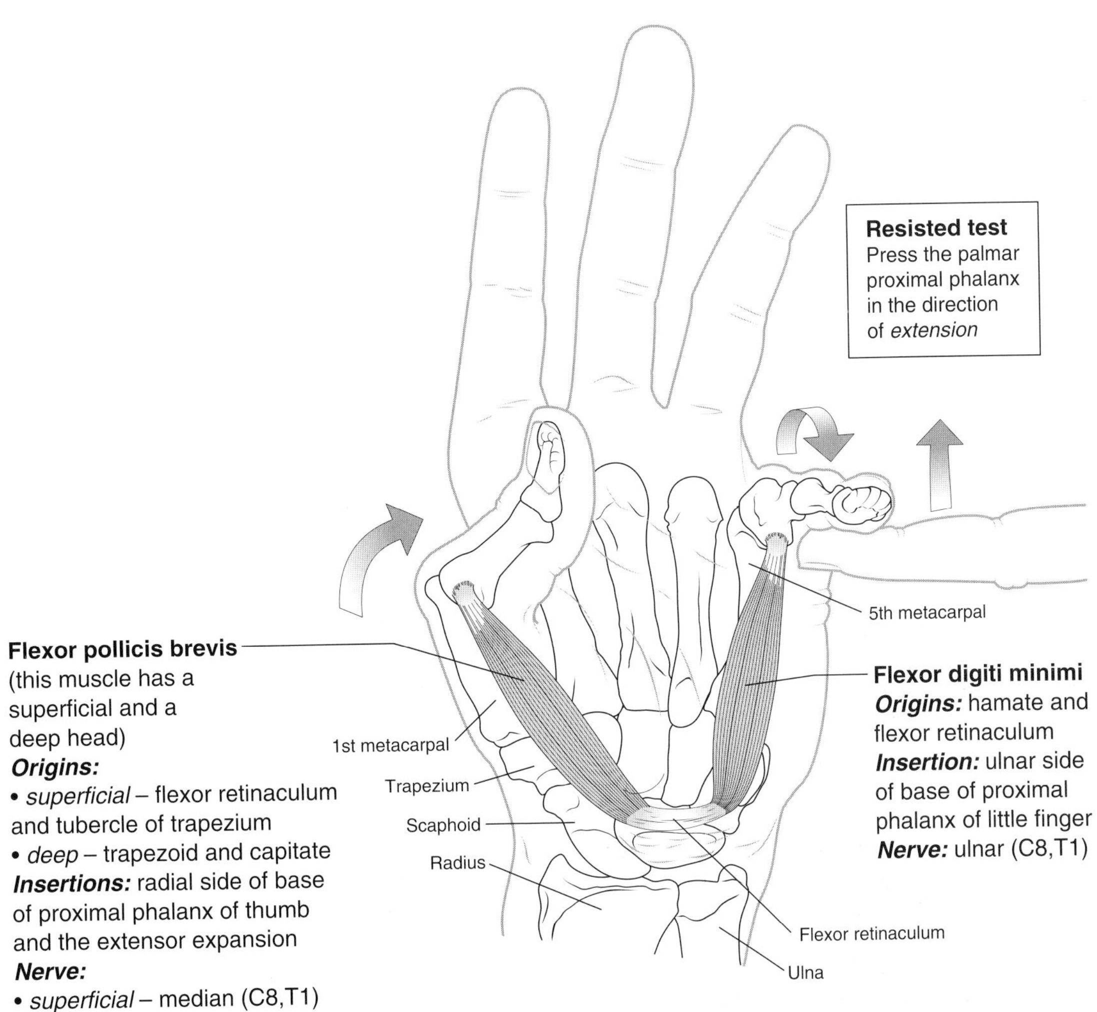

Figure 6.34 The intrinsic flexors.

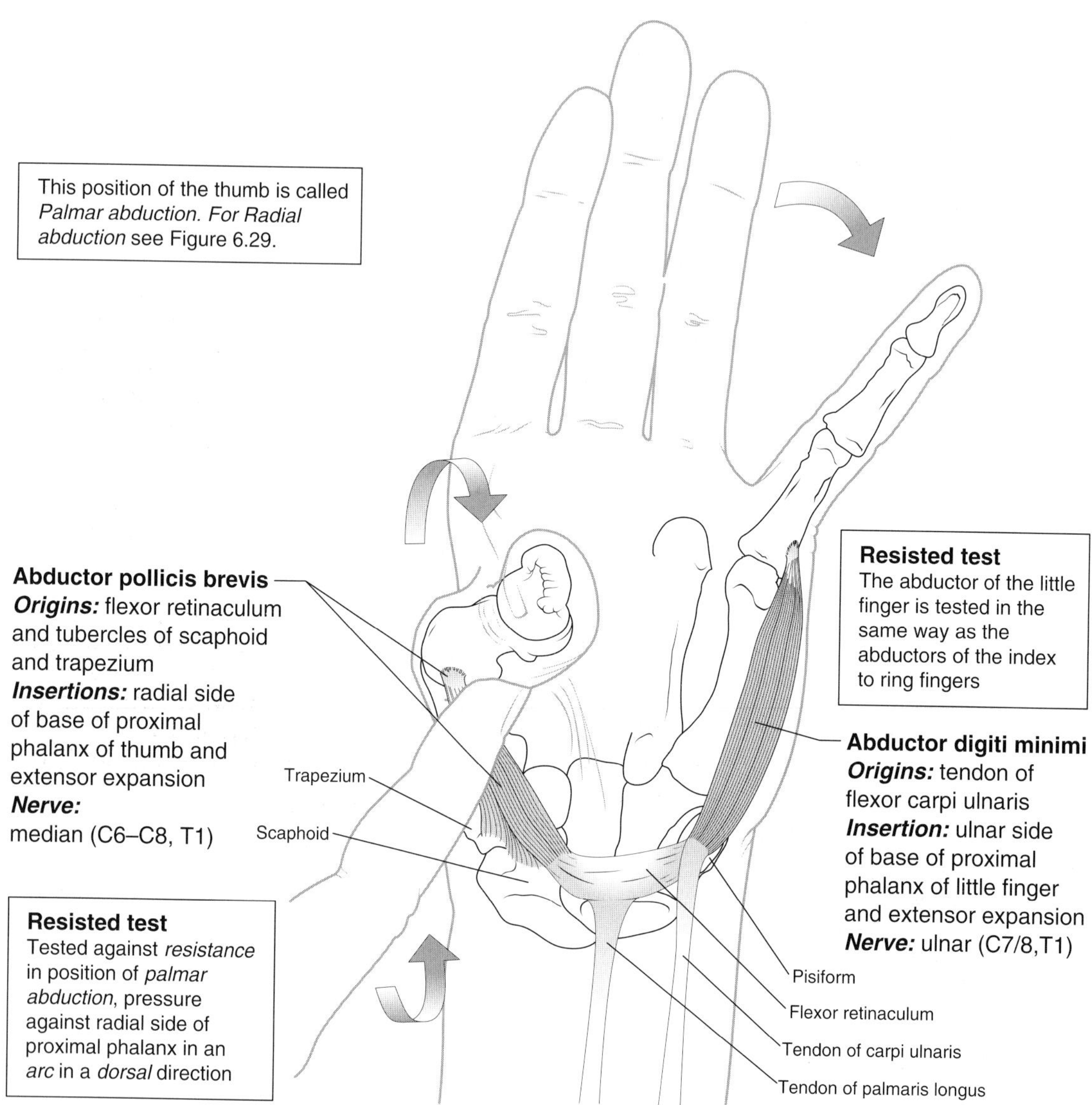

Figure 6.35 The intrinsic abductors.

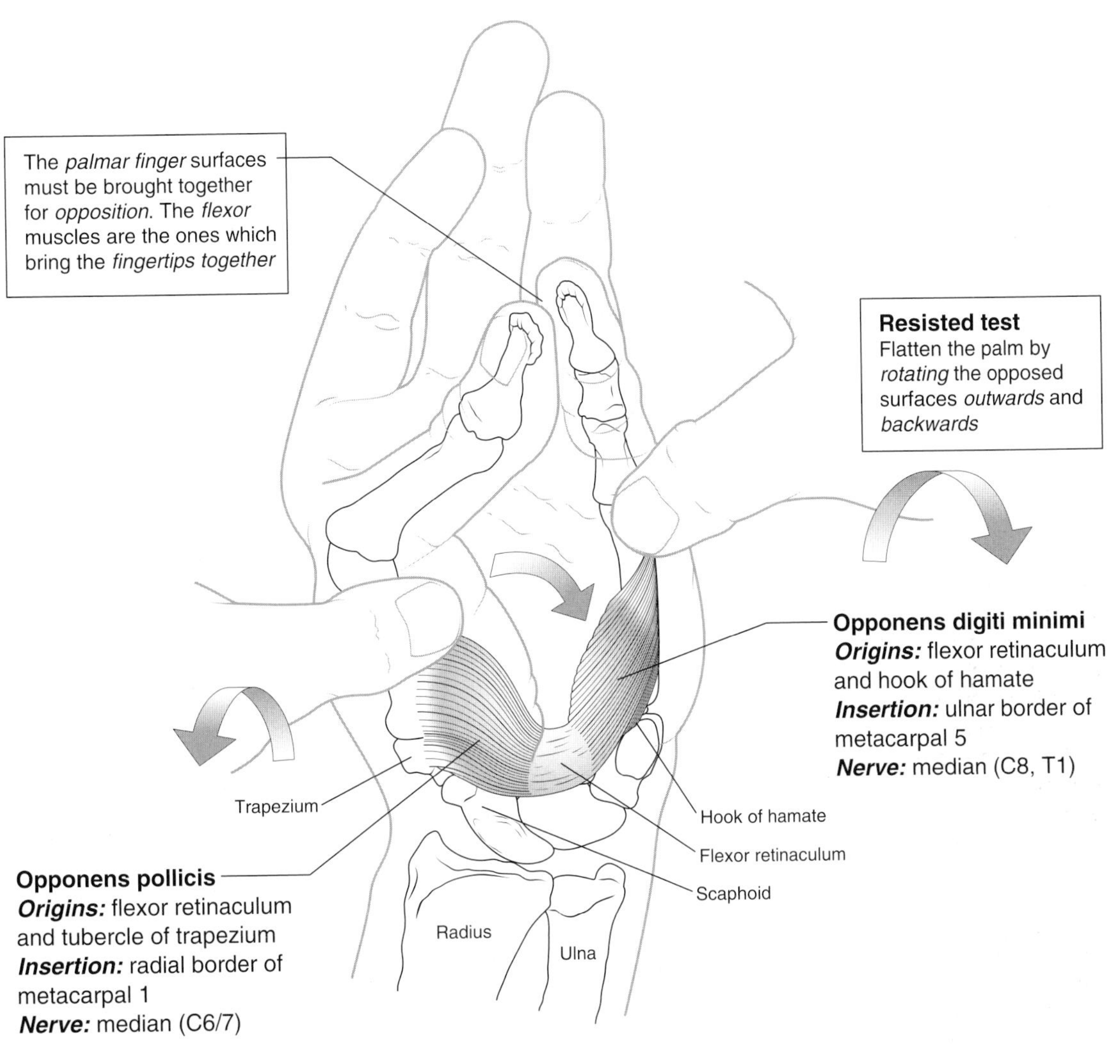

Figure 6.36 The muscles of opposition.

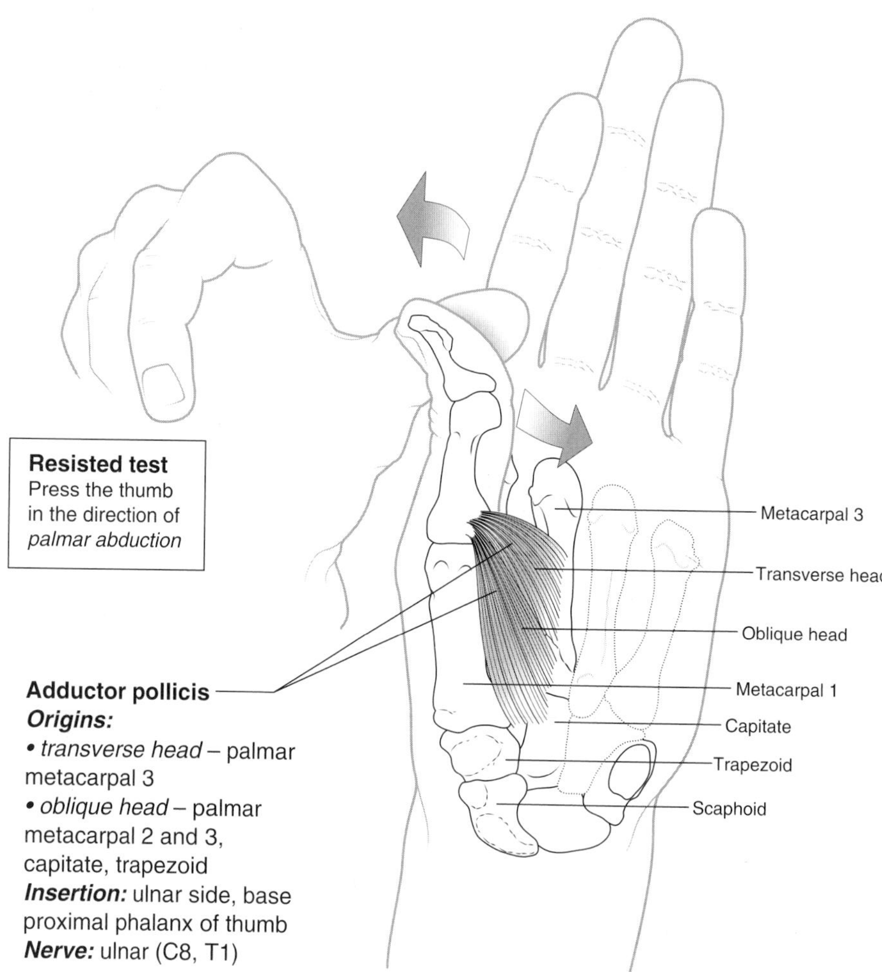

Figure 6.37 **The adductor of the thumb.**

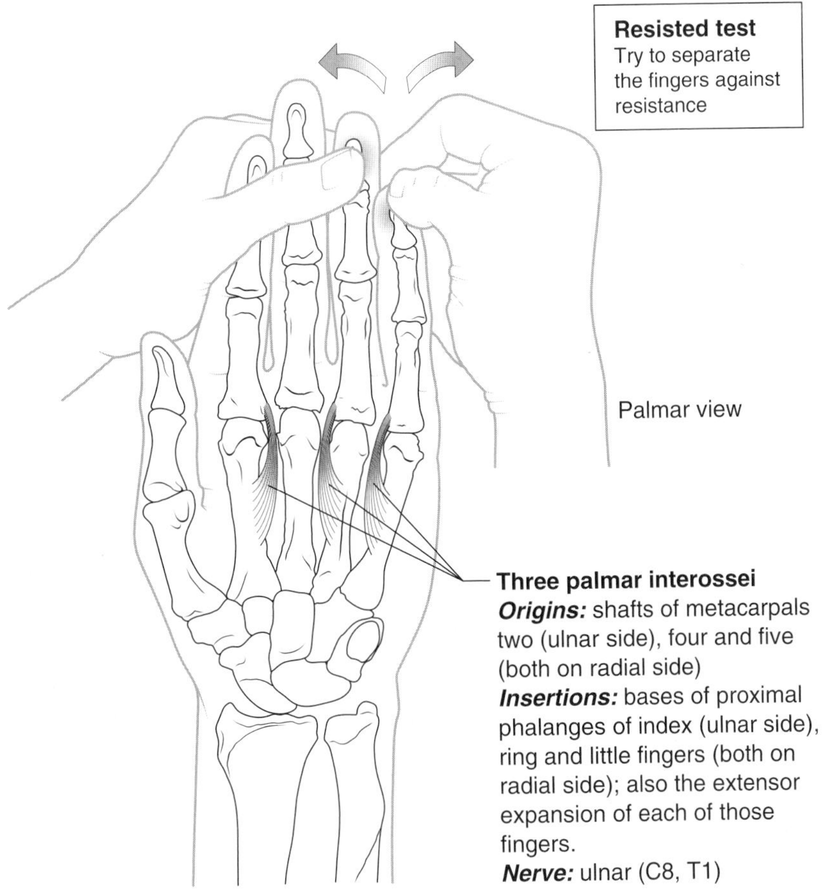

Figure 6.38 The palmar interossei.

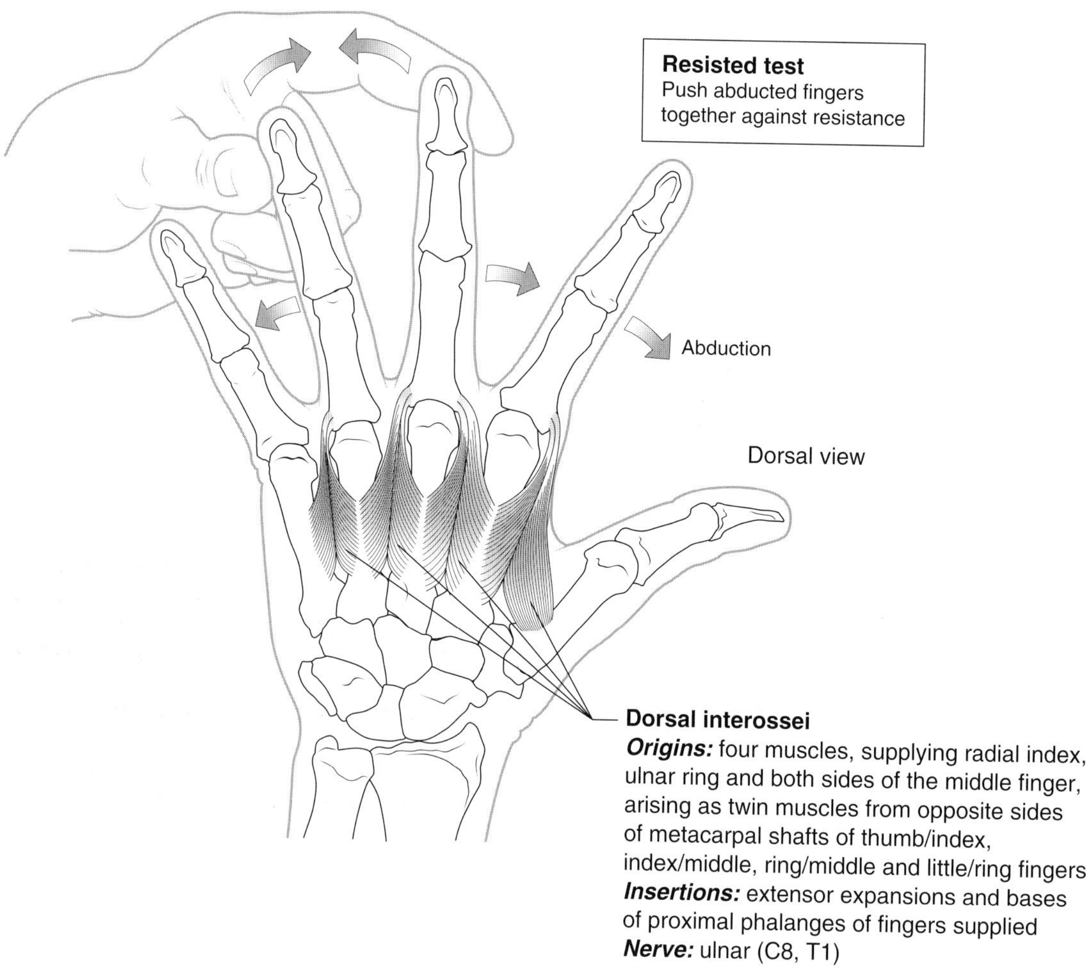

Figure 6.39 The dorsal interossei.

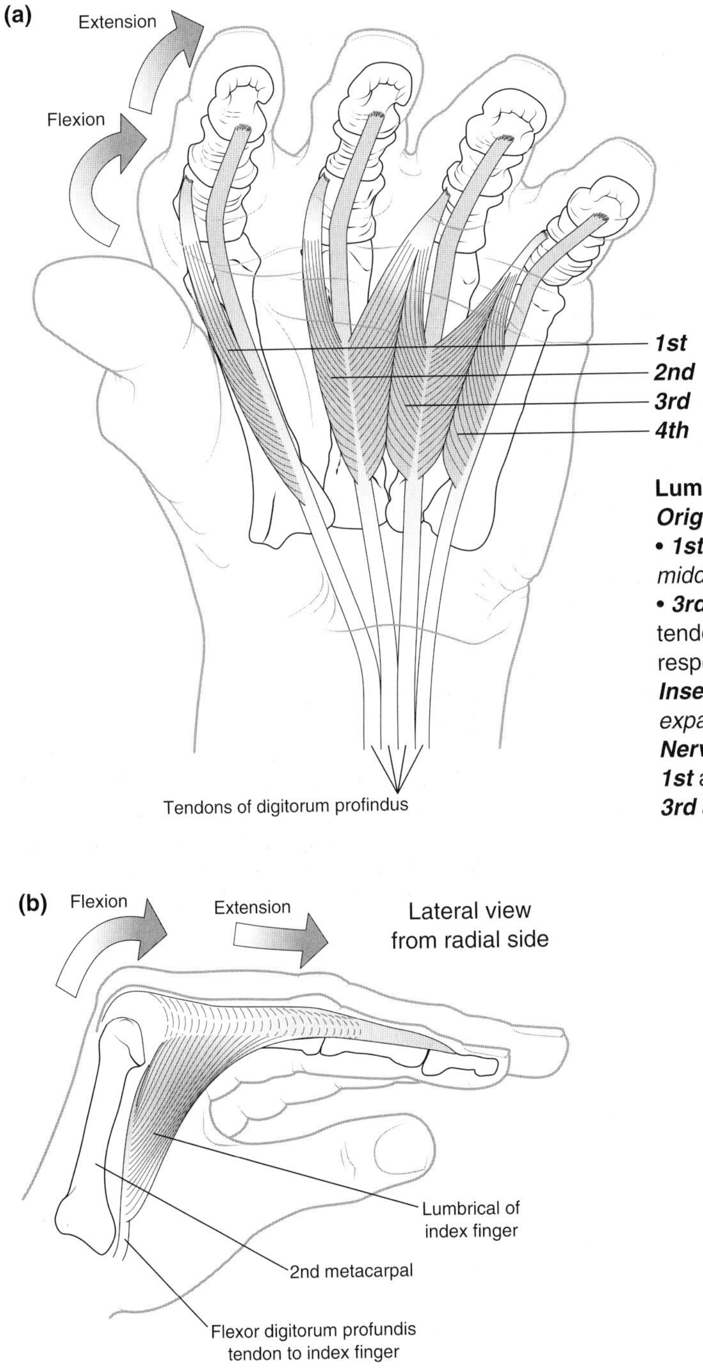

(a)

Extension

Flexion

1st
2nd
3rd
4th

Tendons of digitorum profindus

Lumbricals
Origins:
- ***1st*** and ***2nd*** – radial side of *index* and *middle tendons* of flexor digitorum profundus
- ***3rd*** and ***4th*** – adjacent sides of flexor tendons of middle/ring and ring/little fingers, respectively

Insertions: into *radial side* of *extensor expansion* of each finger
Nerve:
1st and ***2nd*** – median (C6–C8, T1)
3rd and ***4th*** – ulnar (C7/8, T1)

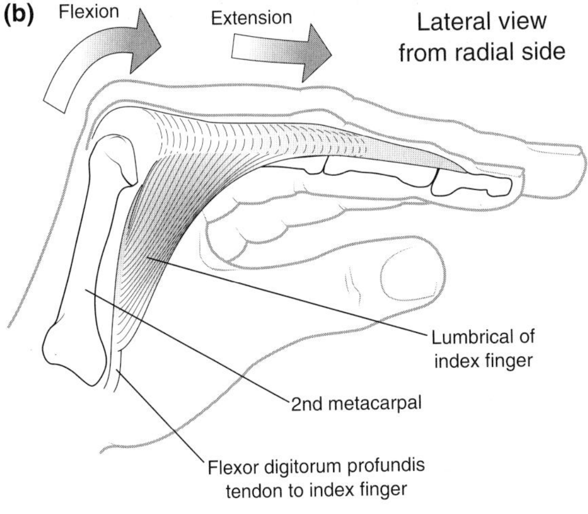

Figure 6.40 The lumbricals.

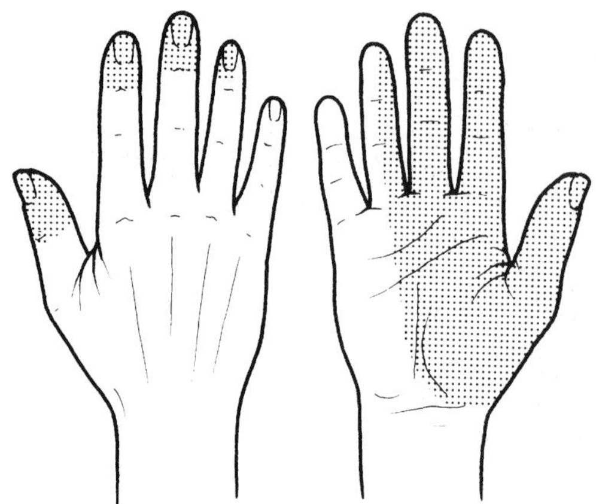

Figure 6.41 **The cutaneous distribution of the median nerve on the front and back of the hand. (Reproduced with kind permission from Dean and Pegington, 1996.)**

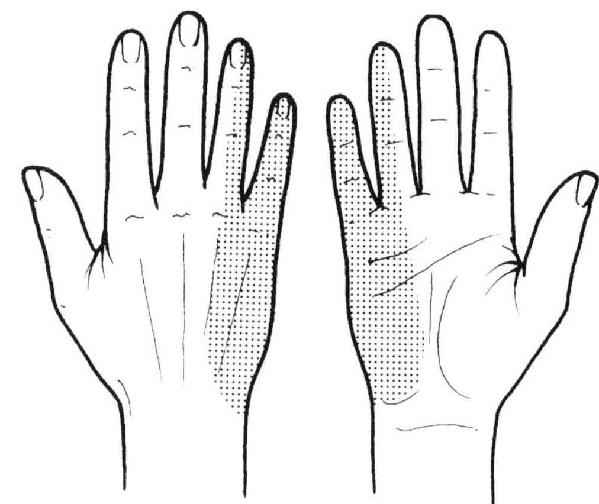

Figure 6.42 **The cutaneous distribution of the ulnar nerve on the front and back of the hand. (Reproduced with kind permission from Dean and Pegington, 1996.)**

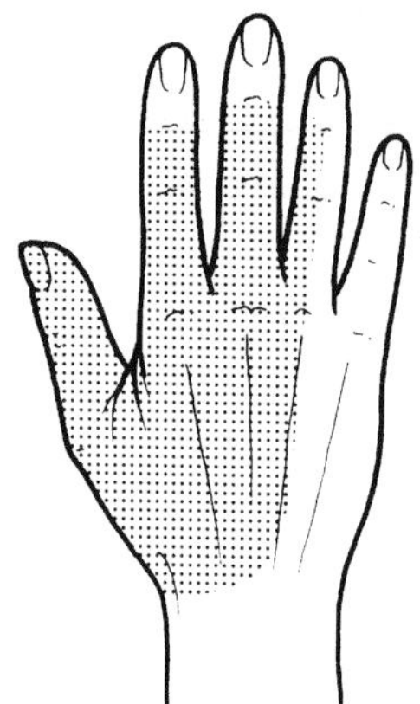

Figure 6.43 **The cutaneous distribution of the superficial branch of the radial nerve on the back of the hand. (Reproduced with kind permission from Dean and Pegington, 1996.)**

Finger fractures

The base of a palmar phalanx is often avulsed by the volar plate when the finger is hyperextended.

Avulsion of the dorsal base of a distal phalanx is often caused by a violent pull on the extensor tendon (an avulsion **Mallet** injury).

Crush injuries are common to the distal phalanges, often caused by closing the finger in a car door. There may be joint or tendon injuries. There is often a subungual haematoma (a bleed under the nail). Trephining this (making a hole in the nail to drain the blood) converts the fracture, technically, to an open injury.

Finger fractures are often treated with buddy strapping, rest and elevation only. They have to be assessed on their merits. The degree of instability, joint involvement, soft tissue damage and neurovascular effects are all important indices of severity. All fractures should be assessed by an orthopaedic specialist, urgently or routinely at a fracture clinic, as they require.

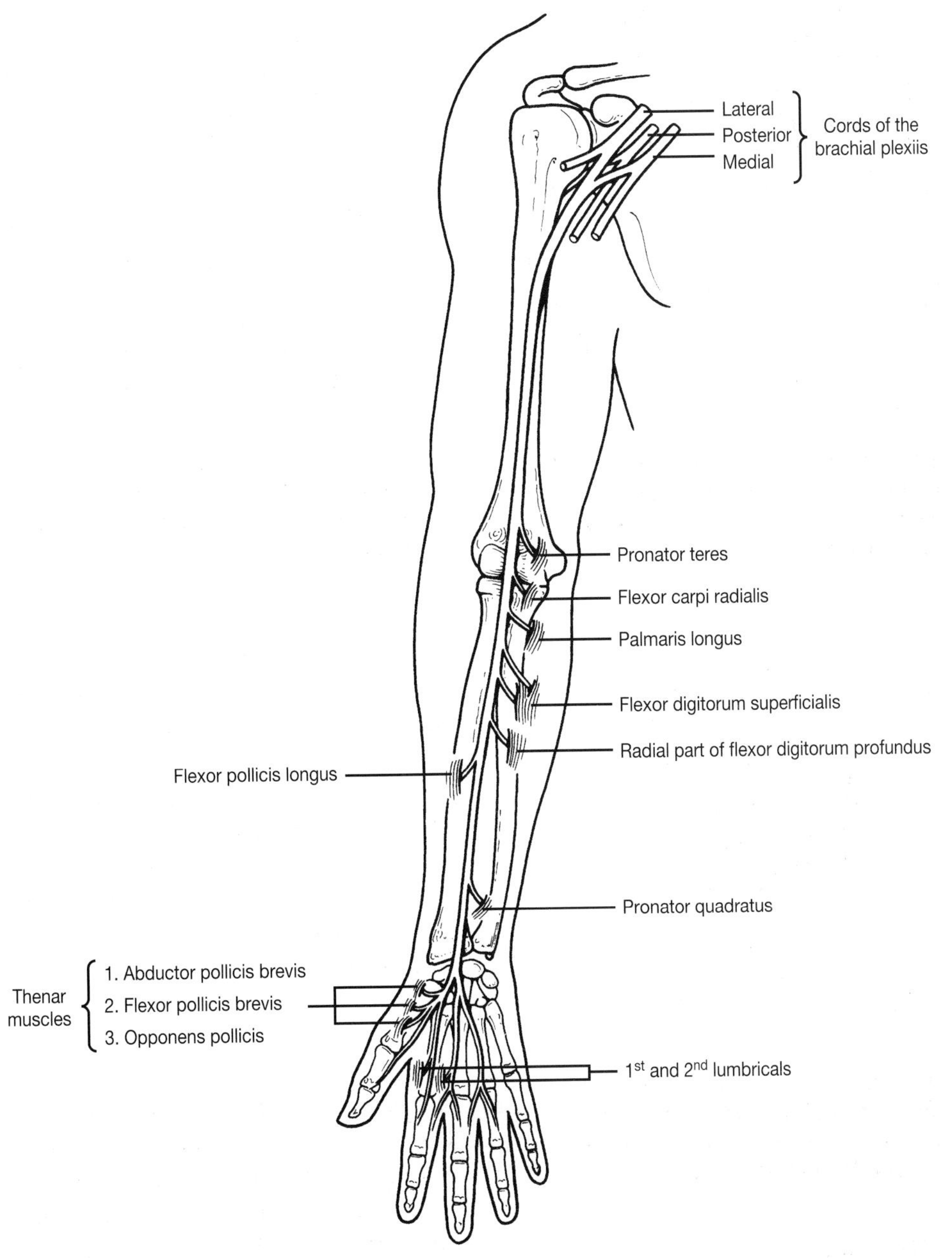

Figure 6.44 The course and distribution of the median nerve in the arm and hand motor supply. (Reproduced with kind permission from Dean and Pegington (1996), after Hollinshead (1982).)

Soft tissue injuries

Skier's (gamekeeper's) thumb

In Skier's thumb, the thumb is forced into abduction, often by a fall while holding a ski stick or by becoming caught in the matting of an artificial ski slope while the patient is falling downhill. The MCPJ is swollen and tender but not fractured. The finger is too painful and restricted for a full soft tissue assessment. A rupture of the ulnar collateral ligament of

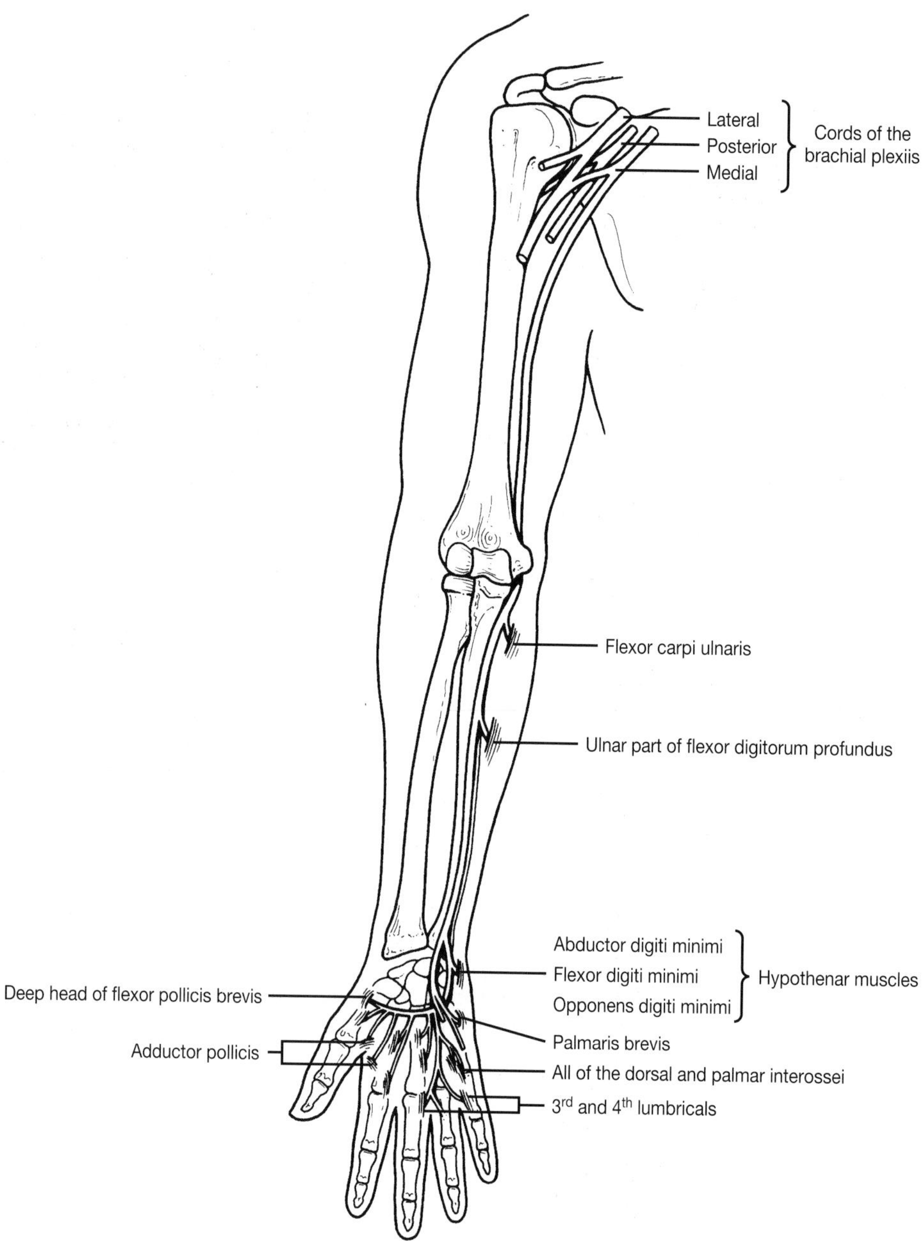

Figure 6.45 The course and distribution of the ulnar nerve in the arm and hand motor supply. (Reproduced with kind permission from Dean and Pegington (1996), after Hollinshead (1982).)

the joint is possible, and this should be excluded by stressing the joint (Fig. 6.47). If examination cannot be carried out at the time, the thumb should be immobilized in an elastoplast spica and reviewed in a few days.

Tendon tears

Complete tears of the extensor slips of the middle and distal phalanges of the fingers both produce characteristic deformities (Fig. 6.48). The tendon is often damaged by an axial

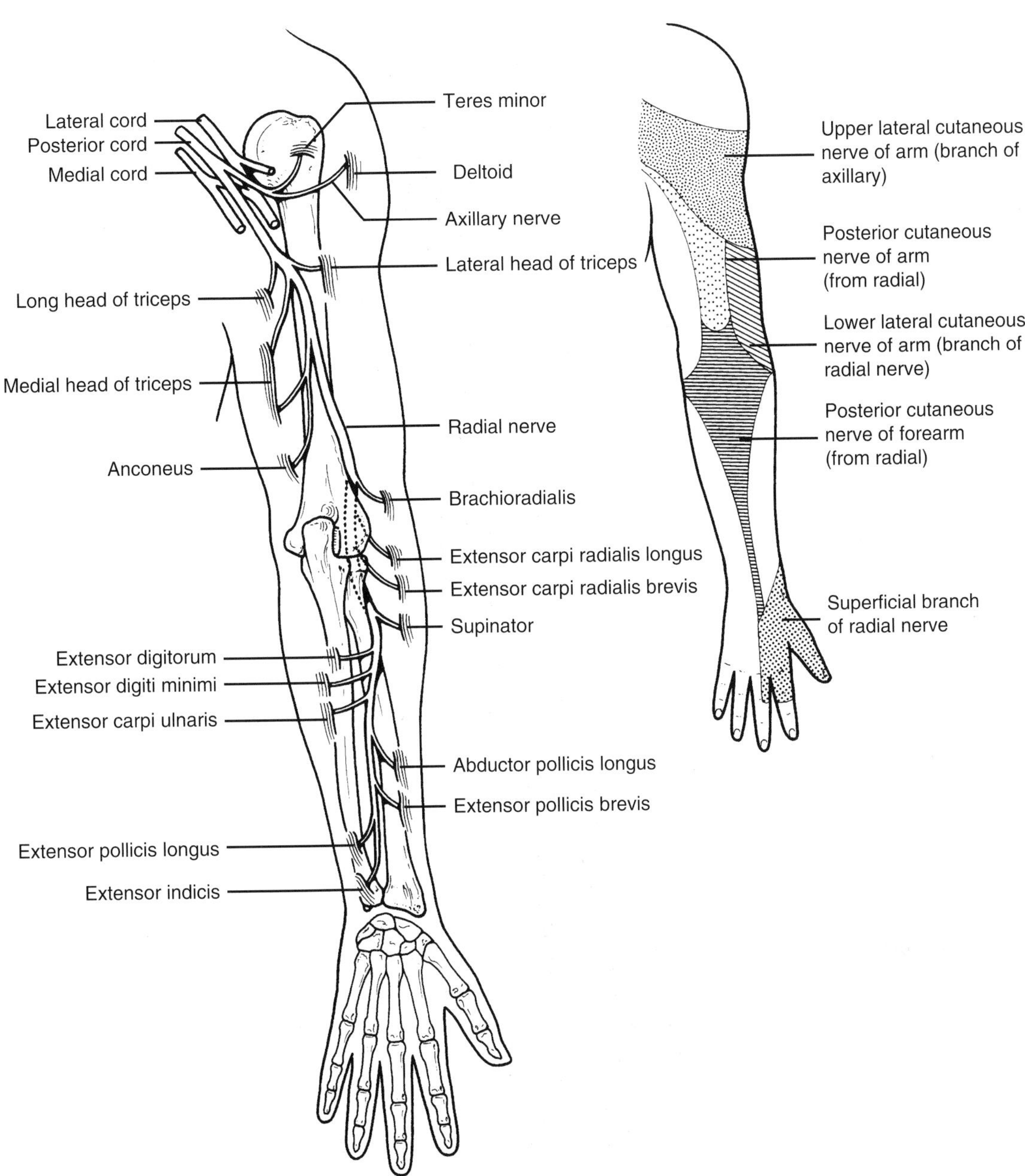

Figure 6.46 Distribution of the radial nerve in the palmar aspect of right arm motor supply. (Reproduced with kind permission from Dean and Pegington (1996), after Hollinshead (1982).)

injury or a crush (or cut) to the insertion of the tendon. The problem with the middle phalanx injury is that the lateral bands of the extensor mechanism may disguise the injury at first. These bands then, in later days, slip towards the palm and cause a fixed flexion deformity at the PIPJ, with forced hyperextension at the DIPJ (a **boutonnière deformity**). At this stage it may be too late to treat the finger. Further advice should be sought for any patient where such an injury is possible.

Rupture of the distal extensor tendon produces an immediate flexion droop at the joint, a **Mallet deformity**, which can be corrected passively. The finger should have an X-ray film taken to exclude an avulsion injury. A Mallet

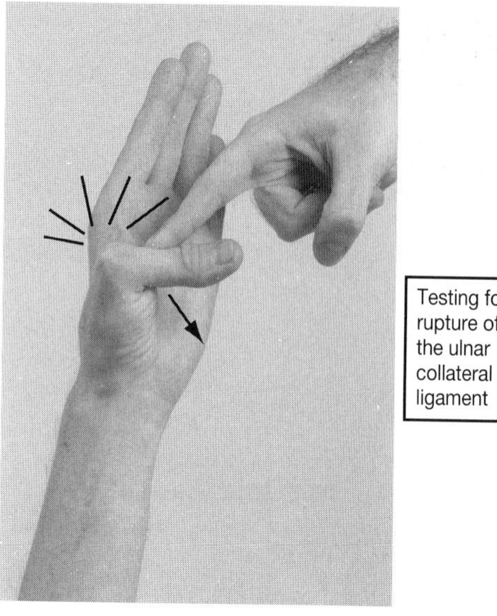

Figure 6.47 The ulnar collateral ligament of the metacarpal phalangeal joint of the thumb. This ligament can be ruptured by violent *radial abduction* of the thumb: so-called skier's thumb.

splint is applied to the finger and the patient is referred for orthopaedic management.

Overuse

Tenosynovitis is common at the wrist, on the thumb side, in the combined tendon passage of the abductor pollicis longus and the extensor pollicis brevis (**de Quervain's tenosynovitis**). There will be pain on movement, crepitations may be present and adduction of the thumb across the palm will cause pain. Rest usually settles the problem.

Infections

Paronychia is the commonest hand infection, usually caused by staphylococci. It sets in at the nail fold and causes a pus-filled painful swelling, and sometimes, a spreading cellulitis. It is usually treated by incision and drainage; it sometimes requires an antibiotic.

Purulent flexor tenosynovitis is a hand infection that requires aggressive treatment. The sheath of the flexor tendon of the finger becomes painful, swollen and tender. The finger tends to curl, and any attempt to extend it passively is painful. It can spread through the whole hand very quickly, and should be treated with intravenous antibiotics.

(a) Mallet – caused by rupture of the extensor tendon of the distal phalanx (or by avulsion of the bony insertion of the tendon)

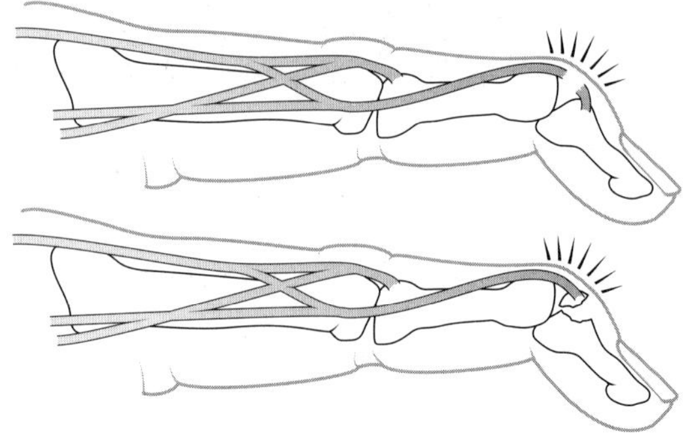

(b) Boutonnière – caused by rupture of the central slip of the extensor tendon of the proximal interphalangeal joint (PIPJ); the radial and ulnar slips move towards the palm, fixing the PIPJ in *flexion* and the distal interphalangeal joint in *extension*

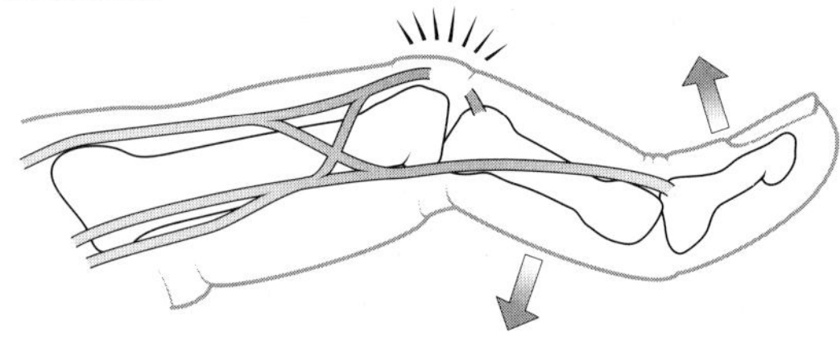

(c) Swan neck – the reverse of the Boutonnière pattern; can be caused by disease, injury to the volar plate of the PIPJ, or a long-standing Mallet injury

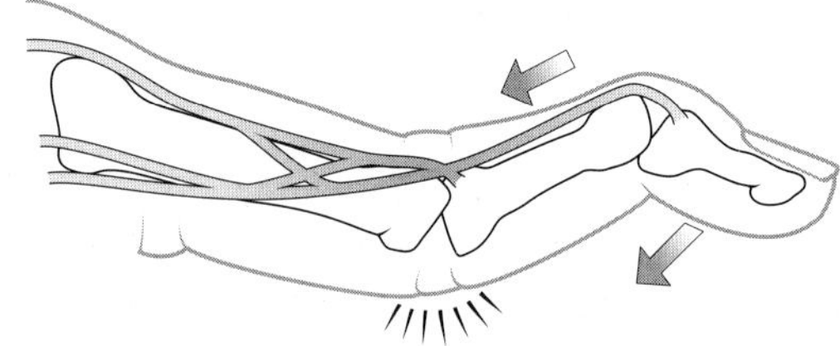

Figure 6.48 Common deformities of the finger.

7 THE BACK AND LOWER LIMBS

CONTENTS

This chapter will look at the lower limbs and the back. As in Chapter 6, the spinal attachment of the leg will be discussed before the leg itself, and problems affecting the ribs and back will be included at that point.

The chest and back are complicated areas where signs and symptoms may herald a serious, even fatal illness. Many chest and back problems are relatively minor but may not be easy to diagnose or treat. The role of the NP will be limited in this area, and accurate assessment of the seriousness of the problem, and swift referral of the patient by prearranged routes, will be a part of that role.

The Chest and Upper Back

It is reasonable, but, as always, subject to local policy, that patients who present with chest pain and a clear history of an injury to the ribcage may be treated by the NP if the injury is uncomplicated. Pain in the upper back or chest, with no history of injury, has to be treated with exceptional caution. Symptoms in the upper back may arise from problems in the neck, or they may be caused by any of the diseases which a doctor has to exclude when a patient complains of 'chest pain'.

Anatomy of the Thoracic Cage

The ribcage is a box-like, bony and cartilaginous, protective structure for vital organs: heart, lungs, liver and spleen and the large vessels of the circulation. In cases of injury to the lower ribs, damage to the kidneys is possible. Like every musculoskeletal structure, it makes concessions to contradictory demands. It cannot be sealed off because its organs serve every part of the body. It cannot be completely rigid because it moves to allow breathing and contributes to the overall mobility of the trunk.

Spine

At the back, in the midline, lies the spine (Fig. 7.1). There are 12 pairs of ribs, and each one of them articulates with one or two of the 12 **thoracic vertebrae**. The thoracic vertebrae are similar to the cervical ones, which were described in Chapter 6. They do not have the transverse foramina of the cervical vertebrae, which carry the vertebral arteries upwards from neck to brain, but they do have facets on the sides of their bodies for articulation with the ribs. The upper thoracic vertebrae are similar in size and appearance to those in the cervical area. They become bigger as they descend, making the transition to the lumbar region, where the vertebrae are large, adapted for bearing the weight of the entire upper body. The spinous processes of the thoracic vertebrae are long and angled downwards.

Sternum

The sternum is the breastbone (Fig. 7.2), a long, irregular plate of superficial bone which lies between the twin mounds of the chest in the frontal midline. It is made up of three bones, one above the other, linked by cartilage joints. The upper one is the **manubrium** (meaning, handle). Marieb (1995) describes it, very appropriately, as looking like the knot in a necktie. At the superior end of the manubrium is a hollow, plainly visible between the medial ends of the clavicles, the **sternal notch**, and there are two **clavicular notches**, divided by the sternal notch, for the clavicular articulations. At the widest part of the 'knot' are two articular facets for the **costal cartilages** (costa means rib) of the first ribs. The **body**, the longest part of the sternum, is joined to the lower end of the manubrium at the **sternal angle**. This is a hinge joint and forms a prominent, horizontal ridge on the upper sternum at the level of the insertion of the costal cartilage of the second rib. It is

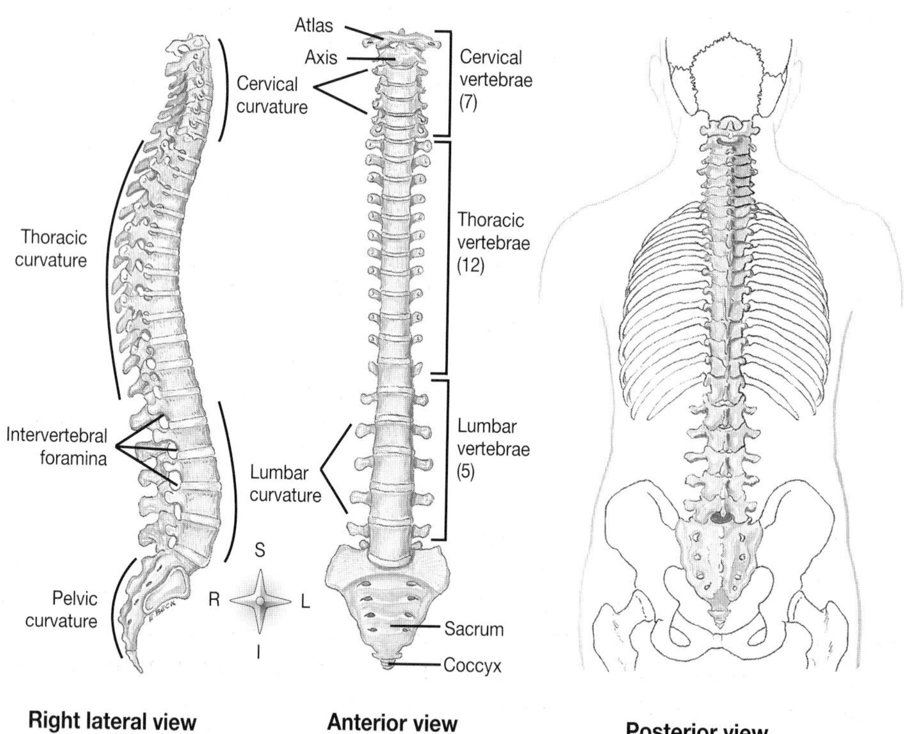

Figure 7.1 The vertebral column. (Reproduced with kind permission from Thibodeau and Patton, 1999.)

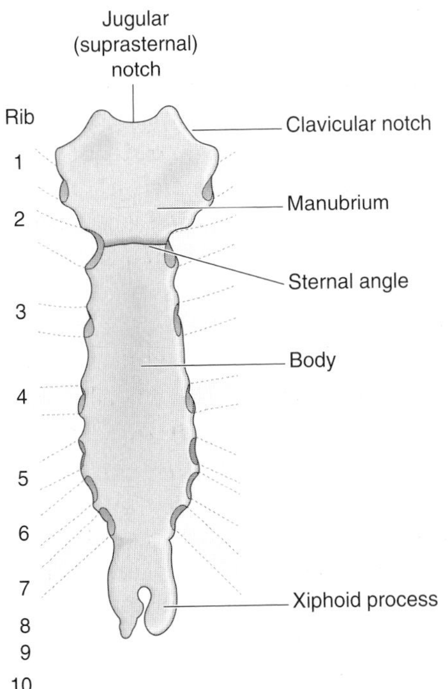

Figure 7.2 The sternum and its attachments. (Reproduced with kind permission from Waugh and Grant, 2001.)

a useful landmark during examination. The body offers insertion points on each side for the second to seventh costal cartilages. The second costal articulations, at the sternal angle, are shared with the manubrium. The third to sixth articulations are notches along the sides of the body. The seventh is at the level of the **xiphisternal joint**, and the xiphoid process shares the articulations with the body. The **xiphoid** (meaning, sword) is a small process at the inferior end of the body which offers attachment to the diaphragm and to muscles of the abdomen.

Ribs

The ribs are bones which ossify from cartilage. They are long, flattened, curving and twisting, having approximately a C-shape when seen from above. They are angled downwards as they curve from the thoracic spine at the back to the sternum at the front. They are variable in appearance, depending on their position in the thorax. There are 12 pairs of ribs, and they form a cage, open at the top and bottom (the **thoracic inlet** and **outlet**), with horizontal bars which constantly separate and come together to allow the lungs to expand and to deflate. The **intercostal spaces** between ribs contain muscles, nerves and blood vessels. The intercostal muscles act to widen the spaces between ribs during inspiration. The intercostal blood vessels may cause a haemothorax if they are injured. A residue of hyaline cartilage is found at the front end of each rib. This costal cartilage links the first seven ribs to the sternum. The costal cartilage of ribs eight to ten merge with that of the seventh rib and are, therefore, only indirectly connected to the sternum. The cartilage of ribs 11 and 12 (short ribs, sometimes called **floating ribs**) merge with the muscles of the abdomen at the front and have no sternal connection. Typical ribs have at the back an area called the **head**; this has two facets for articulation with the sides of the bodies of two neighbouring thoracic vertebrae, the rib's own vertebra and the one directly above.

The costal cartilage is covered with **perichondrium**, a tissue which blends with the periosteum of the ribs. The cartilage can be torn by injury without separation of this outer layer; consequently, there may be a deceptive appearance of integrity in a damaged structure.

Minor Chest Injuries

Minor injuries to the ribs, and to the muscles which relate to them, are the only category of chest problem which a NP will treat.

Triage

Patients with chest pain are in a category where life-threatening illness must be excluded. A patient treated as having a minor rib injury must have a history and a presentation which are consistent with that picture. The history cannot be vague, such as 'I must have injured it'.

From time to time, the NP will be confronted with a patient who is having a heart attack. Myocardial infarctions, and presentations which resemble them, are common. Diagnosis and treatment are time-critical. There must be a system for fast tracking any patient who presents with chest pain without a history of injury, and the nurse must be prepared to initiate resuscitation.

No injury is minor where there is a penetrating chest wound or where the mechanism is severe enough to have caused damage to the thoracic organs.

The minor rib injury

The usual mechanisms for blunt rib injuries are sport in the young and falls, especially in the intoxicated and the elderly. Typical tales are of a blow by an elbow or knee to the chest, a fall with the patient's own elbow trapped against the ribs, a fall in a bath with the arm lifted so that the chest falls against the edge of bath or basin. Patients who have had a chest infection and have been coughing remorselessly will sometimes experience a sudden cracking or tearing in the chest; they will then have the typical pain of those with injured ribs. Assault with blunt objects is another source of rib injury, and injury to the bony spine, the scapulae and the clavicles (as well as other injuries) must be excluded.

The patient will localize a painful spot, which will be very tender. There may not be bruising. The patient may describe feeling abnormal grating or clicking on breathing, and crepitus may be felt when the spot is touched.

Pain is a considerable feature of rib injuries. It is not usually present at rest but is triggered by deep breathing and coughing, and by certain movements. Sleep may be disturbed because it is hard to lie comfortably, and because movement in the bed hurts. Pain tends to worsen, or become more tiring, on successive days for a week or so, and patients will often present, or return, after a week of increasing difficulty, looking grey faced and weary.

The patient often asks for an X-ray. If the injury is not complicated by a severe or dangerous mechanism, the possibility of injury to the organs or medical factors, then the findings on an X-ray film would not influence management. The usual practice is to treat the patient on clinical grounds alone. However, X-ray examination *is* indicated in some cases, and each patient must be assessed fully.

History

Patients should be asked for their occupations as a sickness certificate from the GP may be required.

The patient should be asked if there is a history of any respiratory illnesses, which may predispose to complications, of which chest infection is the most common, after a rib injury. Does the patient have any heart problems? Does the patient take oral steroids or warfarin? Does the patient smoke; if so how much?

The mechanism of injury should be established and whether pain is local to the injury. When did the injury happen? If the injury is days old, why has the patient come now? The patient may be needing help with pain control or may be developing a chest infection. Has the pain changed in location, severity or nature, or in the factors which bring it on? (A patient can have severe pain even though the injury is not complicated.) Does the pain feel as if it is on the surface, or deep, and does it radiate to neck or arm? Is the patient short of breath, as opposed to having pain when breathing deeply? Has the patient coughed or vomited blood? Does the patient feel unwell in any way: sick, dizzy or faint? Does the patient have any symptoms in the abdomen? Is there blood in the urine?

Examination

ABC: airway, breathing and circulation

The examiner needs to look carefully for any sign of a major trauma or illness. ABC describes the basic tenets of checking the **airway**, **breathing** and **circulation**.

Record the patient's vital signs. Look for any systemic signs of lung injury, internal bleeding or chest infection. If the clinic has a pulse oximeter, record the oxygen saturation. If the lower region of the ribs is involved, perform a urinalysis.

Listen to the patient's chest with a stethoscope for equal air entry to all lung fields, and any wheeze or moisture.

Look at the movement of the chest. Is there asymmetry? Are the ribs in the painful area moving with the others?

Stress the ribcage. If the injury is to the lateral part of a rib, compress the cage between your hands, placed over the sternum and the spine. If the injury is to front or back, press the ribs towards the midline, with hands placed at each side. This should elicit pain if there is a fracture.

Palpate the painful area for tenderness, the crepitus of broken ends of bone. If the injury is to the costrochondral junction, tenderness will be felt at the junction of rib to cartilage. Palpate the sternum. A fracture to the sternum may contuse the myocardium. Palpate the spine. An injury would be most likely at the transverse process of a vertebra. Palpate the abdomen and lumbar region. If the patient is tender or the abdomen is rigid, a doctor should exclude injury to liver, spleen or kidneys. The spleen is tucked under the costal margin on the left, and the liver on the right. The kidneys are in the lumbar region.

Radiography

Local policies will lay down protocols or guidelines. These may simply require referral of any patient with a complication to a doctor, or it may be that the NP will be able to request a chest X-ray for those patients as long as a doctor looks at the X-ray film.

X-ray examination will normally be requested if a patient fits the following criteria.

- The mechanism has been severe, including falls from a height, road traffic accidents and injury involving great weight and force, such as may happen with industrial machinery.
- The patient seems to have a multiple rib fracture, or a severe osteochondral separation. Fractures to the first three ribs tend to be the result of a severe injury, and underlying complications are likely, especially injury to nerves and large blood vessels.
- There is any suggestion that the spine is injured.
- There is a possible fracture of the sternum.
- There is any suggestion of a haemo- or pneumothorax, or contusion of the lung.
- There is a history of respiratory illness, or the appearance of respiratory complications.
  A patient would not necessarily have an X-ray because there seemed to be a chest infection. If the patient has no long-standing medical problems, it may be most appropriate to refer to the GP.
- The patient is elderly.

Treatment

Rib injuries are not strapped.

The patient will need pain killers. Ibuprofen is often the drug of choice if the patient has no gastric or renal problems and does not suffer from asthma. Pain is a problem for rib-injured patients, and a NP may see someone who has already tried everything that the minor injury clinic can offer. These patients should be referred to their GPs.

The patient should be told to incorporate several sessions of deep breathing and forced coughing into the routine of pain relief. The injured site is supported with the hands while the patient inhales deeply and breathes out slowly; this is repeated several times, and then the patient should cough. This procedure is repeated six times per day; it will hurt, but it helps to avoid a chest infection. Smoking should be kept to the minimum.

The first 1 or 2 weeks will be the most painful. The patient may have to take time off work and will certainly not be fit for heavy exertion for possibly 6 to 8 weeks. The GP can issue sickness certificates.

The patient who has a discoloured sputum or is feverish should see the GP. However, if the patient develops haemoptysis they should go to A&E.

The Lower Back

Pain in the lower back is rather like the common cold, universal but poorly understood and a source of frustration and misunderstanding between health professionals and patients. This section focuses on the distinctions between emergencies where back pain is a symptom, serious and less-serious neurological presentations, and so-called simple or mechanical back pain. Current guidelines for the treatment of back pain are discussed.

Patients who present with abdominal pain will usually require referral to a doctor. Genuine minor injury presentations with abdominal pain as a main symptom are unusual.

Anatomy of the lumbar spine

The general structure of vertebrae, the arrangement of spinal ligaments and the way in which spinal nerves emerge from the vertebral column has been discussed in Chapter 6. Articulation between the lumbar vertebrae occurs in the same manner as in the higher vertebrae:

- between intervertebral discs and vertebral bodies
- between two facet joints on the inferior aspect of the upper vertebra, and two facet joints on the superior aspect of the one below.

There are five lumbar vertebrae (Fig. 7.1); these are chiefly distinguished from the higher vertebrae by their adaptation for weight bearing. They are large, and their facet joints are directed so that they limit rotation at the lumbar spine (most of the rotation which can be achieved in the trunk occurs in the thoracic spine) for the sake of stability (Box 7.1).

The spinal cord is shorter than the vertebral canal and ends at the level of the first lumbar

Box 7.1 Lumbar Spine Statistics

Capsular pattern equal restriction of side-flexion and rotation, and a lesser degree of loss of extension.

Joint positions close packed is full extension, when the facets meet; loose packed is halfway between flexion and extension.

Flexion up to 60°; end feel is firm, ligament and facet joint capsules.

Extension up to 35°; end feel firm; the posterior bony surfaces meet and the anterior disc, ligaments and muscles are stretched.

Rotation up to 18°; end feel firm; movement is ended by ligaments and atricular processes.

Side-flexion up to 20°; end feel is firm, restricted by the ribs (the facet joints coming together) and stretching of the joint capsules.

vertebra. From there, the nerves, which pass out through the intervertebral foramina of the various lumbar vertebrae, pass down the canal to their exit points as a collection of long strands, called the **cauda equina** (horse's tail).

The ventral nerves from L1 to S4 supply the leg. As at the neck (see the **brachial plexus**; Fig. 6.4), these nerves form networks which permit the exchange of fibres between nerves emerging from the spinal cord and forming peripheral nerves in the limb. There are two networks which are relevant here: the **lumbar plexus** and the **lumbosacral plexus** (Fig. 7.3 and 7.4).

The lumbar vertebrae rest upon, and articulate at L5, with the superior surface of the **sacrum**, a wedge of bone which links the two posterior segments of the pelvis at the **sacro-iliac joints**. The sacrum is the superficial bony surface which can be felt in the midline of the buttocks, just above the cleft. It is considered as a single unit, but it actually comprises five fused vertebrae. It combines three roles. It is the base upon which the vertebral column is stacked, it is the link between the spine and the pelvis, and it is one of the unifying elements between the two halves of the pelvic girdle.

The vertebral canal continues down into the sacrum as the **sacral canal**. On the front surface of the sacrum, there are four **transverse lines**, which mark the fusion of the sacral vertebrae; there are holes at each end of these ridges, **sacral foramina**, which allow the passage of nerves and blood vessels. On the dorsal, convex surface of the sacrum, there is a raised,

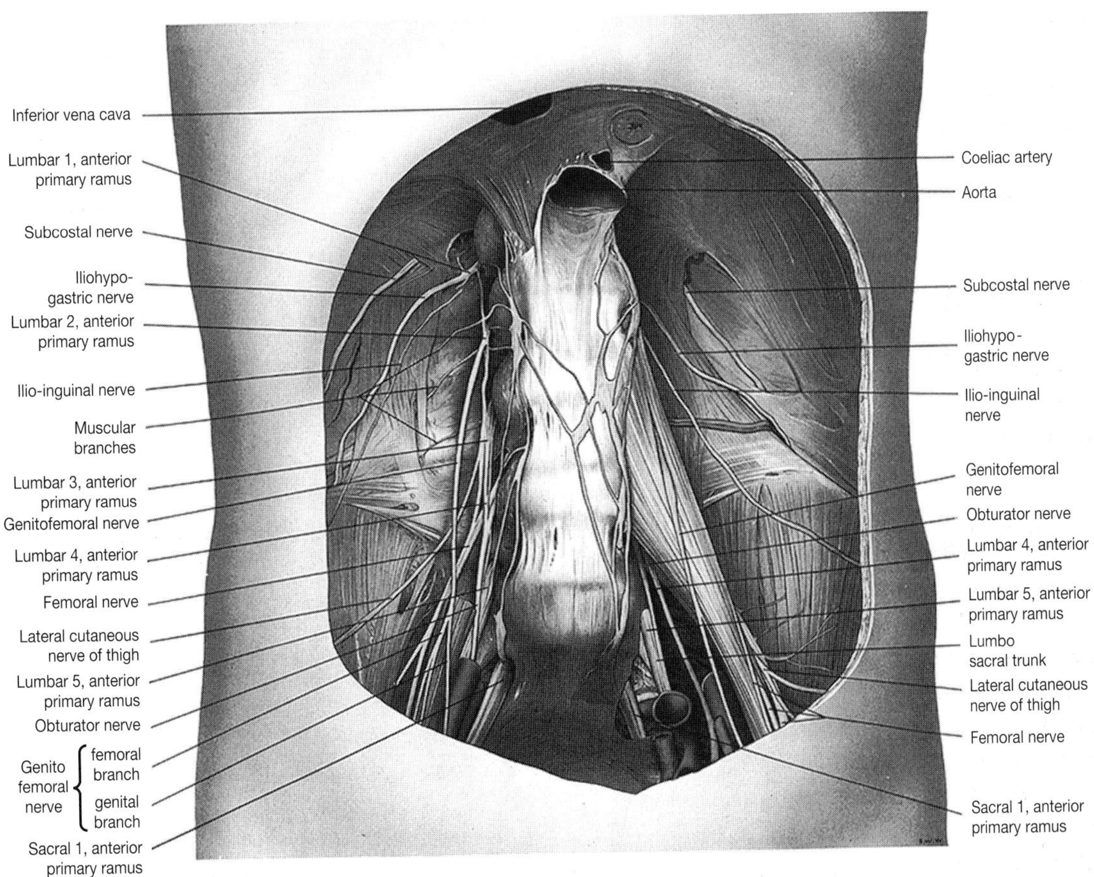

Figure 7.3 The lumbar plexus and sympathetic trunks. In this dissection, the right psoas major has been removed. (Adapted with kind permission from Williams, 1995)

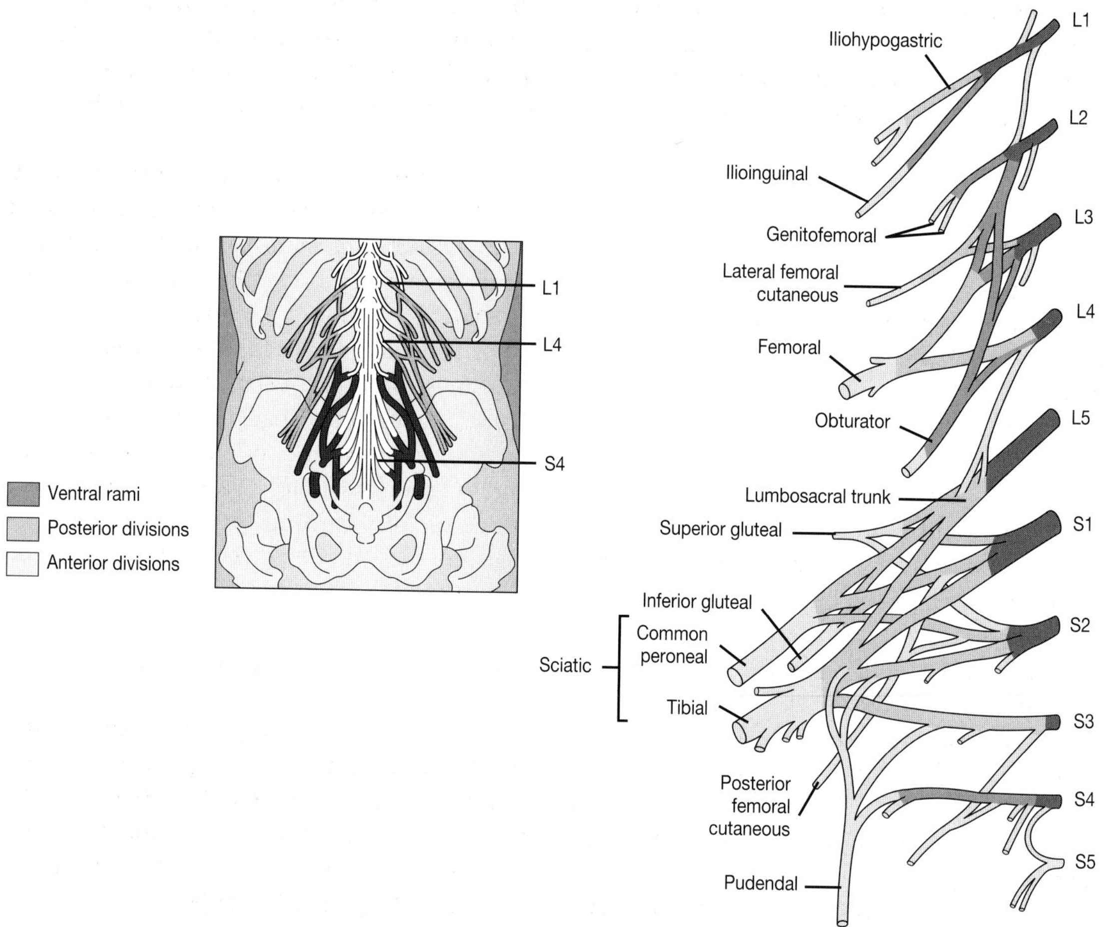

Figure 7.4 The lumbosacral plexus. (Reproduced with kind permission from Thibodeau and Patton, 1999.)

vertical ridge in the midline; this is the vestige of the spinous processes and is called the **median sacral crest**. The ridge is incomplete. The fourth and fifth spinous processes are absent, and, at that part of the midline, there is a small opening, the **sacral hiatus**, which gives access to the sacral canal at its inferior end.

The sacroiliac joints are synovial joints, only slightly moveable, between the sacrum on each side and the articular surfaces of the ilium on each side. These joints close the ring of the pelvis at the back. They are reinforced by interosseus ligaments at the back and front. The posterior ligaments may be torn by injury during the movement of bending forward at the waist.

The sacrum has a small bony tail, the **coccyx**, made of four or five more vertebrae, also fused. The coccyx has no distinct function. It is palpable as a rough, superficial bony surface, just above the anus.

The Patient with Back Pain

Back pain is widely recognized, in the nursing profession as much as anywhere else, as a problem of serious and increasing significance for sufferers, their families and for society at large. In the UK, the number of days lost at work because of back pain has increased from 15 million in 1970 to 106 million in 1994 (Burn,

2000). Many people who suffer from chronic back pain give up their work for good, which is a drain on the health and social security systems and a cause of misery for the individuals and their families.

Triage

It is important that two emergencies are excluded in patients with back pain: lumbar prolapse, which threatens the nerve supply to bladder and bowel, and an abdominal aortic aneurysm.

The patient with a disc prolapse compressing the spinal cord at L1, or the cauda equina in the lower lumbar region, may suffer irreversible damage, and magnetic resonance imaging MRI is the most useful investigation to exclude that diagnosis. The patient may complain of bilateral leg pain (most commonly radiating down the backs of the thighs), paraesthesia and weakness, perianal paraesthesia (in the so-called **saddle area**), a loss of tone of the rectal sphincter, and, possibly, a loss of bowel control or retention of urine. The patient may need emergency surgery (an assessment that would be made by a neurosurgical or an orthopaedic specialist, depending on local arrangements).

A patient with an abdominal aortic aneurysm may present with back pain, which will not be in the pattern of musculoskeletal injury. It will be constant and probably worsening, not improved by a change in position, no better at night. It may radiate into the groin and thigh. There may be a swelling in the abdomen, the classic **pulsatile mass**. This condition is most common in men in later middle age. If this diagnosis is suspected, the patient should be referred as an emergency. The aneurysm may rupture at any time, even if the patient seems well at the moment.

If a patient has suffered a violent mechanism of injury, such as a road traffic accident or a fall from a height, he will need a full assessment at an A&E department. The patient may have rupture of internal organs, with heavy bleeding or spinal, pelvic or hip injuries. Assess (and constantly reassess) in terms of resuscitation and ABC; the patient may require spinal board immobilization and emergency ambulance transfer.

There are other medical problems, including neoplasm, osteomyelitis, osteoarthritis and infections of the genitourinary and gastric tracts, which may cause the patient to present with back pain. There will be no history of injury, the pattern of pain will not be musculoskeletal, and there may be other systemic signs, such as a raised temperature. The patient may have a history of previous cancer, of recent weight loss or may feel generally unwell. The older patient should be considered as a higher risk.

In any case where there is doubt, refer the patient.

Common patterns of back pain

For all that the problem is common and increasing, the causes of, and predisposing factors for, back pain are not well understood. The guidelines which are current for the treatment of patients with back pain do not concentrate on precise diagnosis. The objective is to recognize patterns of presentation, and patterns of outcome, and to make a correct assessment of the *type* of problem, so that the patient is guided along the path which appears, from other patients' experience, to offer the best hope of recovery.

The urgent and serious conditions have been discussed above. Among the less serious, more common presentations, there are two large categories:

- main symptom is pain radiating down one leg
- main symptom is pain in the lower back with no significant radiation to the leg.

The first of these is less common than the second (less than 5% of all patients with back pain according to Burn, 2000). The pain which is referred down the leg because of pressure on a nerve root will follow a dermatomal pattern and will be triggered or increased by a specific test for stretching the nerve (the **sciatic** stretch (Fig. 7.5)).

The second major category of back pain sufferers includes patients who may have pain which radiates to the upper part of the leg (not below the thigh), in a non-dermatomal pattern; this pain does not have a neurological origin. This largest group by far suffer from **simple** or **mechanical** back pain. The pain is triggered by lifting or bending, and there may be either a sudden severe pain or a gradual onset. If the patient experiences muscle spasm at the time of the injury, the back may 'lock' in lumbar flexion. The pain may be felt on one or both sides of the lower back. There may be radiation of pain to the upper part of the leg but not to the foot. The pain will have a musculoskeletal pattern, being aggravated by physical activity and relieved by rest, especially by lying down.

Examination

History

'Simple back pain' is a broad diagnosis, partly arrived at by a process of elimination. The history plays a large part. The patient's age, gender, occupation and general lifestyle will have great bearing on the possible diagnoses and the priorities of treatment.

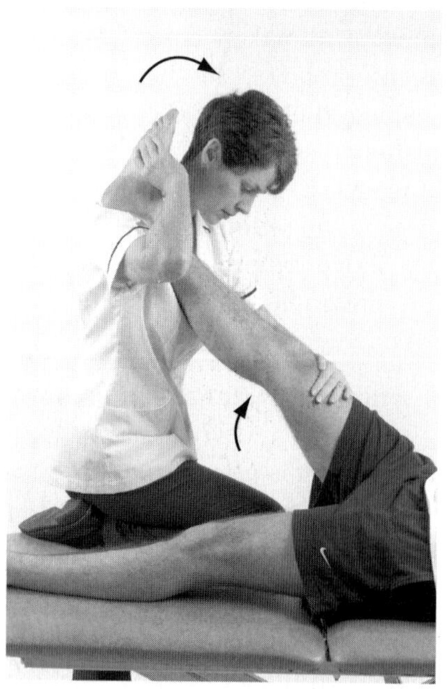

Figure 7.5 **The sciatic nerve stretch test.**

Establish a mechanism of injury. There may not have been a severe force, but the patient will probably recall a recent exertion or may say that the pain began while bending forward. In most cases, there will be some pain at the moment of injury, even if it does not become troublesome until later.

Assess the pattern of pain, its relationship to movement, relieving and aggravating factors, the effects of the pain on sleep, whether it is worse in the morning. Coughing tends to aggravate the pain caused by a lumbar disc prolapse.

Ask about severity of the pain, and whether or not it developed suddenly. Ask where the pain is felt, and whether there is radiation of the pain. If there is pain in the leg, ask if it is more severe than the back pain, which tends to be the case with sciatic pain, and map its pathway on the leg. Ask if there is numbness or tingling.

Ask if the patient feels well, apart from the back pain. Ask about any other symptoms: chest pain, abdominal pain, bilateral leg pain, any weakness or paraesthesia, coordination problems, change in bowel or bladder habit.

Obtain a full medical history, incuding medications and allergies; ask if the patient is taking steroids. Has the patient any history of arthritic disease. Has the patient had any surgery.

Refer the patient to a GP if there are any atypical features, if the patient is describing severe symptoms, or if the history suggest an illness rather than a simple injury.

Look

The patient's ability to stand up and sit, the pattern of walking, the posture and the ability to perform simple tasks, such as tying shoelaces, will give an impression of the pattern of disability and the severity of symptoms. Is the patient limping? The pain and the fatigue which simple back pain causes can be considerable.

Box Sciatic stretch test

A passive straight leg raised above 75° will cause pain and paraesthesia in the leg if there is a disc protrusion at L4 to S1.

To ensure that pain is caused by sciatic nerve, and not hamstring stretch, lower leg slightly until pain stops, then dorsiflex the foot.

The test is positive if the pain returns.

Ask the patient to undress and observe the back and the legs. The patient may have a scoliosis, a lateral curvature of the spine. Scoliosis may exist for different reasons, such as the need to compensate for the angled pelvis which results from having unequal leg lengths, but it may be an acute response, an attempt to relieve the pressure on a compressed nerve root. Look at the pelvis. Is it tilted? You may assess this by checking the levels of the posterior superior iliac spines.

It may be possible to see, on one side of the lumbar spine, the contracted mass of erector muscles of the spine in spasm.

Feel

The lumbar spine is best palpated with the patient prone on a couch. The spinous processes are easy to feel, but the transverse processes may be fairly deep in the erector muscle bulk. Muscle which is in spasm should be both visible and palpable.

Move

Active movement in the back is assessed as:

- the range of movement
- the rhythm of movement
- whether or not there is pain on movement.

The lumbar spine should be tested in flexion, extension and rotation (Figs 7.6–7.8). The sciatic nerve stretch test should also be performed (Fig. 7.5). The straight leg raising test is the most valuable, because it stresses the nerves and their roots from L4 to S1, which are the most likely to suffer the effects of a disc prolapse.

Sensation in the legs is assessed and any deficit mapped. Motor power in the legs can be assessed, using resisted tests

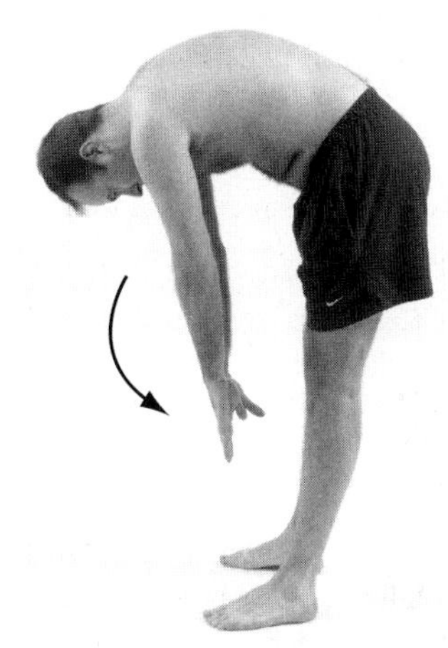

Figure 7.6 Flexion at the waist.

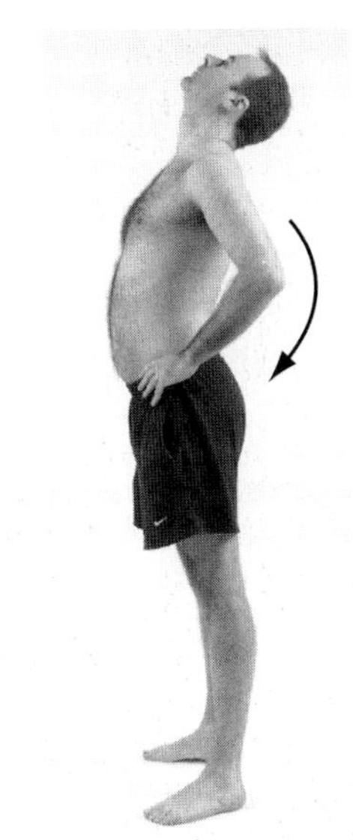

Figure 7.7 Extension at the waist.

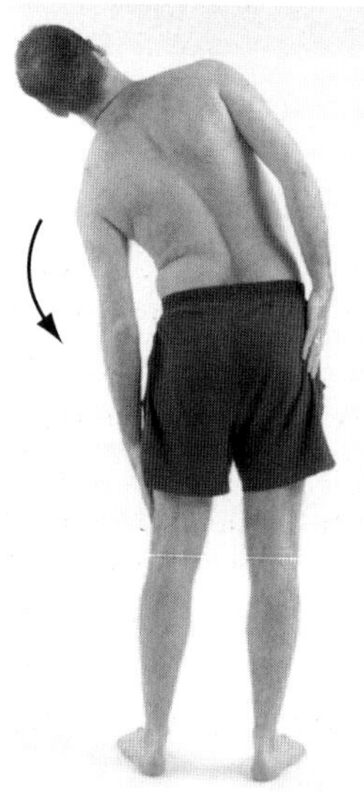

Figure 7.8 **Side flexion at the waist.**

(illustrated in later sections covering joints of the leg) for the following muscles:

L2: hip flexion (iliopsoas; see Fig. 7.10, below)
L3: knee extension (quadriceps; see Fig. 7.20, below)
L4: ankle dorsiflexion and inversion (tibialis anterior; see Fig. 7.30, below)
L5: big toe extension: the patient is asked to dorsiflex the foot and extend the big toe while resistance is offered on the dorsal side of the foot in the direction of flexion of the big toe
S1: ankle plantarflexion (gastrocnemius; see Fig. 7.29, below)
S2: toe flexion (flexors digitorum and hallucis longus): the patient is asked to flex the toes and apply resistance on the plantar side of the foot, in the direction of extension.

Treatment

Patients are referred to a GP if they will need more help with analgesia than can be given in the minor injury clinic. Simple back pain can cause severe pain.

Patients who have sciatic pain should be referred to GPs. The problem may not be quick to settle, adequate pain relief will be needed and, in a few cases, the patient may need orthopaedic treatment.

Current thinking on the treatment of simple back pain, embodied in reports by the Clinical Standards Advisory Group (1994) and the Royal College of General Practitioners (1996), emphasizes two priorities: remain mobile and stay at work. The GP is seen as the lynchpin of management of the condition. Bedrest should be kept to a minimum (ideally, not more than 2 days while the pain is too severe for any other course), except in the case where the pain arises from nerve root problems. Physiotherapists, chiropractors and other specialists in manipulation should be involved if the problem does not settle within a few days. The management of patients with sciatic pain should differ in the length of time spent in bed (up to 2 weeks), but in other ways, the principles are the same as for simple back pain. The patient should move on to a programme of active exercise as soon as possible and should stay at work if possible.

There is a large role for health promotion for patients with back pain. The condition can be recurrent, disabling and depressing. Subjects such as safe lifting, the value of exercise in preventing injuries and in helping recovery are very important.

Box **Hip assessment**

The Nurse Practitioner should be able to assess the hip through its full range of movement, and discriminate between musculoskeletal conditions and other problems.

Palpate and ask the patient to show movement in the lumbar spine (see Figs 7.6–7.8).

The movements of the hip are illustrated.

PASSIVE movements are not shown: they are performed in the same positions as the ACTIVE range, except that the rotations will be performed using only one leg at a time.

The Hip

Anatomy

The **pelvic girdle** relates to the leg as the shoulder girdle does to the arm (Fig. 7.9). The pelvis is also a bilateral and symmetrical structure which connects limb to trunk. It has articular sockets for the heads of the femur. The hip joints are synovial capsules with ligament and muscle reinforcement.

There are, however, significant differences between the pelvic and shoulder girdles. The bones of the pelvic girdle are much more rigid in their unity and correspondingly less mobile. They meet in the midline of the body at the front and form a complete bony ring by articulating at the back, at the slightly moveable **sacroiliac joints**, with the sacrum. Through this articulation, the pelvis is in direct contact with the vertebral column. The upper part of

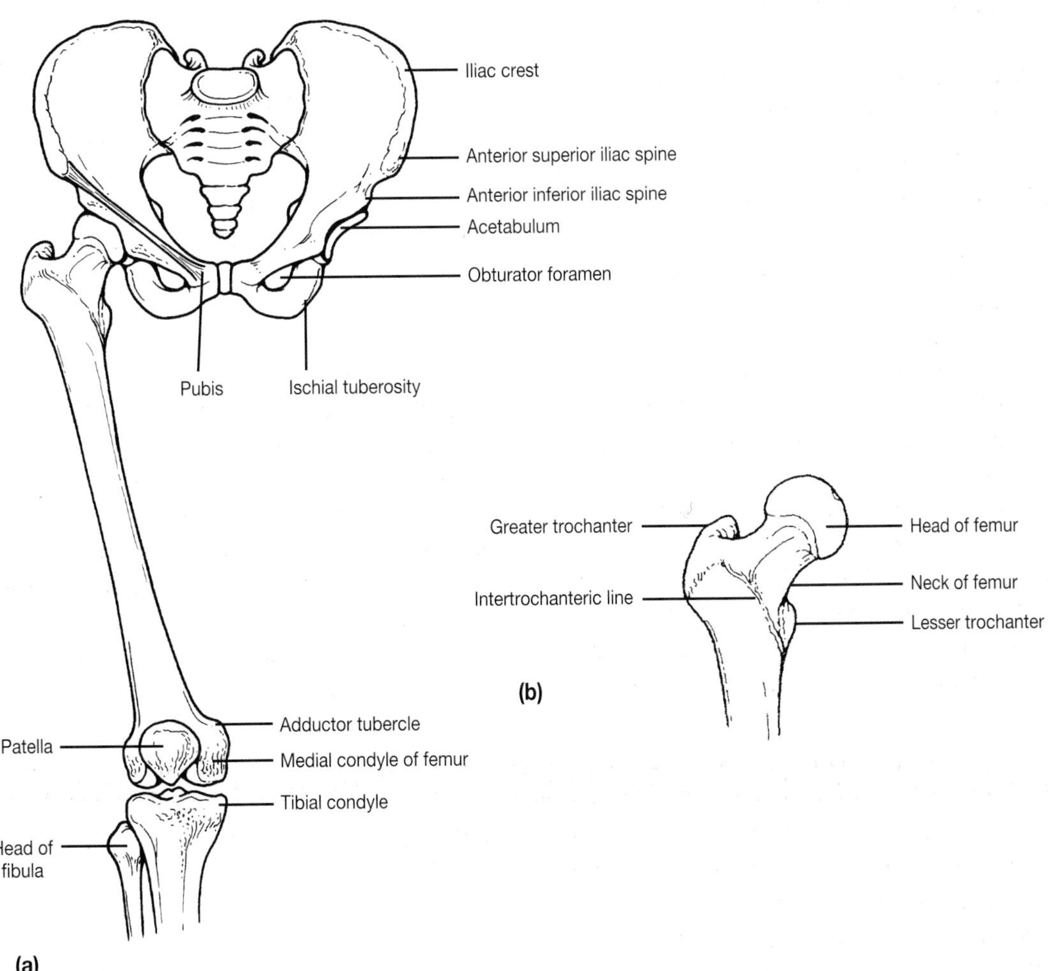

Figure 7.9 The pelvic girdle and femur, anterior view, and the proximal femur, anterior view. (Reproduced with kind permission from Dean and Pegington, 1996.)

the pelvis forms a kind of abdominal basin, holding organs of the gastrointestinal, reproductive and urological systems. The lower part forms a channel, the pelvic canal, through which these organs have outlets for their external functions.

The **hip joint** itself reflects the major difference in the functions of arm and leg. Both limbs are concerned with movement. The arm places the hand in space. The leg carries the weight of the whole body through space and also, in coordination with the upper body stabilizes the body both at rest (especially when standing) and in motion. The hip joint is, consequently, larger and much more stable in its deep ball-and-socket structure. It permits a smaller range of movement, with a greater emphasis on basic flexion and extension, than the shoulder joint. The bones and muscles of the leg are larger than those of the arm, adapted for weight bearing and power rather than fine movement. The hips are closer together than the shoulders. The legs are central pillars that meet in the midline of the body while the shoulders are widely spaced so that the arms are lateral appendages.

The pelvic girdle is an assembly of three pairs of closely united bones: the **ilium**, the **ischium** and the **pubis**, combined with the **sacrum**. The ilium, ischium and pubis are collectively named the **innominate** (nameless) **bone**. The innominate, seen from the front, looks slightly like a human ear, with the iliac crest as the upper ridge, the helix, and the arches of pubis and ischium as the lobe. The place where the three bones of the innominate meet and fuse is called the **acetabulum**. The acetabulum is the socket which articulates with the **head of the femur** to form the hip joint.

Ilium

The ilium is the upper pelvic bone, an expanded, cupped dish. It meets the sacrum on its medial border with the pubis below to the front and the ischium below to the back. Its main inner surface, called the **iliac fossa**, forms the pelvic basin, which supports the abdomen. Behind the fossa, the ilium articulates on its inner, medial surface with the sacrum and offers attachment for the sacroiliac ligaments. It has a semicircular **iliac crest** as its upper border, which passes from front to back and can be felt, and usually seen, just below waist level. The crest ends in two prominences, one at the front and the other at the back: the **anterior superior iliac spine** and the **posterior superior iliac spine**, respectively. Below each of these spines, both of which are palpable, lie lower, deeper spines separated from the upper ones by a notch. These are the **anterior inferior iliac spine** and the **posterior inferior iliac spine**. The acetabulum, of which the ilium forms the upper section, is found on the outer face of the ilium, at the lowest part of the bone.

Pubic bones

The two pubic bones meet in the midline at the front, at the angle where the abdomen ends and the genitals emerge, at a non-synovial, cartilaginous joint called the **symphysis pubis**. From here, each pubic bone divides into two fingers of bone, both of which travel backwards and outwards. The upper one, the **superior ramus** (meaning upper branch), fuses with the ilium and ischium at the acetabulum. The lower branch, the **inferior ramus**, fuses with the ischium at the **ischial ramus**.

Ischial bones

The two ischial bones form the lower, rear part of the pelvis. They do not meet in the midline like the pubic bones. The space between them is part of the canal of the pelvis. The circle of the pelvic girdle is only closed at a higher point at the rear, at the sacroiliac joints. The lowest and most posterior part of the ischium, the **ischial tuberosity** (the bone in the buttock which contacts the chair when sitting), is angled in a similar way to the pubis, travelling upwards to its fusion at the acetabulum and inwards and forward as the ischial ramus, to the inferior pubic ramus. An irregular oval area called the **obturator foramen** (a foramen is a passage, usually a channel through a bony structure) is enclosed by the ischial–pubic ramus below and the meeting of the ischium and pubis at the acetabulum above.

Femur

The femur is the thigh bone. It is the longest bone in the body. At its proximal end, it forms the ball of the ball-and-socket hip joint. In comparison with the humerus, it has a more completely spherical **head** and a much longer **neck**. The head is covered in hyaline cartilage and has a small hole on its medial surface through which it is connected to a ligament inside the acetabulum. The neck is angled upwards towards the pelvis, at approximately 125 degrees from the shaft of the femur. The shaft expands at the point of union with the neck, with two processes on its lateral and medial sides. The large, lateral one is the **greater trochanter** and the medial one, under the angle of the neck, is the **lesser trochanter** (Fig. 7.9).

Ligaments

There are three stabilizing ligaments, which are of special importance at the hip because they limit extension and help to maintain the upright position with a minimum of muscle effort. These are the **iliofemoral**, the **pubofemoral** and the **ischiofemoral ligaments**. Of these, the iliofemoral or Y ligament is the strongest and most significant in the limiting of extension. It lies in front of the joint and runs from the anterior inferior iliac spine to the intertrochanteric line of the femur.

Examination

Figures 7.10–7.15 illustrate the relevant muscular anatomy of the hip for different hip motions and the methods of testing for these functions.

Hip pain and injury

Patients who present complaining of pain at the hip should be assessed with particular care, especially if they do not have a history of injury. The joint is large and stable and, from the point of view of the nurse in a minor injury clinic, is relatively uneventful. Complaints of injury are much more common at the other limb joints. The injury which is probably the most common at the hip in an older or frail adult, a femoral neck fracture after a fall, will not be seen often in a minor injury area.

Trauma violent enough to produce fracture or dislocation at the hip in a young person, at work or in sport, would disable the patient

Box 7.2 Hip Statistics

Capsular pattern equal loss in flexion, abduction and internal rotation.
Joint position loose packed is 30° flexion, 30° abduction and a small degree of external rotation; close packed is full extension and internal rotation, with a small element of abduction.
Flexion 0–120°; end feel tissue approximation of thigh and abdominal muscles.
Extension 0–30°; end feel firm, stretch of capsule, ligaments and muscles.
Abduction 0–45°; end feel firm, stretch of capsule, ligament and muscle.
Adduction 0–30°; end feel firm, stretch of abductor muscles.
Lateral rotation 0–45°; end feel firm, stretch of capsule, ligaments and muscles.
Medial rotation 0–45°; end feel firm, stretch of capsule, ligaments and muscles.

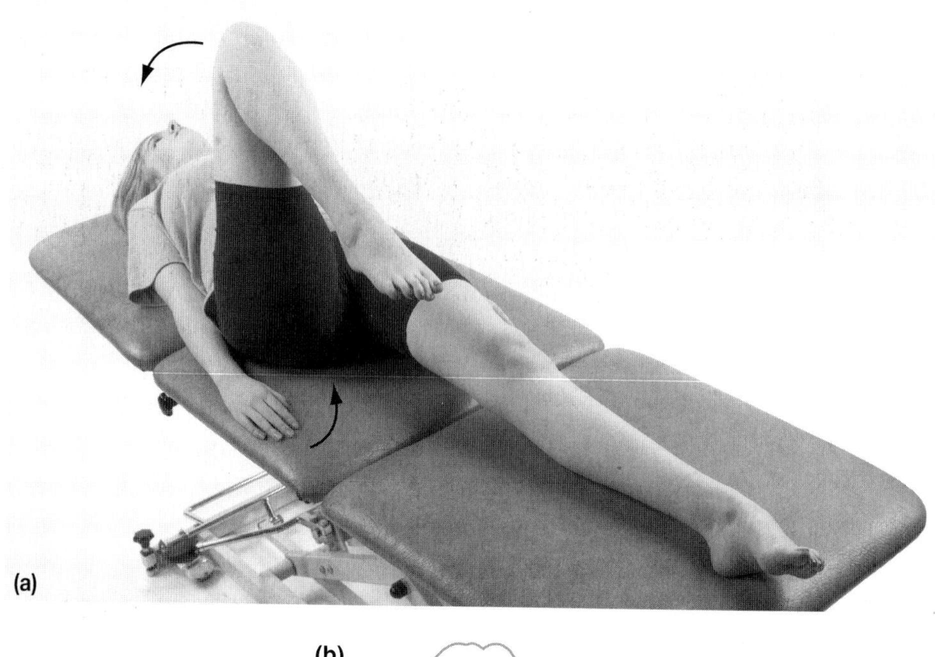

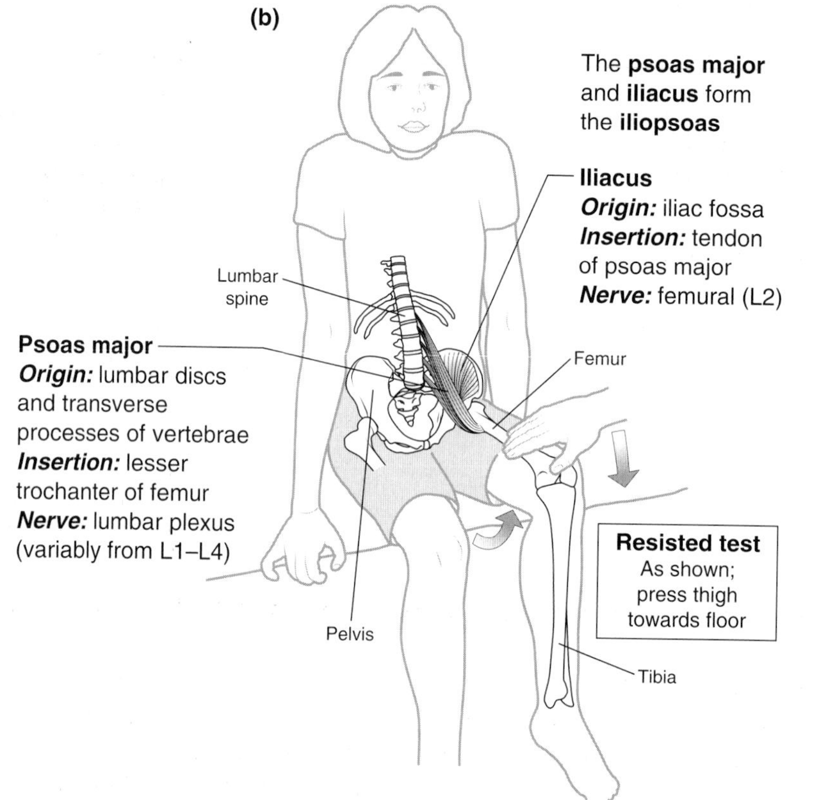

Figure 7.10 **(a) Active flexion of the hip. (b) Resisted flexion of the hip, showing the flexor muscles.**

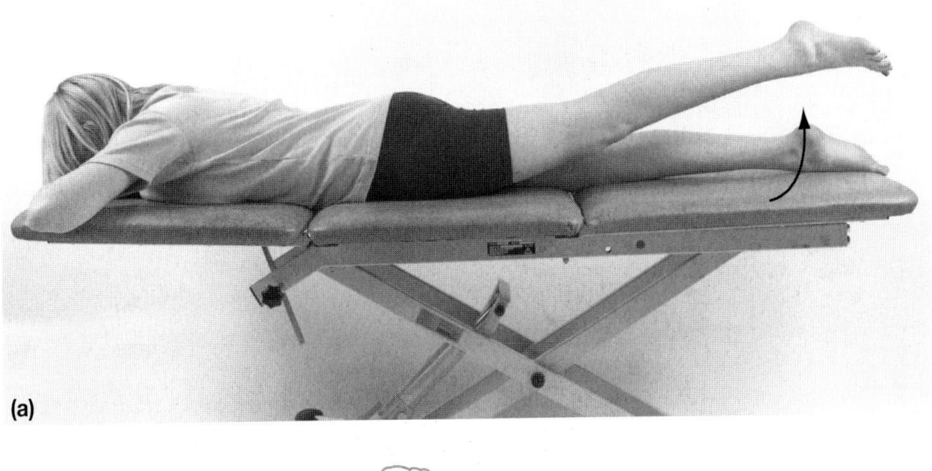

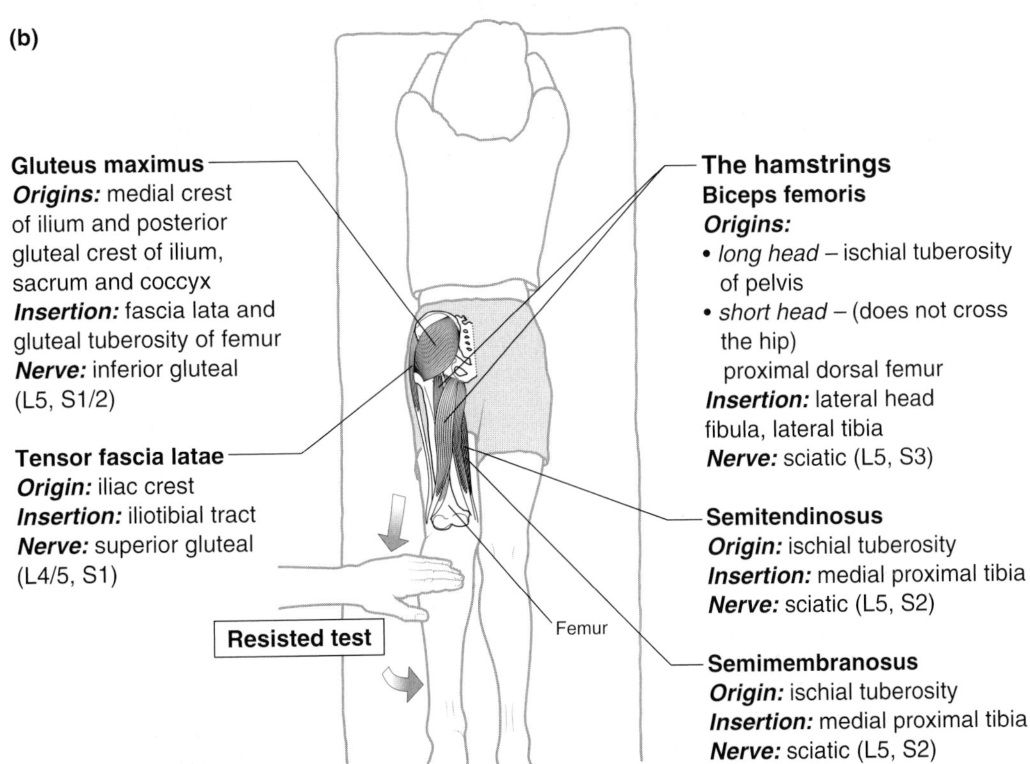

Figure 7.11 (a) Active extension of the hip. (b) Resisted extension of the hip showing extensor muscles.

and cause considerable pain and shock. An ambulance would almost certainly be called, and the patient transferred to a major trauma team.

The close relationship between the pelvis and the abdominal organs and the spine means that there are several local suspects as the source of any unexplained pain, and illness and referral from a lumbar spine problem must be excluded. As well as diseases of the main organs, symptoms can arise from problems such as hernias, especially inguinal and femoral, and various kinds of abscesses, fistulae and sinuses.

Children with painful hips (or painful knees, which may be caused by referral from the hip), a limp or a reluctance or inability to weight-bear should be referred for medical assessment.

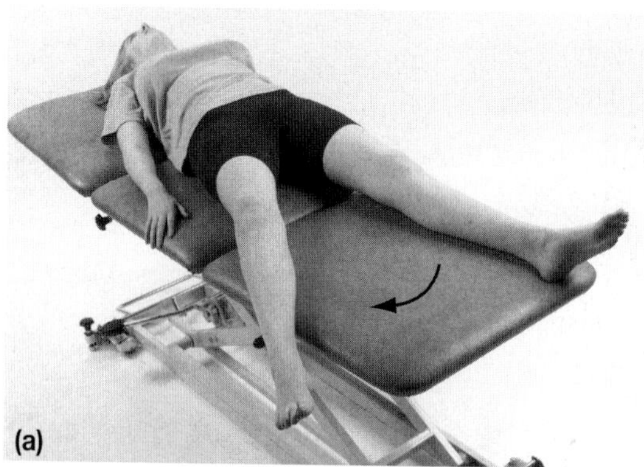

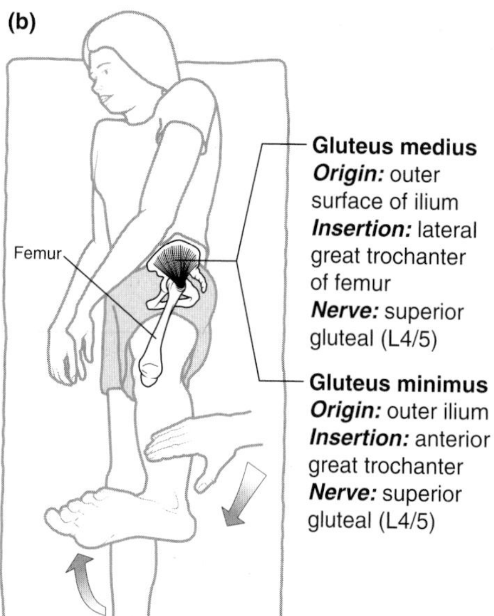

Figure 7.12 (a) Active abduction of the hip. (b) Resisted abduction of the hip showing the abductor muscles.

Possible diagnoses include a transient irritable hip in those under 7 years of age, Perthes' disease (an avascular necrosis of the epiphysis of the head of the femur) in those under 10 years and slipped femoral epiphysis in adolescent patients. Osteomyelitis and joint infection can also occur.

In sporty adolescents, especially after a growth spurt when the strength of bone has not kept pace with the development of muscle power, muscles around the hip may avulse bone at one of their insertion points. This can happen, for example, at a hamstring origin at the ischial tuberosity, at the origin of the rectus femoris (a quadriceps muscle) at the anterior inferior iliac spine and at the femoral insertion of the iliopsoas, the flexor of the hip. Patients of that age who present with apparent muscle strains, especially if they are tender at the bony insertion of the muscle, need a specialist assessment and X-ray. Be suspicious if a young patient with an apparent muscle strain presents late because he or she is not recovering.

Muscle strains at the hip

Any muscle can suffer injury but, at the hip, certain muscles are particularly prone to injury by inflammation, caused by overuse, and by strain and complete rupture, especially in the sportsman.

In the case of overuse, the pain follows the inflammation pattern of settling once activity is underway but returning after a rest; the pain gradually worsens if not treated and eventually becoming an established 'cycle of pain'. The standard treatment for acute episodes is rest, perhaps with ibuprofen if the patient can tolerate it, and the use of ice.

Muscle tears are treated by strict rest and ice in the initial phase and rehabilitation, which is dictated by the severity of the tear.

The muscles described below are the ones that are most prone, at the hip, to overload injuries. A compression force, a blow which crushes a muscle against bone, can happen at any site. In that case, the deeper muscles are most likely to suffer damage.

The adductor longus

The adductor longus brings the leg to the body from the side.

If the muscle is inflamed, there is groin pain on movement, often with tenderness at the pubic origin of the muscle, symptoms elicited by resisted adduction and passive abduction (Figs 7.12 and 7.13).

If there is a strain, a sharp pain will be felt, followed by the symptoms of muscle injury,

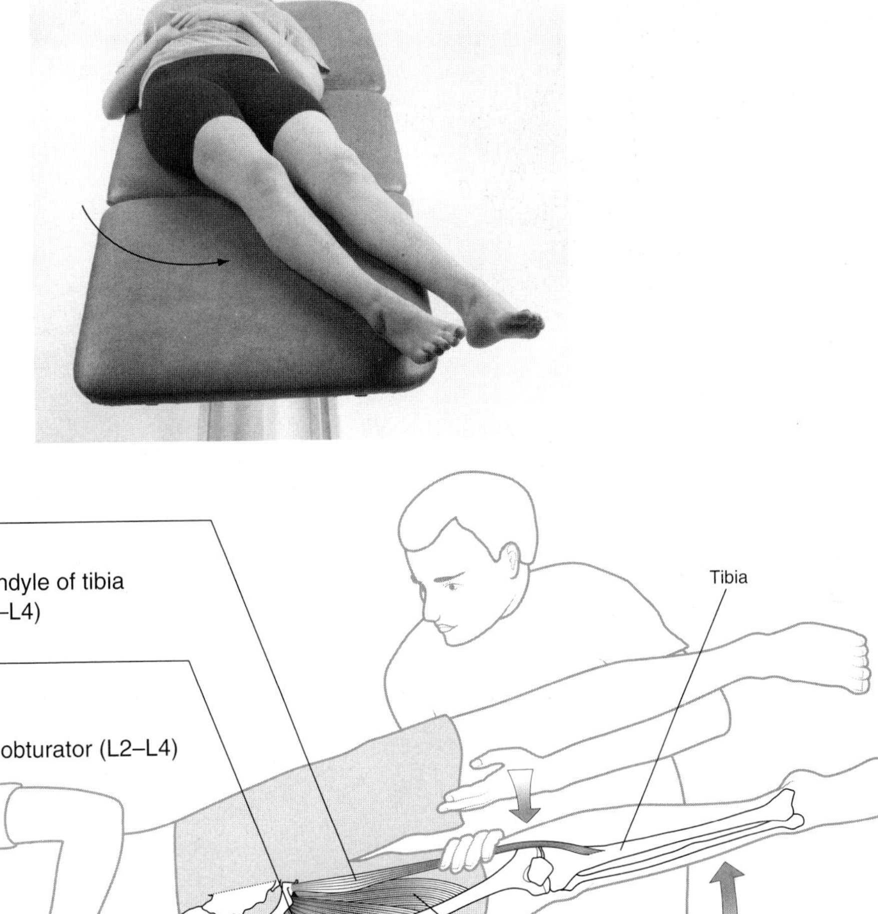

Figure 7.13 **(a) Active adduction of the hip. (This movement is sometimes shown with adducted limb crossing over the other.) (b) Resisted adduction of the hip showing muscles of adduction.**

which may be pain and/or loss of function depending on how severe the tear is. The mechanism may be a sudden block of the inside of the foot as it kicks a ball across the front of the body. There may, with complete rupture, be a palpable defect in the muscle.

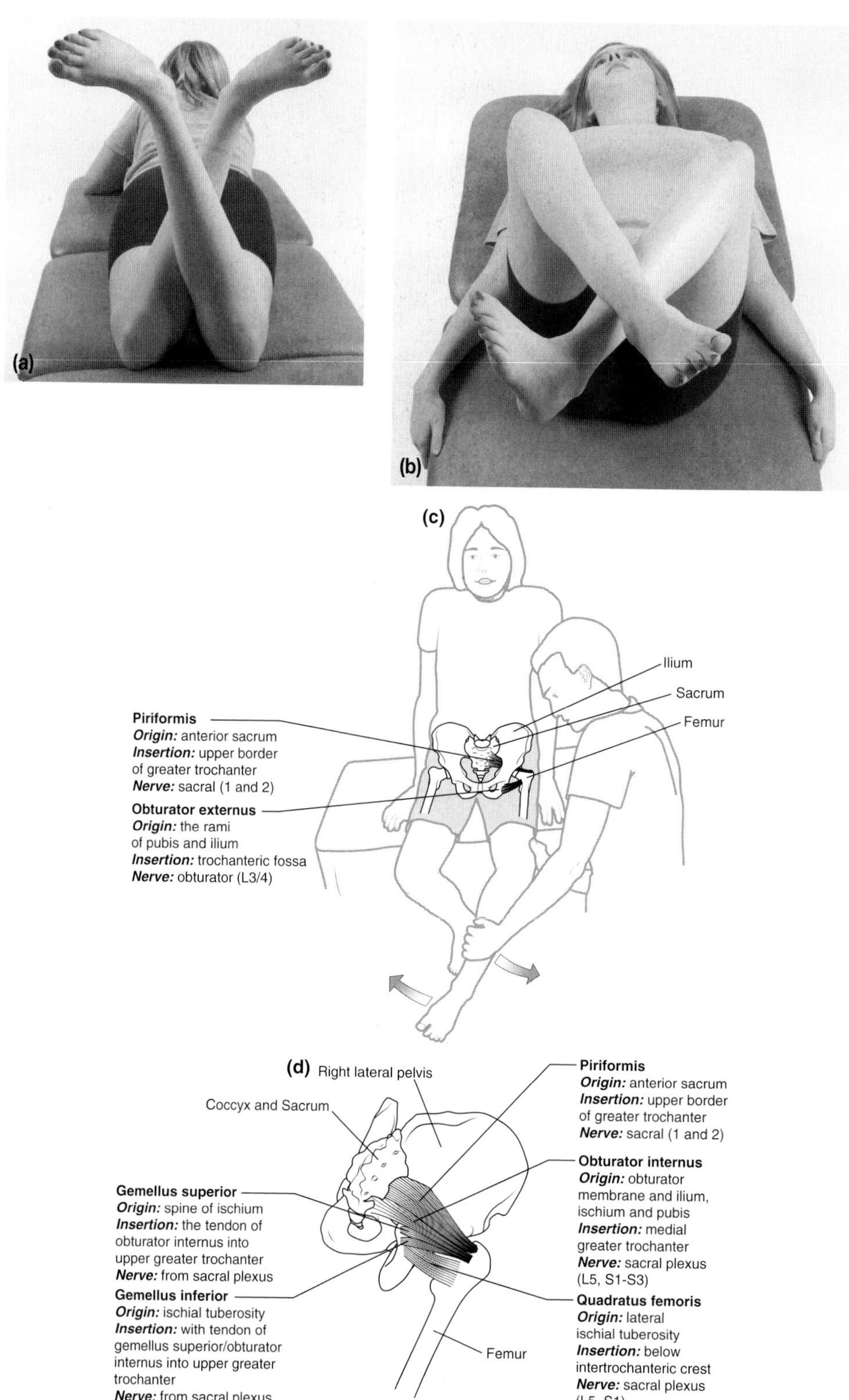

Figure 7.14 (a), (b) Active lateral rotation with hip at 0° flexion and at 90° flexion. (c) Resisted lateral rotation showing muscles of lateral rotation. (d) Muscles of lateral rotation of hip.

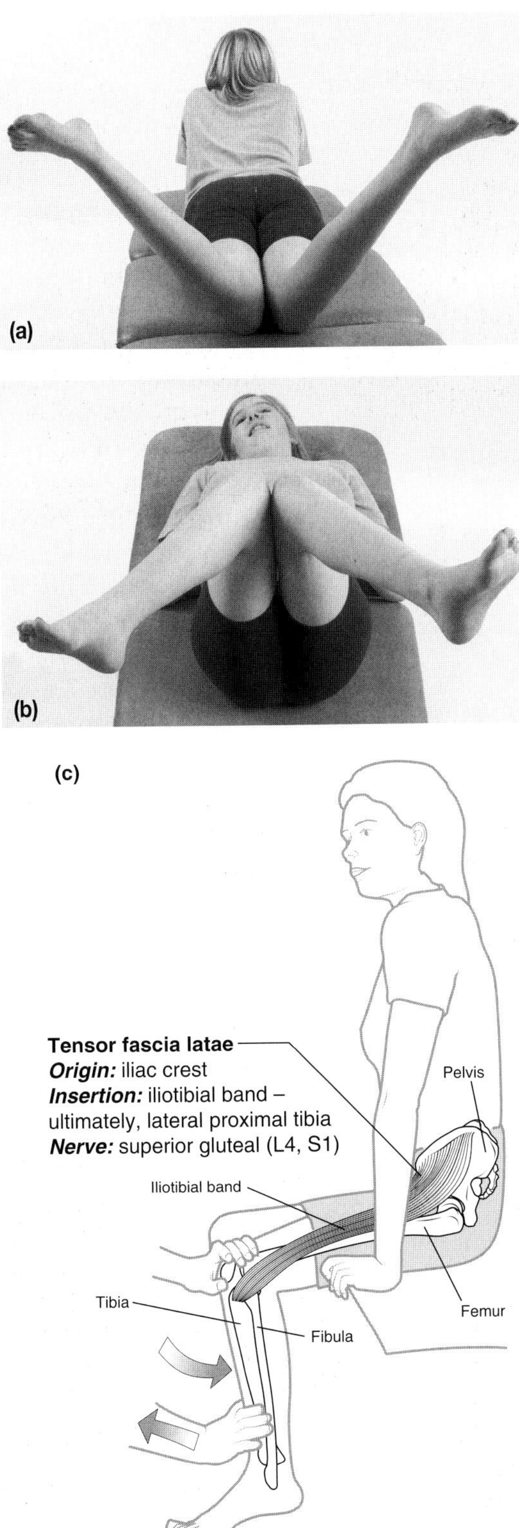

Figure 7.15 (a) Active medial rotation of hip with hip at 0° flexion. (b) Active medial rotation of hip with hip at 90° flexion. (c) Resisted medial rotation of hip showing muscles of medial rotation.

The Hip

The iliopsoas

The iliopsoas is the main flexor of the hip.

Inflammation can arise from overuse caused by any one of a variety of movements which involve raising the leg or sitting up, especially if weights are used. The pain is usually felt at the insertion of the combined tendon of the iliopsoas into the lesser trochanter of the femur. Note that there is a bursa under this tendon, and bursitis at this site would cause similar symptoms to tendon inflammation.

Strain might occur at the femoral insertion of the muscle, with pain at the time of injury, reproduced on examination by resisted hip flexion and passive stretching of the muscle with the hip in extension (Figs 7.10 and 7.11).

Piriformis syndrome

In a minority of people, the common peroneal branch of the sciatic nerve may be prone to compression by the piriformis muscle because the nerve passes through the muscle, instead of passing under it, into the back of the thigh. This may cause buttock pain, with referred numbness and weakness in the leg, which would seem to suggest a problem in the lumbar spine. The piriformis involvement can be demonstrated by stressing the muscle, which is a lateral rotator and abductor of the hip, in a resisted test or passive stretch (Fig. 7.14), and increasing the symptoms.

Quadriceps tears

The muscles on the front of the thigh, the quadriceps, are extensors of the knee. Three of the quadriceps muscles do not cross the hip joint and are less prone to the sudden overload that 'two joint muscles' can suffer. The fourth muscle, the rectus femoris, may suffer a partial or complete tear during a violent hip flexion or knee extension. Flexion of the knee to 45 degrees will stress the rectus femoris during hip flexion, and a resisted test can be done in this position. Pain will indicate a strain, and weakness may suggest a complete rupture. A defect may also be felt in the muscle if there is a severe tear. Passive flexion of the knee will be increasingly painful as the muscle is stretched.

Hamstring tears

Three of the four hamstrings are 'two joint muscles' (only the short head of the biceps has a femoral origin, the others arise from the tuberosity of the ischium) and their twin roles are extension of the hip and flexion of the knee. Injury can be caused by violent contraction of the muscle or overstretching, which is more likely in a 'two joint muscle'. Passive stretching, in the direction of knee extension and hip flexion, may elicit pain in a partial tear. Resisted knee flexion will be painful in a partial tear, and weak if the tear is large. There are various sites on both sides of the posterior thigh which can be affected. Hamstring injuries are very prone to recurrence.

Bursitis at the hip

Overuse may also cause bursitis at the hip, and three sites are recognized.

1. The bursa of the greater trochanter. This lies between the femur at the widest point of the hip and the fascia of the iliotibial band which travels down the outer side of the thigh to below the knee. Adducting the hip compresses the bursa. This can be caused by running on a cambered road or the distortions of movement caused by flat feet. Pain will be felt in the lateral hip, and may travel down the outer leg. Active and resisted abduction of the hip will elicit the pain.
2. The iliopsoas bursa. This has been mentioned in relation to iliopsoas muscle inflammation.
3. The ischial bursa. This bursa, at the ischial tuberosity, can suffer direct trauma, usually from a fall.

The Knee

Anatomy

The weight-bearing function of the leg requires a good deal of stability in its joints (Fig. 7.16). The precarious balancing of the two big knuckles of the **condyles** of the **femur** on the shallow hollows of the **tibial plateau** seems surprising. The third member of the bony assembly of the knee, the **patella**, is essentially a sesamoid implanted in the quadriceps tendon. It brings no extra sense of stability.

The joint is largely stabilized by soft tissues, with duplication of some of those tasks by a dynamic arrangement of muscles (in which the patella plays its part) as well as inert tissues such as the **meniscus**, the synovial capsule and the ligaments of the knee (Figs 7.17 and 7.18).

The joint has a small but important capacity to rotate. Its main movements are flexion and extension, often while weight bearing and always in coordination with the movements of

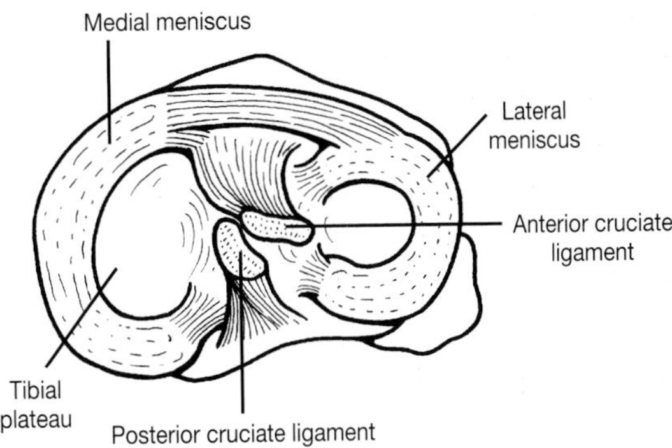

Figure 7.17 The tibial plateau showing the menisci and the tibial insertions of the cruciate ligaments. (Adapted with kind permission from Dean and Pegington 1996.)

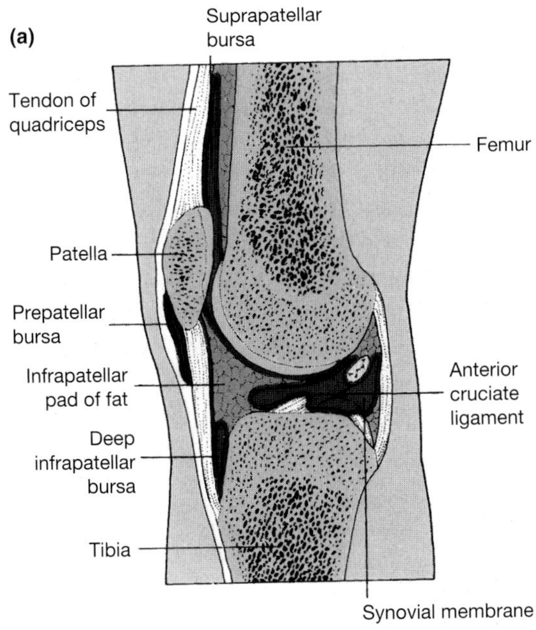

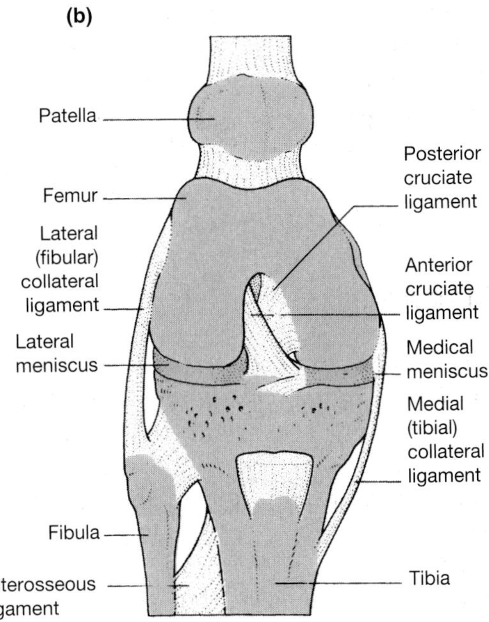

Figure 7.16 The knee joint. (a) Section through the left knee from the side. (b) A front view with the patella tendon cut and the patella displaced to show the underlying structures. (Reproduced with kind permission from Rutishauser (1994) after Rogers (1992).)

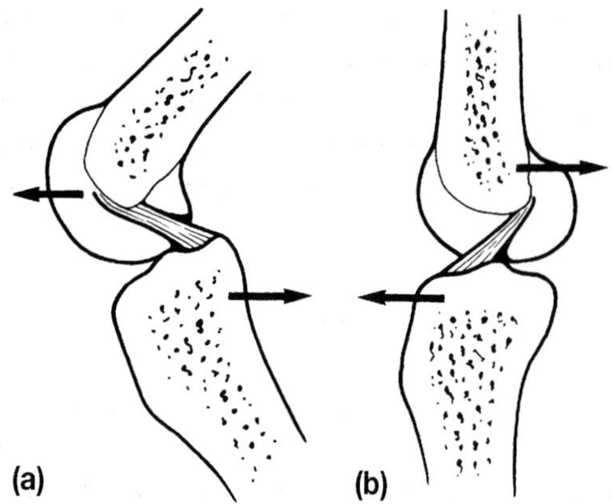

Figure 7.18 The cruciate ligaments limit rotational strain at the knee. (a) The posterior ligament prevents slippage forward of the femur on the tibia, especially in a flexed knee. (b) The anterior ligament prevents posterior displacement on an extended knee. (Reproduced with kind permission from Dean and Pegington, 1996.)

the hip, ankle and foot, with which joints the knee shares muscles (Box 7.3).

The knee can suffer injury in all the usual ways but is particularly vulnerable to destabilizing injuries of the soft tissues of the joint. The knee can be attacked from all four sides and often is during sports like rugby and football. It is often put under undue pressure while carrying the weight of the body or while in extreme positions (such as the forced extension which occurs during a sliding tackle at football). It may, therefore, suffer violent angulations. Injuries which include an element of rotation can be particularly destructive to ligaments and meniscus.

Femur

The shaft of the femur is angled inwards to the knee and expands into two large bulbous condyles at its distal end. The medial and the lateral condyles curve backwards behind the line of the bone and outwards to either side. The condyles are coated with articular cartilage over a much larger area than that which touches the tibia at any one moment. This allows smooth contact over the whole range of movement. The front of the femur has a **patellofemoral groove** between its condyles, which articulates with the patella as it moves up and down during flexion and extension. This surface is covered with cartilage. Between the condyles on the back and underside is a hollow, the **intercondylar fossa**, which allows passage of the cruciate ligaments and their attachment at their upper ends.

Tibia and fibula

The tibia and fibula, the two long bones of the lower leg, are linked along their length by ligament and fascia in a manner resembling the radius–ulna pairing in the forearm. However in the leg the unit is much less dynamic. The fibula plays no part in the knee joint except as an attachment point for structures like the **lateral collateral ligament**. It has a greater role at the ankle joint. The tibia is the larger bone, and the main weight bearer of the lower leg. At the knee it presents an expanded, very flat superior surface, which, like the femoral condyles, projects backwards behind the line of the shaft. This is the tibial plateau. It articulates with the condyles of the femur. Seen from above, the tibial plateau (Fig. 7.17) has two irregular areas, one on the medial side and one on the lateral, which are the top surfaces of the **medial** and **lateral**

Box 7.3 Knee Statistics

Capsular pattern greater loss of flexion than extension, with no loss of rotation.
Joint positions loose packed midflexion; close packed full extension.
Flexion 0–140°; end feel tissue approximation of calf on hamstrings.
Extension 0° but 10° of hyperextension possible; end feel firm, posterior capsular stretch.
Rotation of tibia 0–30° medial, 0–40° lateral; end-feel firm, capsular and ligament stretch.

condyles of the tibia. The medial and lateral menisci lie on these plateau surfaces and articulate with the condyles of the femur. Also on the plateau is a central ridge between the meniscal surfaces, called the **intercondylar eminence**. In the central area of the plateau, at the front, the **anterior horns** of both menisci are attached, as is the lower part of the anterior cruciate ligament. Similarly, the **posterior horns** of the two menisci, and the lower attachment of the posterior cruciate ligament, are attached to the back of the tibial plateau in this central area. In front of the tibia in the midline, just distal to the plateau, is a bulge called the **tibial tuberosity**, which is the insertion of the tendon (or ligament) of the patella. This is the point which offers attachment at the lower leg to the whole extensor mechanism of the quadriceps. From the front, the two condyles of the tibia can be seen bulging out to either side, beyond the line of the shaft of the tibia.

Patella

The patella is a sesamoid bone, offering a focal point for the forces exerted by the quadriceps muscle before they are transmitted to the lower leg. It is of variable shape. It tends to be roughly oval, but with a flattened top and pointed base. On its patellofemoral surface, it is thickly coated with cartilage to withstand the tremendous forces to which it is subjected during, in particular, weight-bearing flexion and extension of the knee.

Meniscus

The menisci are similar in makeup (collagen with a small amount of elastin) to ligament. They lie on the tibial plateau, one medial and one lateral. They are crescent shaped, with their openings facing towards the central ridge of the plateau and each other. They deepen the articular surface of the tibia for the femoral condyles. They are shock absorbers. They stabilize and guide the movement of the femur on the tibia. The pulling and compressing forces in the joint can cause tears in the meniscus, especially during rotation. No extreme movement is necessary to tear the meniscus, and the mechanism of injury can seem slight to the patient.

Collateral ligaments

The knee has two **collateral ligaments**, one **lateral** and one **medial**, which fasten the femur to the head of the fibula on the outer side and to the tibia on the inner side. The medial ligament has a deep layer which is joined to the medial meniscus, and it can be difficult on examination to discriminate between injury to one or other; indeed, sometimes they are both injured (the 'unhappy triad' is a combined injury to medial ligament, meniscus and the anterior cruciate ligament caused by a violent valgus stress to the knee). These ligaments take a part in stabilizing the knee, but their main function is to limit varus and valgus movement, respectively. They are usually injured by a blow to the opposite side of the knee during sport.

Cruciate ligaments

The **anterior** and **posterior cruciate ligaments** are so called because they cross in the middle of the knee joint (Fig. 7.18). Each one prevents slippage of the tibia on the femur; by tightening around each other during movement, they limit the range of internal rotation. The anterior cruciate travels from the front of the tibia, on the medial side, to the rear lateral condyle of the femur, to which it is joined on its medial side. It tightens as the tibia is pulled forward from under the femur, and this is the movement which it limits (Fig. 7.18a). The posterior cruciate, travelling backwards from the lateral side of the medial condyle of the femur and inserting into the rear edge of the tibial plateau, slightly to the outer side, limits the reverse movement, backward slippage of the tibia on the femur (Fig 7.18b).

Bursae

There are several bursae around the knee. The one which commonly causes symptoms is the **prepatellar bursa**, which lies over the front of the patella. Inflammation there is widely known as **housemaid's knee**. The other bursa which can cause problems is the **infrapatellar bursa**, which is directly below the patella, over its ligament. Inflammation there is called **clergyman's knee**.

Examination

The knee should be examined carefully for swelling. Swelling is most easily seen in the medial hollow of the knee and the suprapatellar area. A localized, soft swelling anterior to the patella, with redness, heat and tenderness, may be a prepatellar bursitis. Check the patient's temperature and assess the possibility of infection.

When taking a history from an injured patient with a swollen knee, ask how quickly the swelling developed. A swelling which developed within minutes of injury, rather than hours, is probably caused by bleeding, a **haemarthrosis**. This needs medical assessment. The blood may need aspiration from the joint, and the severity of the injury may be considerable.

Many of the injuries which cause pain in or around the knee will cause patients to alter their gait. Often patients avoid straightening the knee. This prevents painful stretching of many of the joint tissues and muscles. Try to decide why the patient will not extend the knee. If the joint is 'locked' by a meniscal obstruction, the patient may need surgery. If the joint is not locked, the patient's gait is tiring, potentially unsafe and will not make for good healing. Provide a walking aid until the patient can extend the knee.

On palpation, assess the patellofemoral joint with the knee straight, and assess the menisci, at the tibial plateau, with the knee in flexion. The lateral collateral ligament is more easily felt with the leg in a 'figure four position' (i.e., the outer ankle of the injured leg lying across the other shin and the knee bent).

Figures 7.19–7.27 show the basic examination of an injured knee, selectively stressing muscles, ligaments and the joint surfaces.

Fractures

Fractures require orthopaedic assessment.

Patellar injuries, and injuries to the extensor mechanism

A direct blow or a violent contraction of the quadriceps may fracture the patella. This may also tear the quadriceps tendon, the patellar ligament or fracture the tubercle of the tibia. In a child, a patellar subluxation may avulse a part of the patella. Direct trauma to the patellar ligament when the knee is flexed (e.g. falling, with the knee bent, on a hard edge such as a step or low wall) may rupture it.

The patient will be unable to walk or extend the knee, either because of pain or weakness, and there may be bruising, swelling and local tenderness.

Fracture of the tibial plateau

The tibial plateau can fracture through a valgus stress of the knee, the mechanism which causes a medial collateral ligament tear. This depression fracture presents as a painful knee which has swelled rapidly, with bruising and inability to walk. The knee may remain in a valgus deformity.

Soft tissue injuries

Ligament tears

One or more ligaments can be torn by a violent angulation or rotation, a blocking blow to the front of the tibia (such as hitting a car dashboard in a crash) or a violent hyperextension or flexion. The history will normally be of a very painful injury, and the more severe injuries may cause haemarthrosis and avulsion or other fractures (such as tibial plateau depression). The knee may be unstable in a varus/valgus direction (collateral ligaments), anterior/posterior direction (cruciates), or there may be rotational subluxation. When examining a patient with a history of injury to the knee, the collateral and cruciate ligaments should always be stressed to establish that they are patent (Figs 7.23–7.26).

Box

Observe the patients gait. Is there a 'lag'? (Is he walking on the ball of his foot to avoid straightening his knee?)

Ask the patient to expose both legs from thigh to foot.

Ask the patient to lie supine on a trolley and to extend both knees.

Assess distal sensation and circulation.

- **LOOK** for swelling, redness, bruising or deformity. If there is an effusion (most clearly seen in the medial hollow and suprapatellar areas)? Did it develop within moments of injury (a haemarthrosis) or more slowly? Is there wasting of the thigh muscles? Is the patient avoiding full extension of the knee? On the back, is there popliteal swelling?
- **FEEL** the patella and move it in the femoral groove with the knee extended and relaxed. Feel the quadriceps. Flex the knee to 90° to feel the joint and related structures. Feel the tibial tuberosity and the patellar tendon. Move laterally over lateral meniscus and femoral condyle, the lateral collateral ligament and the head of the fibula. Assess the medial meniscus and femoral condyle and the medial collateral ligament. Feel the popliteal fossa and the tendons of the hamstrings.
- **MOVE** (these test are shown in the following illustrations). Passive extension of the knee will clear the joint. Note the endfeel. A displaced meniscal tear will have a springy endfeel. Active and resisted extension will assess the quadriceps and patella. Assess active, resisted and passive flexion. Assess rotation passively. Stress four ligaments by stretching them, look for pain or laxity. If you suspect meniscal locking, the McMurray's test is designed to assess the joint surfaces by compressing them and moving them against each other.

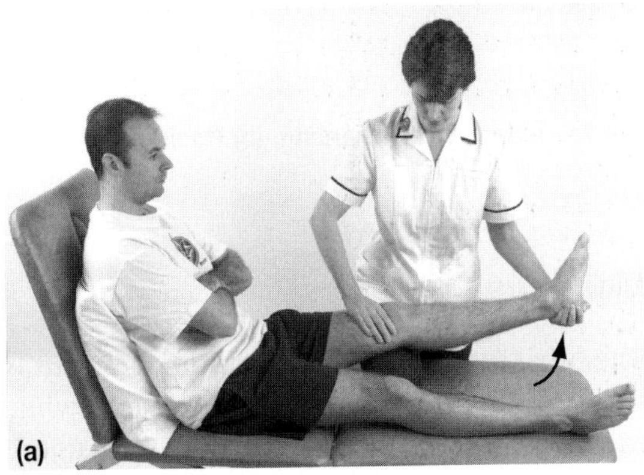

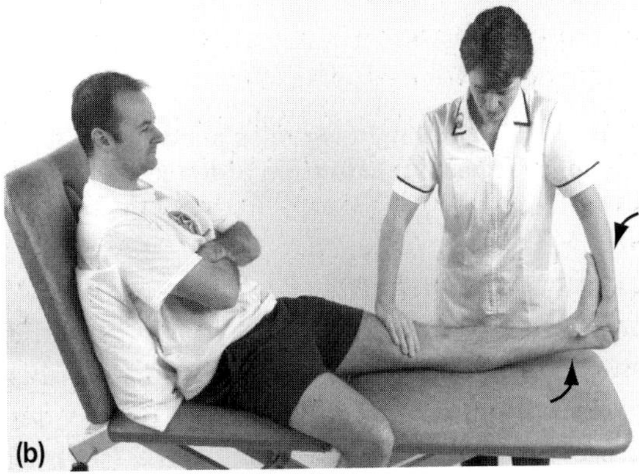

Figure 7.19 (a) Passive extension of the knee. Does the knee extend fully? Is the endfeel firm, or is there a springy obstruction? (b) Active extension of the knee. Dorsiflex the foot to expose any hypertension in the knee. Compare the two sides to decide what is normal for the patient.

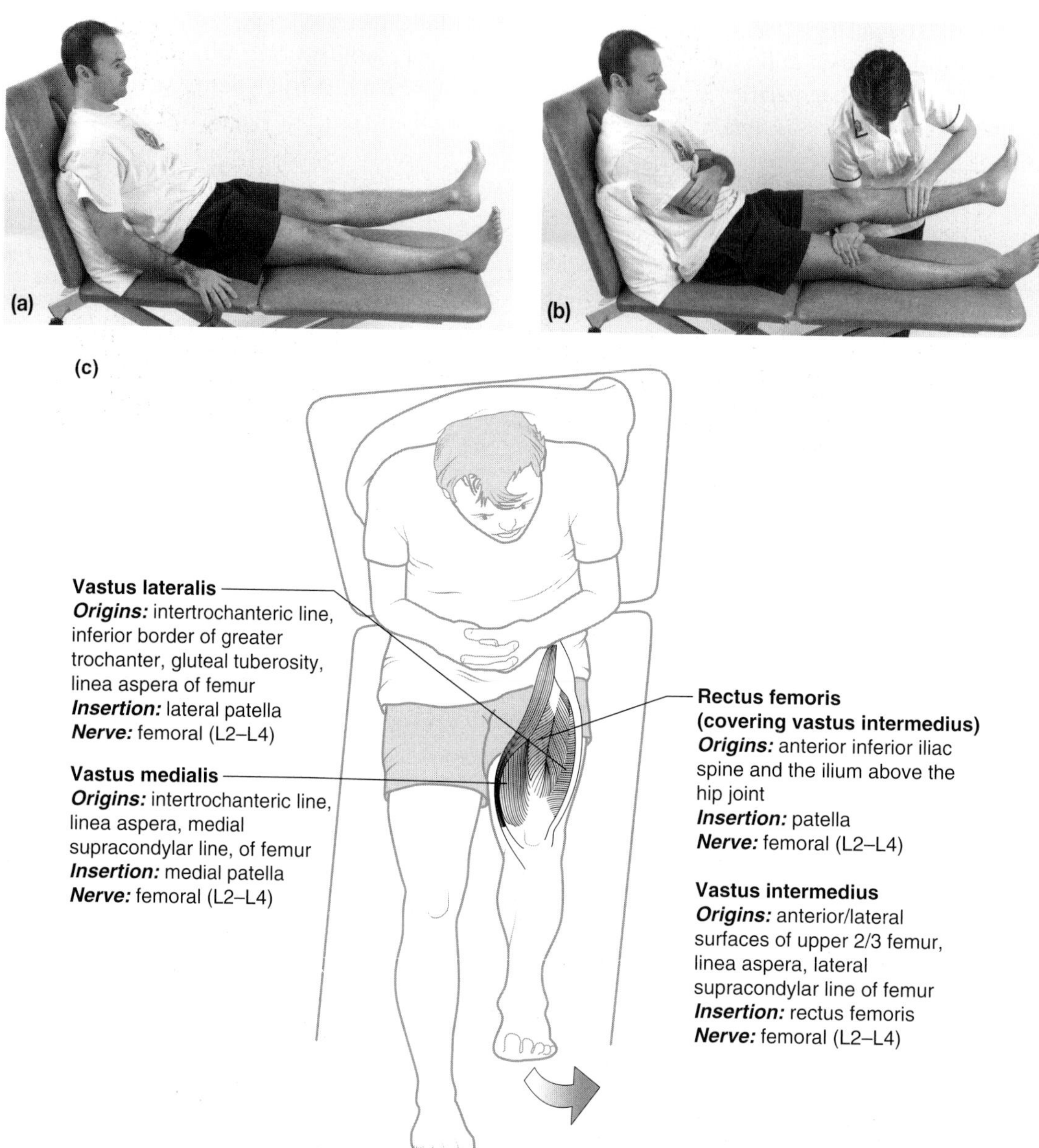

Figure 7.20 **(a) Straight leg raise shows good function of the extensor mechanism. (b) Resisted extension of the knee. (c) Extensors of the knee.**

Any injury where there is laxity in the collateral ligaments or a possible injury to either cruciate ligament should be assessed by a doctor. A painful collateral ligament which is not lax and has no other worrying signs (such as haemarthrosis) can be treated on its merits, with physiotherapy if possible for grade 2 sprains.

Meniscus

The usual mechanism by which the meniscus is torn is rotation of the knee, particularly while flexed, as often happens at football. The injury will be painful but not necessarily violent. The problem is more common at the medial meniscus. There may be obstruction of the joint

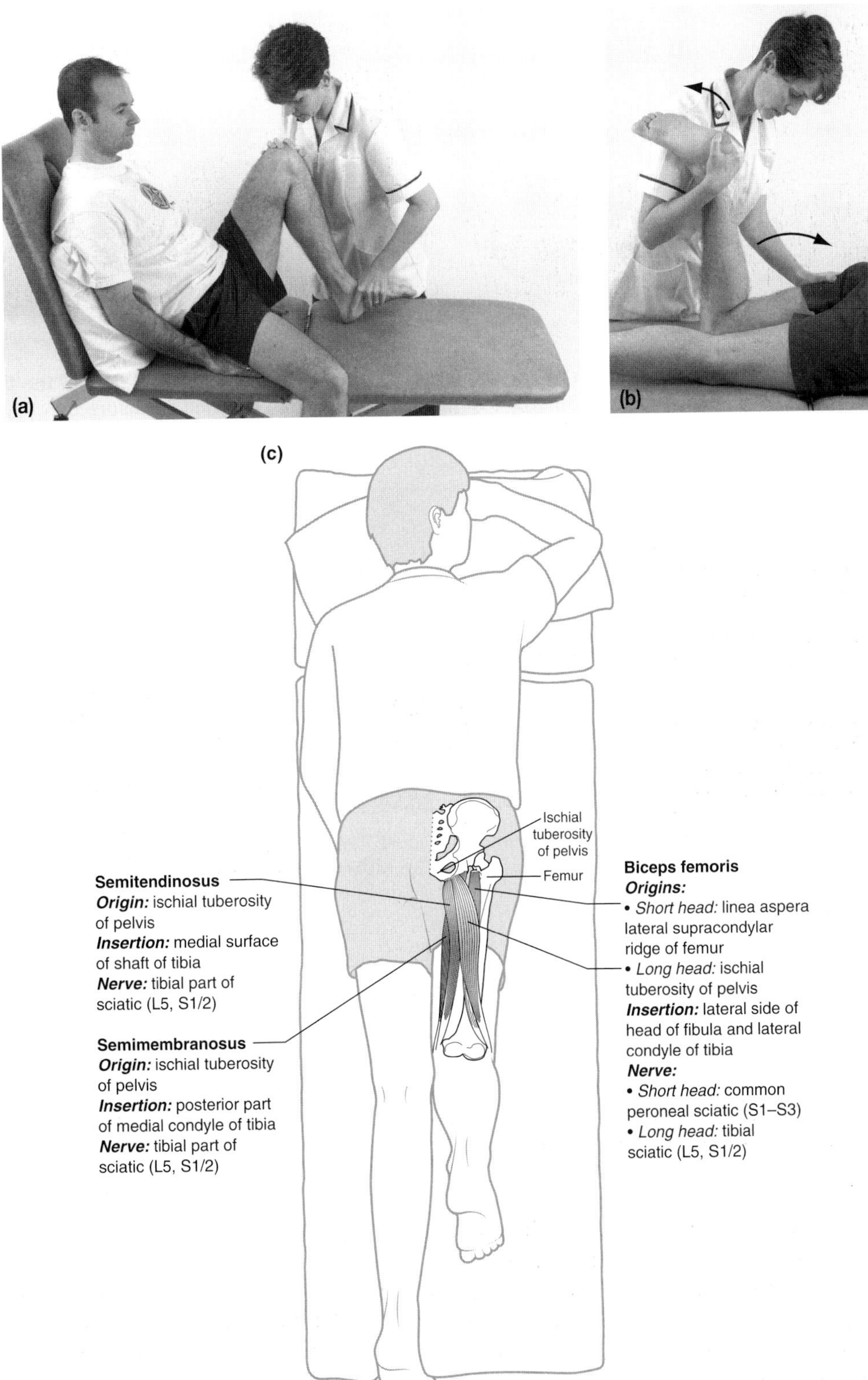

Figure 7.21 **(a) Active flexion of the knee. If the patient has a full range, passively overpress the knee to clear the joint. (b) Resisted flexion of the knee. (c) Flexors of the knee.**

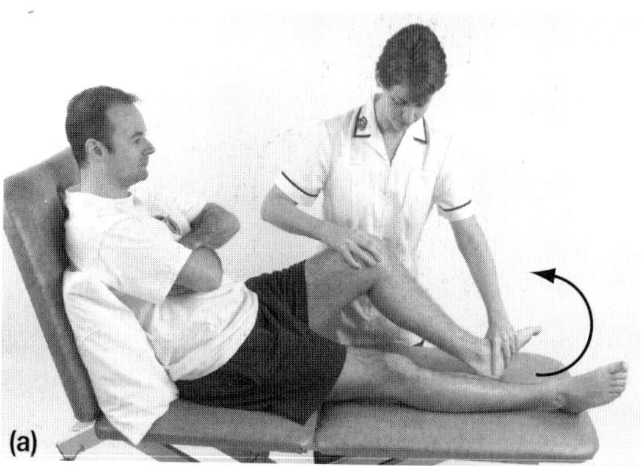

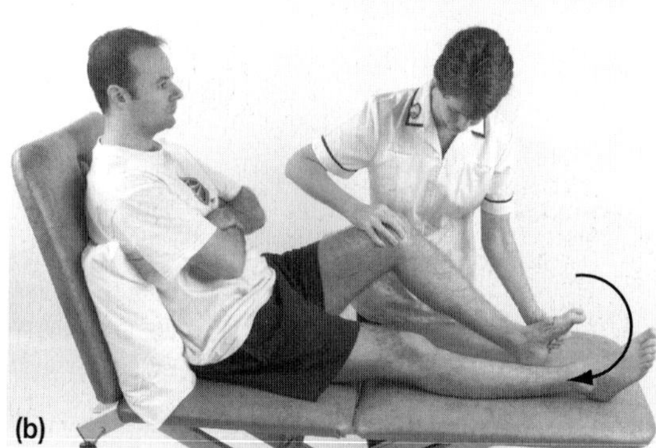

Figure 7.22 **(a) Passive lateral rotation of the tibia at the knee. (b) Passive medial rotation of the tibia at the knee. Note the tester's hand positions. Feel the knee and watch the shin to ensure that foot is not rotating instead of lower leg.**

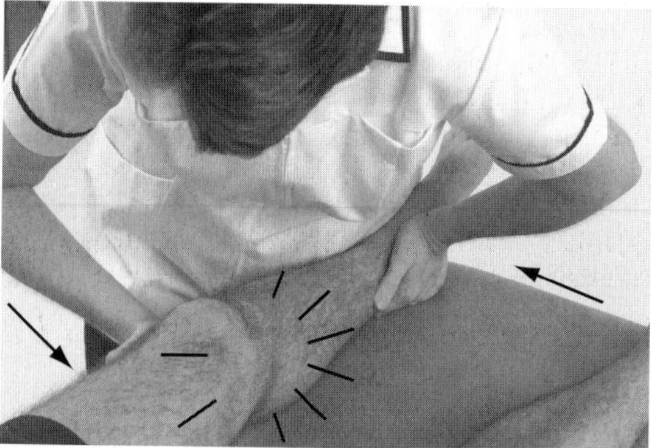

Figure 7.23 **Stress of medial collateral ligament. Pressure is applied to lateral knee to stress medial side. Patient has to relax with knee in slight flexion. Pain or laxity are positive.**

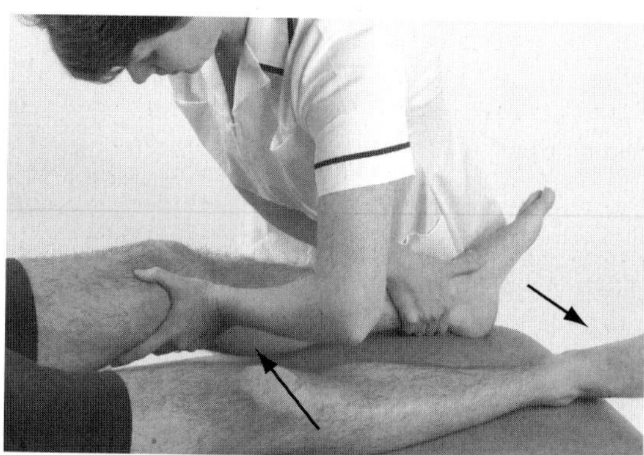

Figure 7.24 **Stress of lateral collateral ligament. The reverse of Figure 7.23.**

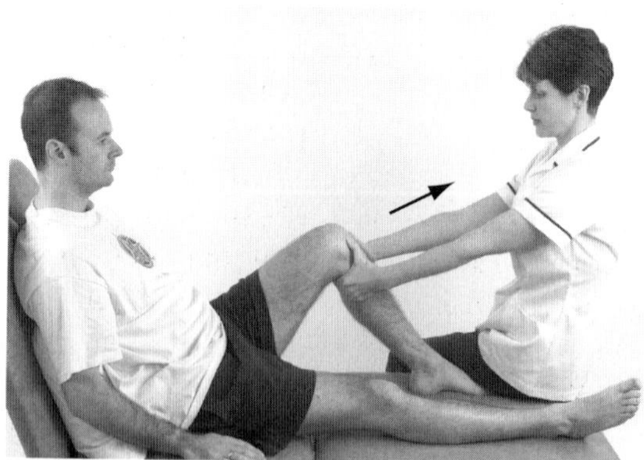

Figure 7.25 **Anterior cruciate drawer test. Knee flexed to approximately 90°. Stabilise it by sitting on patients foot. Ensure that hamstrings are lax by putting index fingers against them. Put thumbs on knee joint line to feel any laxity. Use hands on calf to pull tibia forward; lean back with straight arms to ensure good power. Compare both sides. Laxity or pain are positive.**

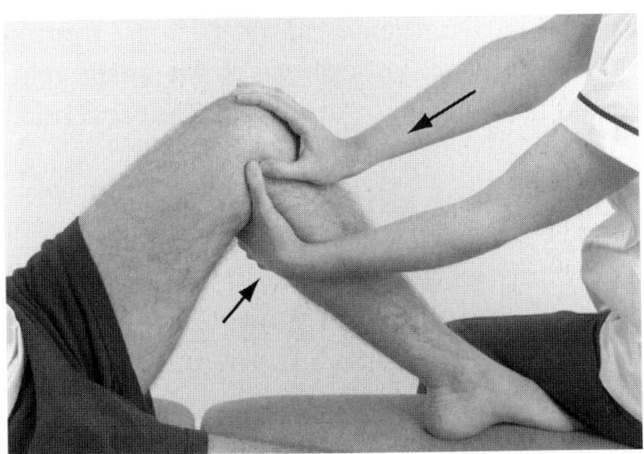

Figure 7.26 **(see Fig 7.25) Continue by testing posterior cruciate ligament. Support tibia at calf with one hand (to ensure that, if posterior cruciate *is* lax, that tibia has not already fallen backwards). Use the same thumb to feel the joint line. Put the other hand on the tibial tuberosity (it is a common fault to place the hand over the patella). With arm straight, push the tibia backwards. Feel for laxity. Compare both sides.**

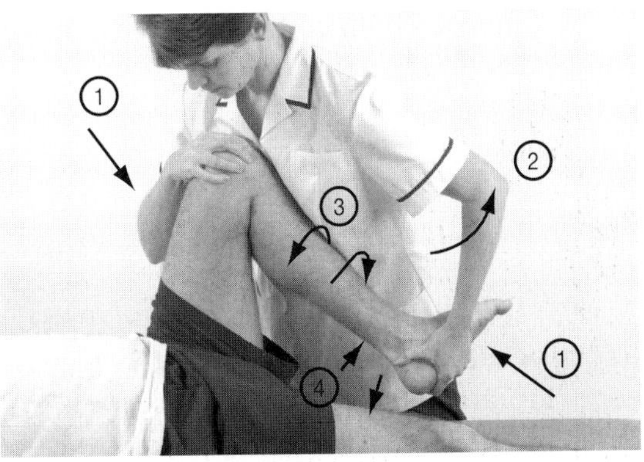

Figure 7.27 **The McMurray's test for meniscal obstruction. This is a difficult test to perform. The joint surfaces are tested by grinding them against each other in every position they can attain. The knee moves passively in: 1. Compression of tibia against femur; 2. Full flexion to almost full extension; 3. Lateral–medial–lateral rotations of joint. 4. Lateral–midline–medial angulations of joint. Pain alone is not a positive result. Grating or clicking in the joint is positive.**

(locking) by a torn piece of meniscus; this may resolve itself (sometimes suddenly during examination) or it may require surgery. If the problem settles, the patient may have no more than general signs of injury, swelling, tibial plateau tenderness and pain on full extension of the knee. However, healing tends to be poor in the menisci, and there may be a recurrence.

The Ankle and Foot

Anatomy

The bones of the lower leg, ankle and foot and the main ligaments are shown in Figure 7.28.

Tibia

Below the knee, the shaft of the tibia narrows and is relatively slender until it reaches the ankle joint, where it broadens again. Seen in cross-section, the tibial shaft is triangular, with the base of the triangle at the back of the leg, covered by the calf muscles. The apex is at the front. This front ridge of the tibia curves down and inwards to the **medial malleolus**, the bulging inner ankle. The medial surface of the triangular section of the tibia is the shin. It is superficial from knee to inner ankle. The lateral border of the tibial shaft has an **interosseus border** with the fibula. This side of the bone is clothed in extrinsic muscles of the foot and ankle, which arise from the proximal tibia and fibula. (This is unlike the situation in the upper limb, where many of the extrinsic muscles arise from the humerus and cross the elbow as well as the wrist. In the lower leg, only the gastrocnemius and plantaris muscles of the calf cross the knee joint.)

The medial malleolus points downwards as a styloid process. The **deltoid ligaments** emerge from it in a fan shape, attaching to bones of the hindfoot and midfoot to stabilize the inner ankle.

The union of tibia and fibula at the ankle will be described below.

Fibula

The fibula is similarly expanded at top and bottom, with a long, slender shaft between. The head of the fibula articulates with the tibia on its lateral side, tucked under the bulging lateral condyle and taking no part in the bony articulation of the knee. The shaft passes down the lateral side of the tibia, but lying behind its posterior margin for most of its length. It expands at its base into the **lateral malleolus**, or outer ankle bone, and unites with the distal tibia to form the mortise of the ankle joint. The head is palpable and the lateral malleolus is superficial, but most of the shaft is buried in muscle.

Ligaments of the lower leg

The tibia and fibula are linked by ligaments and a fibrous **interosseus membrane**, which binds the bones along their whole length. The membrane is strengthened at its base to form a fibrous joint or **syndesmosis** at the ankle, reinforced by the distal ligaments at front and back.

Bones of the foot

The bones of the foot are described in two ways, by zones, the **hindfoot**, the **midfoot** and the **forefoot**, and by groupings of bones (analagous to the groupings of the bones of the wrist and hand). The **tarsal** bones lie in the hindfoot and comprise the **calcaneus** (the heel bone), the **talus** (the bone of the ankle joint) and the five midfoot bones: **cuboid**, **navicular**, and three **cunieform** bones. In the forefoot, the **metatarsals** correspond to the metacarpals of the hand, five in number, each one shaped like a digit but disguised by the flesh of the foot, and each one supporting one of the five toes. Each toe has phalanges, two for the big toe and three for the others. Unlike the hand, the largest digit of the foot, the big toe, lies on the inner side. It absorbs weight and acts as a kick-off point for movement.

Box Lower leg/foot

Observe the patient's gait.

If the history suggests a tear of the Achilles tendon, seat the patient to avoid extending the injury. Ask the patient to expose both legs from below the knees.

Assess distal sensation and circulation.

- **LOOK** for any bruise, swelling, redness or deformity.
- **FEEL** all structures below the knee. Key sites include the head of the fibula, the calf, the Achilles tendon, the heel, the malleoli and the base of the 5th metatarsal.
- **MOVE** the basic combined foot and ankle movement as illustrated. The movements which are tested will depend on the patient's complaint (e.g. it is pointless to assess resisted ankle/foot movements with a freshly swollen ankle sprain).

Special test for Achilles tendon tear: the Simmons' (calf squeeze) test. Ask the patient to kneel facing backwards on a chair with both feet hanging over the seat. Look at the injured side: Does the foot sit square at the ankle, lacking normal plantar flexion? Squeeze the calf. This should move the foot into plantar flexion. Compare both sides. If the foot fails to move, the test is positive.

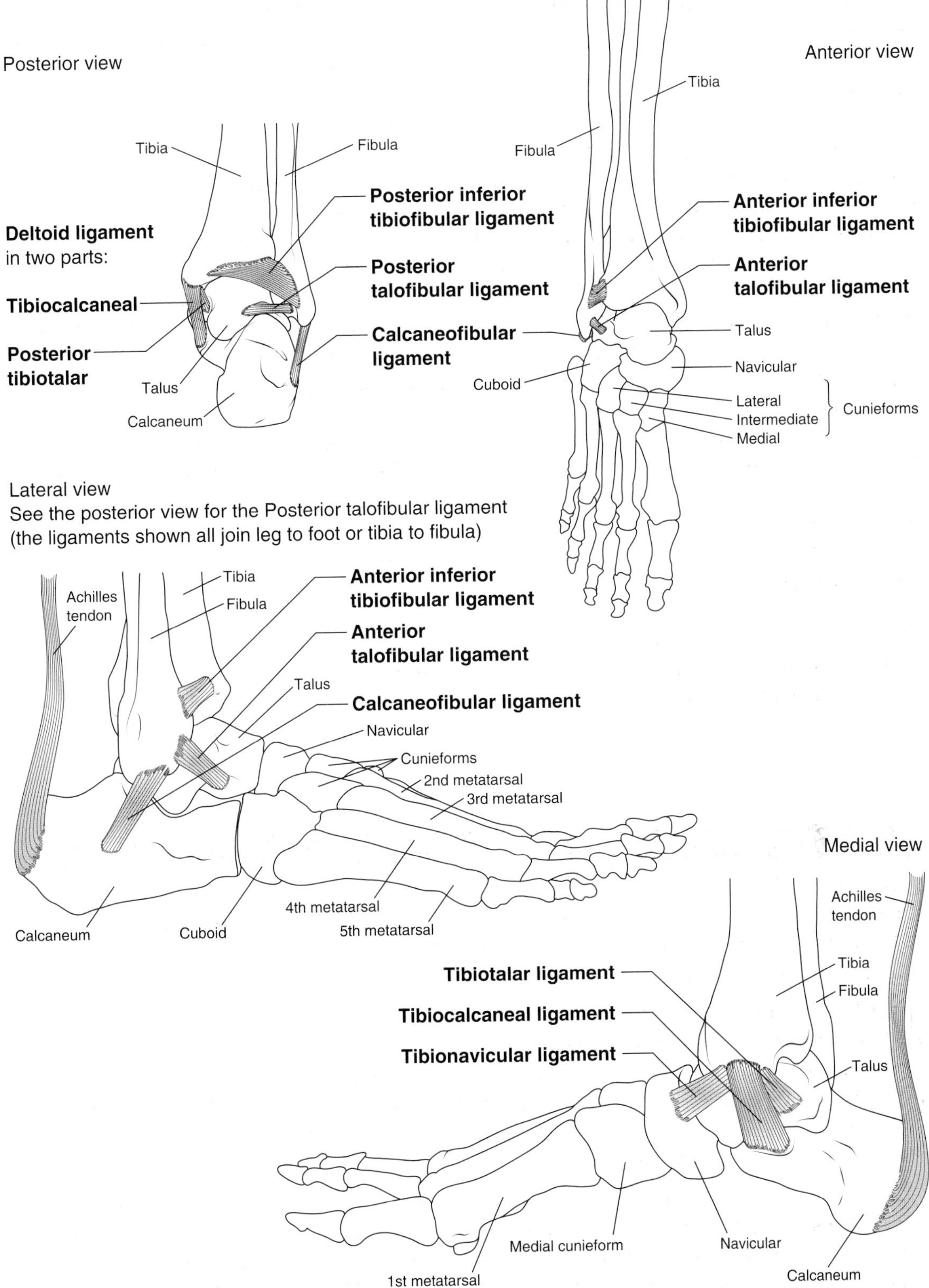

Figure 7.28 The bones of the lower leg, ankle and foot with the main ligaments.

The arrangement of the bones may also be seen in terms of medial and lateral groupings. The talus articulates, in a sequence which proceeds distally, with the navicular, the three cunieforms, metatarsals one to three, and the first three toes. The calcaneus articulates with the cuboid, the fourth and fifth metatarsals, and the fourth and fifth toes.

The calcaneus lies under the ankle bone, the talus, in a vertical line with the tibia and angles down and backwards from that line to form the posterior projection of the heel. At the front and inner surfaces, it articulates with the cuboid. The rounded back of the bone receives the insertion of the Achilles tendon from above. On its plantar surface, it has tubercles for the attachment of various structures including the medial tubercle insertion of the plantar fascia, which can be a site of inflammation (plantar fasciitis).

On the medial side of the calcaneus is a projection called the **sustentaculum tali** (meaning support of the talus), which is the origin of the **plantar calcaneonavicular ligament**, also called the **spring ligament**. This ligament is a part of the soft tissue support of the medial longitudinal arch of the foot. The talus has no bony underpinning at its navicular articulation and is subject to downward pressure from the weight of the body, through the leg to the foot. This is resisted by a soft tissue sling of tendons and ligaments, including the spring ligament. If posture collapses at this arch, **pes planus** can develop (the form of flat-foot caused by excessive pronation of the foot). This can cause stresses in the leg and hip and painful fixed deformities of the foot.

On top of the sustentaculum tali is one of the articular surfaces of the calcaneus for the talus.

The talus articulates with the tibia at its superior **trochlear surface**, which forms the top surface of the **body** of the talus, and the fibular lateral malleolus on its lateral side, to make the ankle joint. It rests upon the calcaneus. The **neck** of the talus passes forwards, downwards and to the inner side of the foot to the point where its **head** articulates with the navicular. Thus, it accepts the weight of the body through the ankle joint and transmits it down and back to the heel through its calcaneal articulations, and forward to the foot through its navicular articulation.

The ankle joint and the joints of the foot

The ankle joint, also known as the **talocrural joint**, is shaped like a mortise and tenon, with the distal tibia and fibula forming the inverted U-shaped ceiling over the body of the talus. The medial malleolus sits slightly in front of the lateral, so that the foot sits in slight outward rotation. The joint permits the movements of **plantarflexion** (pointing the toes downwards) and **dorsiflexion** (bringing the dorsal foot back towards the shin).

The main parts at which movement of the whole foot occur are the **subtalar joint** (between talus and calcaneus, where inversion and eversion occur) and the **midtarsal** (the combined action of the calcaneocuboid saddle joint and the talonavicular condyloid joint allow inversion and eversion, abduction and adduction, and plantarflexion and dorsiflexion).

Movements of the ankle and foot are usually compound. Dorsiflexion combines with abduction and eversion, and plantarflexion combines with adduction and inversion (Box 7.4).

Collateral ligaments of the ankle

The lateral ankle is secured to the foot by a collateral ligament, which is divided into three parts, the **anterior talofibular ligament**, the central **calcaneofibular ligament** and the **posterior talofibular ligament**. The anterior talofibular ligament is a vital part of ankle joint stability, and also the ligament most likely to be damaged by an inversion injury.

Box 7.4 Ankle Statistics

Capsular pattern talocrural joint is plantarflexion more limited than dorsiflexion; subtalar joint is inversion more limited than eversion.
Joint positions close packed position full dorsiflexion; loose packed 10° plantarflexion, halfway between inversion and eversion.
Dorsiflexion 20°; firm end feel caused by tension in capsule, ligament and tendon.
Plantarflexion 50°; firm end feel caused by tension in capsule, ligament and tendon.
Inversion 30°; firm end feel caused by lateral capsule and ligaments.
Eversion 10°; firm end feel caused by tension in the medial capsule, ligaments and the posterior tibialis muscle.

The medial ankle's collateral ligament is also divided into several bands, collectively called the **deltoid**, and is stronger and less prone to injury than the lateral group. The deltoid is related to the spring ligament and has deep layers formed by the **anterior talotibial** and **posterior talotibial** bands and the more superficial **naviculotibial** ligament. As with the lateral ankle, there is a **calcaneotibial** band.

Examination

Palpation of the lower leg and foot should begin at the head of the fibula and include the calf, Achilles tendon, the bones of the lower leg, both malleoli, the anterior and posterior aspects of the ankle and the bones of the foot. Figures 7.29–7.33 show the basic assessment of the muscles and ligaments of the lower leg and ankle.

Lower leg fractures

Tibia

With the exception of two types of injury, it is unlikely that a patient who has suffered a tibial fracture will present at a minor injury clinic. The tibia is a large weight-bearing bone and the patient will be shocked and unable to walk. The injuries which may be seen are to the medial malleolus and a stress fracture to the shaft of the bone caused by running.

Major tibial fractures usually happen in one of three ways, perhaps while

- twisting, perhaps while skiing
- a fall from a height onto the feet (a mechanism which may also produce bimalleolar fracture/dislocation at the ankle, calcaneal fracture and injury to the spine)
- by a direct blow, especially to the superfical shin.

Open fractures are common at the shin, and severe blood loss is likely. Damage to nerve and blood vessels is possible. There is a large risk of complication, which is assessed not only on the severity of the fracture but also by the soft tissue damage and contamination of the wound.

Record the patient's vital signs. Assess perfusion and innervation distal to the injury. Control bleeding and dress any wound. Give pain relief. Obtain intravenous access as soon as that is practicable. The priority is a prompt transfer to the orthopaedic surgeons.

Fibula

The fibula may suffer a combined fracture with the tibia (although the injury may be at a different level of the bone).

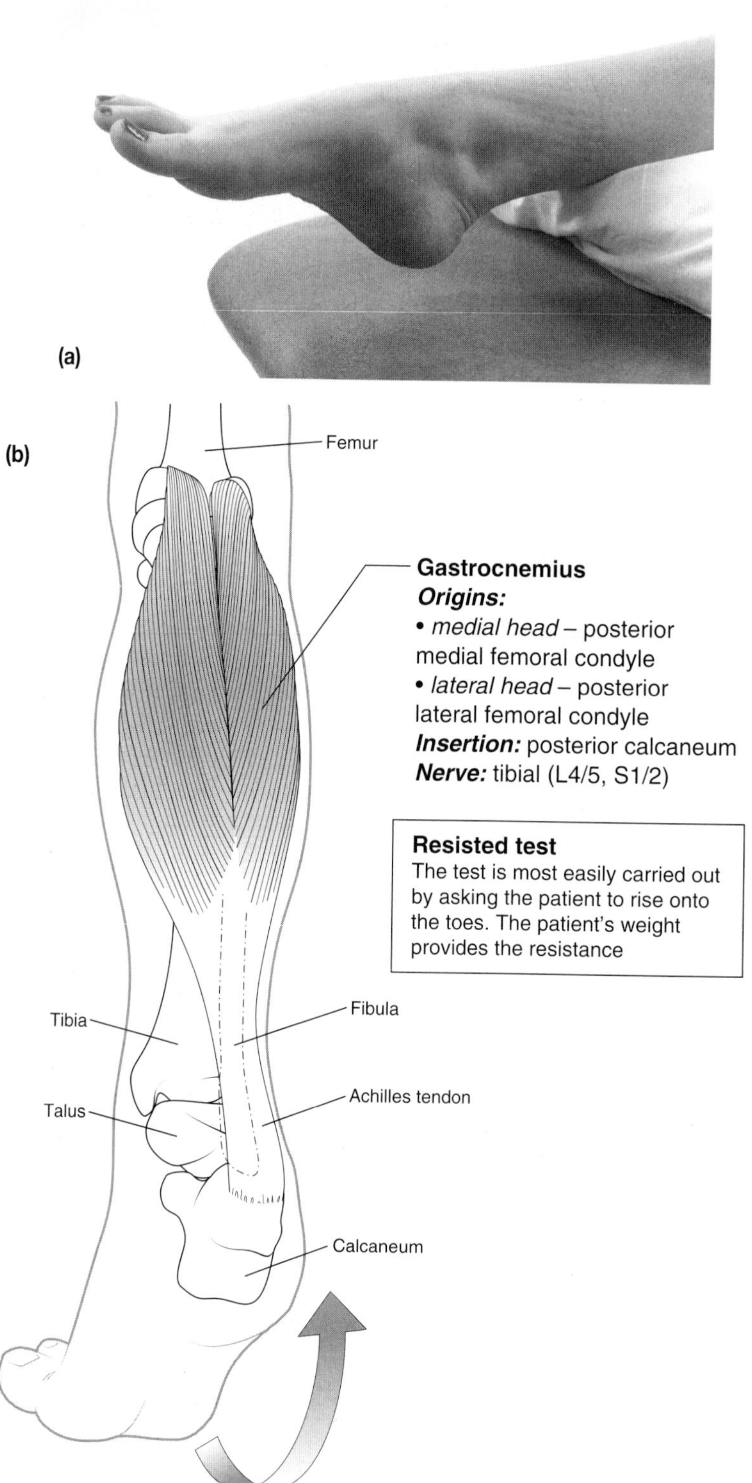

Figure 7.29 **(a) Active plantar flexion of the ankle. (b) Resisted plantar flexion showing muscles of plantar flexion.**

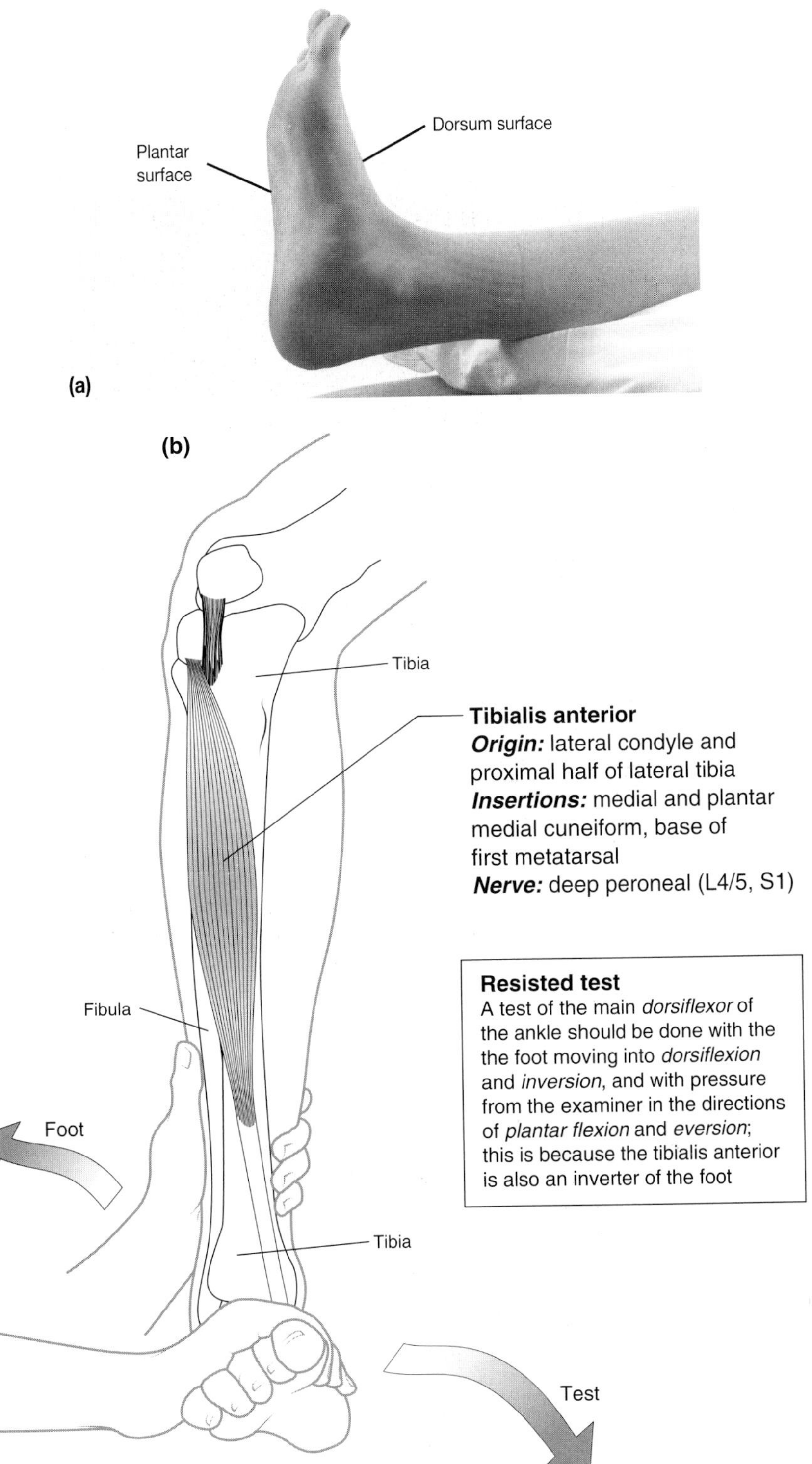

Figure 7.30 (a) Active dorsiflexion. (b) Resisted dorsiflexion of ankle with muscles of dorsiflexion.

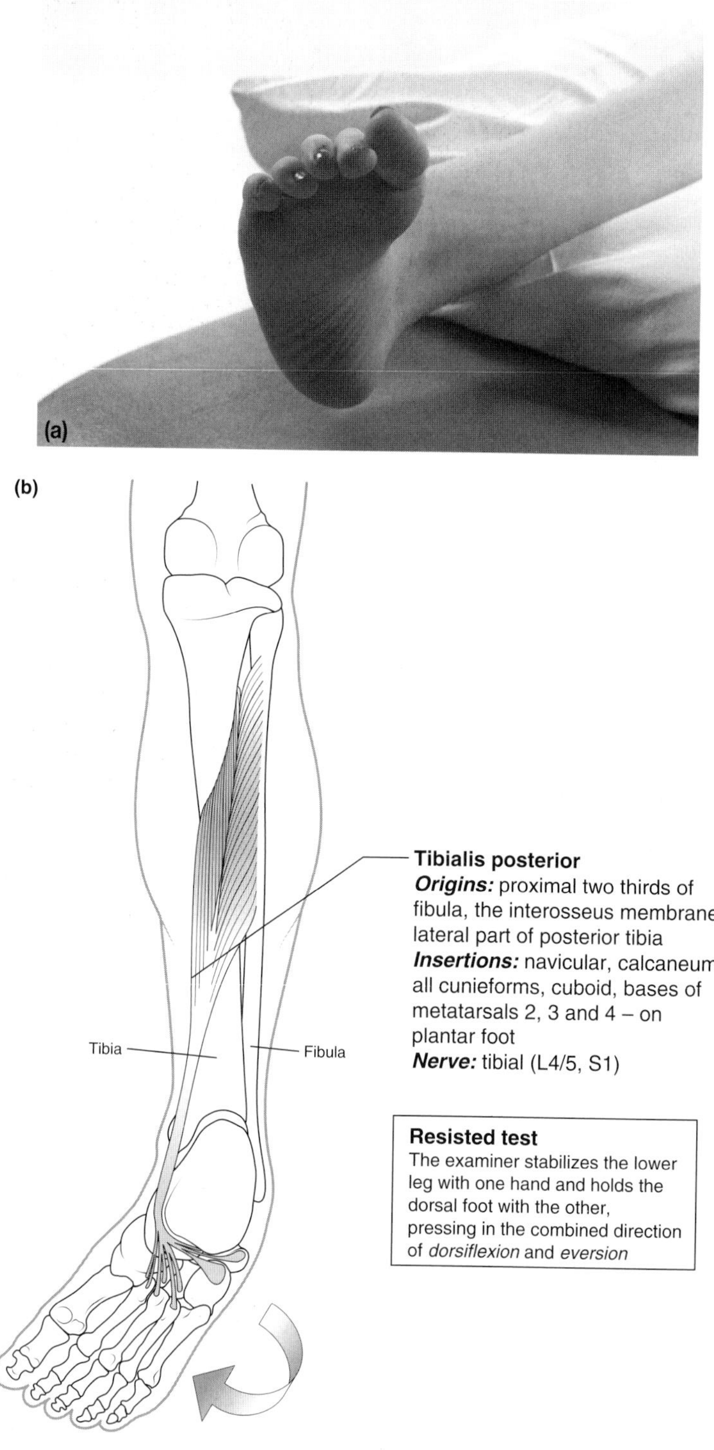

Figure 7.31 (a) Active inversion. (b) Muscles of inversion.

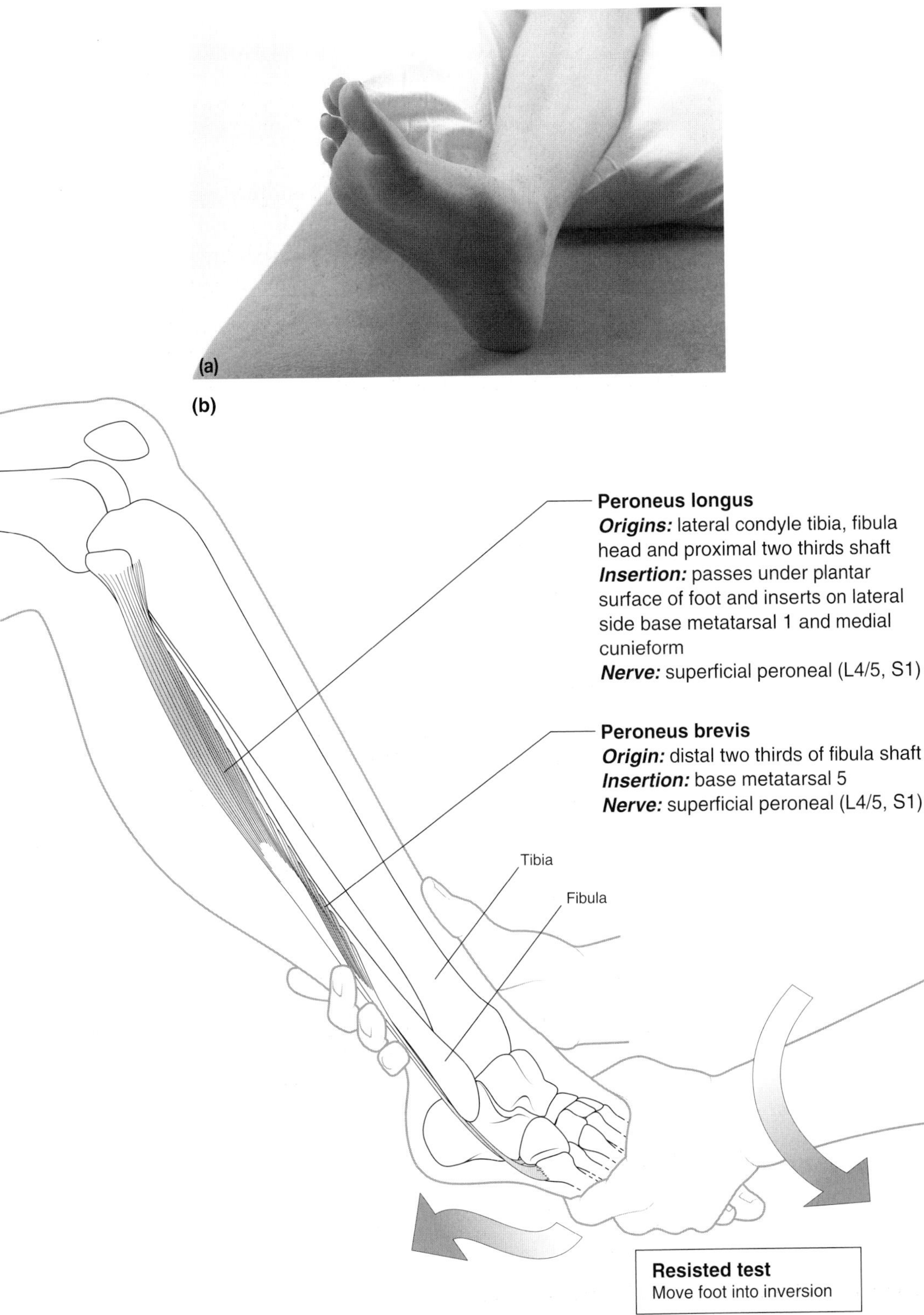

Figure 7.32 **(a) Active eversion. (b) Resisted eversion of foot and ankle with muscles of eversion.**

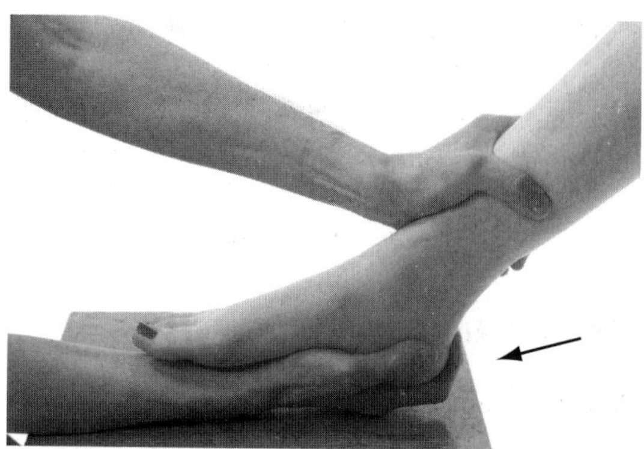

Figure 7.33 The anterior drawer test for the ankle stresses the anterior talofibular ligament: the foot should be in slight plantar flexion for this test.

The fibula does not bear weight at the knee. An isolated fibular fracture is often inflicted by a direct force, such as a kick at football, or by a twisting force at the ankle. It may not stop the patient from walking and the patient may not present for treatment right away. An undisplaced and uncomplicated injury may require no active treatment in any case. However, a fracture to the fibula may affect the tibiofibular syndemosis and ligaments, and the ankle joint requires careful assessment. Conversely, an ankle injury, especially in cases where there is a twisting force applied to the foot, may injure the fibula anywhere along its shaft or at the proximal tibiofibular articulation. Examination of the ankle must include the whole fibula. Fractures at the distal end of the fibula, caused by injury at the ankle, may destabilize the ankle joint. Stress fractures may happen in the fibula in the young and sporting or in the elderly and osteoporotic.

Lower leg pain

Compartment syndromes

Compartment syndrome has been discussed. **Chronic compartment syndrome** may occur in the lower leg. The two forms of compartment syndrome are linked by the fact that their symptoms are caused by an increase in pressure within one of the fascia-wrapped muscle compartments which exceeds the ability of the inelastic tissue to accommodate it. The conditions are not alike in their progress, severity or urgency. Chronic compartment syndrome is caused by overdevelopment of the muscles for the space inside the compartment. The patient feels pain when the muscle enlarges during heavy activity. This condition is distinguished by the relationship between exertion and pain in the way that symptoms begin and cease.

Medial leg pain

Possible causes of pain in the medial lower leg among sportsmen include stress fracture of the tibia, acute and chronic compartment syndrome and periostitis. A patient who presents with pain in the medial lower leg which is induced by exercise and settles with rest may have chronic compartment syndrome or periostitis. If the problem is inflammation over the surface of the periosteum of the tibia, there should be tenderness on the anterior surface of the distal shin. Radiography may identify a stress fracture of the tibia but a negative result will not completely exclude a stress fracture. The term 'shin splints' is often used for pain in this area, but clinicians vary in their definition of it. It is inherently vague.

Each of these conditions signals overuse or problems in training technique. The sportsman should rest and review the training programme.

Tibialis anterior injury

The tibialis anterior muscle may suffer two forms of injury, commonest among athletes, which should be carefully discriminated: acute compartment syndrome and inflammation of its tendon sheath. (Chronic compartment syndrome is also possible at this site.) Acute compartment syndrome can be caused by direct trauma or overtraining. A severe increase in pressure in this compartment threatens the blood supply to the foot, and surgery is sometimes needed.

Tendon inflammation is an overuse injury and symptoms such as crepitus in the sheath are common.

Patients with either condition will have severe difficulty walking, pain on active dorsiflexion and passive plantarflexion of the ankle. The tendon problem should produce signs in the distal, tendinous area of the muscle, sometimes heat, redness and swelling. The signs of the compartment syndrome will be at the muscle belly, and there may be paraesthesia in the foot. If there is any doubt about the diagnosis, the patient should be referred for medical assessment.

For tendonitis of this kind, strapping of the foot may reduce the pain caused by movement and allow rest. The patient may need crutches and should rest and use ice.

Calf pain and injury

A gastrocnemius tear is a common sports injury; it often occurs at the medial head at its widest point, or at the Achilles musculotendinous junction. The patient will describe a sudden 'blow' to the calf while lunging forward. Stretching of the muscle will hurt and the patient will walk on the ball of the foot with the knee bent. There will be tenderness at the tear, and bruising, swelling and a palpable gap in the tissue are possible. Passive dorsiflexion will hurt. The patient should rest and use ice to allow bleeding to settle. It is preferable with all but the smallest injuries to refer to a physiotherapist. Advise the use of orthopaedic felt to raise the heel to avoid stress on the tear. The patient may need crutches.

Other causes of calf pain include acute and chronic compartment syndromes. The risk of a deep vein thrombosis must be assessed in any patient who presents with calf pain with no history of injury. The absence of the classic signs, redness, heat and swelling, do not exclude the possibility. A ruptured Baker's cyst may mimic the appearance of deep vein thrombosis; this cyst is a herniated sac of synovial fluid in the popliteal area of the knee, which may open and drain into the calf. Ischaemic artery disease may cause pain in the lower leg, but it is unlikely that the undiagnosed condition would present in a minor injury clinic. Infection, superficial or deep, in the lower leg should be excluded.

The Achilles tendon

The Achilles tendon is prone to two injuries: overuse inflammation and rupture. The first may predispose to the second.

Achilles tendonitis is common among sportsmen, especially such groups as long-distance runners. Pain is felt at the back of the heel. There may be swelling, tenderness, crepitus, redness and heat, and there will be disability in all but the mildest cases. The pain will be felt on movement, and the inflammatory pattern of pain and stiffness on rising in the morning will be present.

Management is the same as for any tendon inflammation, but this type of tendonitis can easily become chronic. The patient may need crutches at first, and a physiotherapist may apply ankle strapping.

Achilles tendon rupture occurs by a similar mechanism of injury to that for a calf muscle tear, but the presentation and clinical appearance are different. The patient is unlikely to favour a plantarflexed gait. Patients are often middle aged, returning to sport or exercising irregularly. The rupture may be partial or complete.

The patient feels a sudden 'crack' over the tendon and will probably collapse. Even if the patient feels that walking is possible, the sense of having poor control of the foot makes patients wary of trying.

The patient should kneel up on a chair with the feet hanging over the front of the seat. If the calf is squeezed this will mimic contraction of the gastrocnemius and should plantarflex the foot if the tendon is intact. Comparing the result with the uninjured side will show the injured foot looking flat across the back of the ankle. It will rest in dorsiflexion. The uninjured foot will have a concavity at the back of the heel and will sit in slight plantarflexion. There may be a bruise and swelling at the rupture site, and a gap which is palpable or visible.

This injury needs orthopaedic treatment. Keep patients off their feet. If the tear is not complete, walking may extend it.

Ankle injuries

The inversion injury of the ankle, 'going over on it', is the commonest injury seen in minor injury clinics. The patient feels the ankle forced into inversion. Sometimes the mechanism is violent; sometimes it is trivial. The injury may be aggravated by extra force, if the patient is running, jumping, falling from a height or if the weight of another person is added. Patients who have had previous ankle injuries may be predisposed to further injury.

There is sickening pain. The patient usually has to sit or lie down and may feel faint and dizzy. There may be a sudden, immediate swelling, sometimes an 'egg' over the lateral malleolus, or swelling and bruising over a matter of hours. If swelling is large, the ankle may move into its loose-packed position. The patient may feel pain at the lateral ankle, over the lateral foot, tingling in the foot and shooting pains along the dorsal foot to the shin.

If the injury is a displaced fracture, there may be deformity consistent with dislocation or widening of the ankle joint, and the patient may need urgent orthopaedic treatment to reduce and stabilize the injury. The injury should be splinted, with a box splint if that is possible, constantly reassessing the distal innervation and circulation. The patient should be transferred as soon as possible.

Walking is always affected, and the severity of the injury may be partly assessed by the history of the patient's ability to walk from the time of injury until seen at the clinic. The common result of the inversion injury is to overstretch the soft tissues on the lateral side of the ankle – skin, tendons, joint capsule and ligaments – and to cause a sprain. The same mechanism may cause an avulsion fracture from the base of the lateral malleolus.

Another fracture, often seen in women of over middle age, is avulsion from the base of the fifth metatarsal of the foot at the insertion of the peroneus brevis muscle. This fracture, if it is uncomplicated, is often treated by rest, tubigrip and crutches. If the foot is very violently inverted, the tip of the medial malleolus may also be crushed.

If the pattern of injury has not been typical (if, for instance, there has been a rotation or eversion injury), there may be injury to ligaments other than those at the lateral ankle, and any patient who has a severe-looking injury should have further review. This may be immediate, from a doctor, for stress radiographs or soft tissue scanning, or later, from a physiotherapist, when the ankle is easier to examine. Some severe ligament injuries require treatment in plaster of Paris and even, on occasion, surgery.

Pain may be considerable in the first 1 to 2 days. Recommend analgesia (ibuprofen is often advocated if the patient can tolerate it), crutches may be required and the patient should be warned that it is common to have pain for six weeks or longer.

If the patient is discharged in the expectation that walking will improve rapidly, advice to return in a week if it is not improving should also be given.

Some foot problems

There are a number of foot problems that may be seen in the minor injury clinic.

1. The heel is unlikely to suffer fracture from a slight injury. Fracture is usually caused by falling onto the feet from a considerable height, and the force which fractures the heel may also injure the spine. Assess the patient fully.
2. Plantar fasciitis is often found in older people. Heel pain is felt as morning pain and on weight bearing, with no history of

injury. There will be tenderness at the medial tubercle on the plantar heel. X-ray film may show a bony spur at that site, although the relationship between the spur and the pain is not clear. The painful spot is the insertion point for the plantar aponeurosis. This passes forward along the sole of the foot to the connective tissues at the toes. The pain may be difficult to treat. Treatments which GPs try include heel pads to relieve the pressure, ultrasound from a physiotherapist and hydrocortisone injections.

3. Crush injuries to the foot from a heavy weight. These are painful with poor walking and a risk of fracture and acute compartment syndrome. The foot should be X-rayed to exclude bone injury. Passive toe movements will hurt if compartment syndrome is present. If in doubt, the patient should be referred for orthopaedic review. A patient who is discharged should take painkillers and use ice and elevation to reduce swelling and, perhaps, crutches. Advise the patient to return if the pain is worse or if circulation or sensation to the toes is reduced.
4. Tendinitis is common in the ankle and foot because of too much walking or running. It often occurs on the dorsum in the extensor tendons of the toes as they cross the anterior ankle. Pain will follow the inflammatory pattern. There may be crepitus. Immediate treatment is rest and ibuprofen if the patient can tolerate it. Gentle activity should be resumed when the symptoms have settled.
5. Paronychia may occur around the nail of the toes, in a similar manner to those of the hand (Ch. 6).
6. It is common to see a patient with sudden pain, redness and swelling in the big toe at the metatarsophalangeal joint and no history of injury. The patient should see a GP, but the NP should check that there is no sign of infection: temperature, systemic signs of infection (such as feverishness) and a possible break in the skin. If there is any suggestion of infection, refer for orthopaedic assessment. Osteoarthritis and gout are common causes for acute non-infective episodes of this kind.
7. Stubbed toes are very painful. Patients present with bruised swollen toes and pain on walking. They ask for an X-ray. If there is no obvious deformity of the toe, it is unlikely that X-ray film will influence management. The toes require buddy-strapping, ice and elevation; the patient should use pain killers, and the pain will usually be more managable in a day or two.

3

Part 3
OTHER MINOR INJURIES

8 MINOR WOUNDS AND BURNS

CONTENTS

Initial Presentation with Wounds

Triage

Patients with superficial wounds often believe that their injuries are more serious than they are. Conversely, patients will underestimate certain wounds, for instance where there is painless damage to tendons or where there is the potential for a vigorous infection. This probably owes much to the different impressions created by the frightening, visible aspect of a wound, the torn skin and the blood, and its quiet depths. Nevertheless, serious injuries are usually obvious, from the history of a severe mechanism, from the evidence of the wound itself and from the shocked appearance of the patient. Routinely patients do not sit in the waiting area of a minor injury clinic with unannounced, life-threatening wounds. There are, however, some situations where a NP will give an urgent priority to the patient.

Potential neurological damage

Many patients with wounds to face and head have superficial and easily treated injuries. However, the neurological situation should always be assessed before the wound is dealt with. If a patient is bleeding from the canal of the ear or from the nose (or if there is a discharge of pale fluid which tests positive to sugar on a urinalysis stick) after a blow to the head, the differential diagnosis includes fracture of the base of the skull. Consider the possibility of a depressed skull fracture with scalp lacerations, especially where the history is of blunt injury, where there are indications of neurological disturbance in the history or the examination, where there is a large haematoma, or where the bone surface does not feel smooth. Full-thickness scalp lacerations may need closure in layers.

Penetrating Wounds

Any patient with a penetrating wound, or any wound where the base of the lesion cannot be seen, over the neck, chest or abdomen is a potential emergency even if the patient seems uncompromised. The patient should be assessed for resuscitation (ABC: airways, breathing, circulation), monitor vital signs and transfer the patient to the appropriate medical team. Surgical exploration of the injury may be required.

Potential HIV infection

If a patient has just suffered a needlestick injury or a human bite and there is a possibility that HIV (human immunodeficiency virus) prophylaxis will be given, treatment is time critical. Do not lose a minute in contacting the responsible doctor. There are Department of Health guidelines (1997) on the treatment of needlestick injuries to health workers and there should be a local policy based on them and contact numbers for advice. The assessment of a patient who has suffered a human bite wound will be covered by local guidelines or protocols. In practice, given the common hazards which accompany human bites – tendon and joint injuries, hepatitis B infection, aerobic and anaerobic bacterial infections, as well as the risk of HIV – every such patient may be referred to a doctor or, at the least, there should be a very low threshold for doing so.

Initial Problems

A patient will usually have a minor wound under control when arriving at the clinic. There will be a rough pressure dressing on the wound, controlling the **bleeding** and reducing the **pain**. The patient will not be likely to **faint** if the dressing is not touched and dressings should not be touched in a waiting area. It can never be known what will be seen, and bystanders will not be pleased with the chance to see or be splashed by blood. Bring the patient to a treatment area to lie down on a trolley.

Bleeding

Bleeding will stop if some swabs are put over the wound and direct pressure is applied with a gloved hand. In the case of a limb wound, elevation will reduce the flow of blood. An arterial bleed, with pulsing, spurting blood rather than a venous ooze, means that you are not dealing with a minor wound. Bleeding will stop with direct pressure, but it may be necessary to maintain pressure indefinitely to control the flow. Such bleeding may require surgery.

If there is heavy bleeding and glass or metal can be seen in the wound, do not remove the object, press on it or otherwise disturb it. Put swabs around the object and apply pressure proximal to it.

Bleeding is a factor throughout the treatment of a wound, and it can make exploration and closure difficult. With a hand wound, elevating the bleeding part often solves the problem. If the protocols or guidelines for the clinic do not allow use of a local anaesthetic with epinephrine (adrenaline; which causes vasoconstriction and thereby reduces bleeding at the wound), the patient can be referred for treatment by a doctor. A surgeon also has the option of using a tourniquet to provide a bloodless field for certain procedures.

Pain

A patient with a minor wound does not usually complain of pain until the wound is examined. Any pain which is caused during examination will settle if treatment is completed rapidly.

Most experts emphasize adequate anaesthesia, local or general, before embarking on cleaning and exploration.

In a minor injury clinic, many patients have small, superficial wounds (1 cm or less), which are painful to treat but which have a tiny risk of complications. The patient's reason for coming is that 'it wouldn't stop bleeding'. (Usually, by then, it has stopped, and the NP starts it again.) It is unpleasant to receive a local anaesthetic, and, in some sites such as the hand, it can be as painful as treatment. It is, therefore, reasonable to ask the patient to put up with the discomfort if the NP can predict that a small flap wound will be cleaned, explored and closed with steristrips in a matter of a minute or two.

If the wound is not complicated by any injury to deep structures, but needs suture (wounds with a Stanley knife to the fatty tissue of the thigh are a common example), a local anaesthetic is necessary and there is no point in cleaning or exploring the wound before it is given.

The most difficult situations arise when the patient has a wound which needs suture but when there is also a risk that exploration will reveal a complicating injury to a deep structure such as a tendon. This is often the case with wounds to the hand. The NP may not be sure at the outset that it will be possible to complete the treatment and may not wish to anaesthetize the injury until it is assessed. The exploration of a wound which is bleeding and painful cannot be done with any certainty of a correct result if it is not done under optimum conditions. The patient should be referred sooner rather than later. A wound which is both dirty and deep makes referral mandatory.

The time factor

The treatment of wounds, especially in cases where closure is an option, is time critical. Details of management are given below. The management of problems such as infection and deep structure injury is hampered if the wound is closed before those possibilities have been fully considered. Inappropriate closure of a wound may cause the patient harm. These factors mean that a patient with a wound requires management which is both prompt and accurate (in contrast, for example, to a sprain, where full assessment might be deferred until it is easier). If there is any doubt about a wound, the patient should be referred at once.

Faint

If it takes a few minutes to clean, explore and close a small hand wound, the patient is likely to feel faint. There is no reason not to lie all patients with wounds on a trolley. Some patients are happy to lie flat while the nurse work. Others resist this. Do not assume that a patient who sits up and watches everything you are doing will not faint. Watch the patient and make sure the backrest can be reached easily. Patients become pale before they faint. If patients lie down at this stage, they will soon feel better. Relatives in the treatment room may also faint.

Blood-borne infection

A wound is a potential hazard to any health worker who comes into contact with it because of the risk of blood-borne infection.

Nurses run the risk of contracting hepatitis B and HIV. A nurse is treating a stranger with a wound, in a setting where only what the patient chooses to tell about the medical history is known. This means that nurses must be rigorous in their precautions against contact with the patient's body fluids. The patient may also have concerns in this situation. Nurses work in a high-risk environment, and the patient is entitled to know that there is also protection from the *nurse* who is touching his bleeding wound. Always use gloves, and a visor if there is a risk of a splash.

Occupational health departments have policies for staff protection, covering a variety of matters such as protective equipment, immunizations against hepatitis B, the cleaning up of contaminated spillage, and needlestick injuries.

Definition of a Minor Wound

A wound is a break in the skin. Wounds occur under many circumstances and require different responses. The wounds which concern us here are those caused by trauma.

Types of wound

A traumatic wound can be one of several types. The distinctions between them are important for assessment and treatment. Describe the wound accurately in the notes. The following terms are used to describe wounds.

Cut

A cut is a break which has been **incised** into the skin by something with a sharp edge such as a knife, razor blade or glass. These wounds look neat and tend to be relatively easy to close. The main concern with cuts is the ease with which deep structures like nerves, tendons and blood vessels may be divided.

Laceration

A laceration is a break in the skin caused by blunt force. The skin has been burst rather than cut. It will look more ragged than an incised wound. It may be **contused** (bruised). Blunt violence may complicate treatment. There may be brain injury or damage to any vital organ; there may be fracture. Swelling causes pain and compromises distal parts and makes suture inadvisable. Dirt and devitalized tissue carries a high risk of infection.

Penetrating wound

A penetrating wound is caused by something long, pointed and narrow. The term **puncture** is often used to describe penetrating wounds on the hand or sole of foot by nails, garden rakes or fence spikes. A penetrating wound looks like the least of wounds. The lurid, superficial signs are usually absent. There may be no external bleeding or bruising, and only the tiniest break in the skin.

The problem is that the base of a wound cannot be seen. It is impossible to assess the damage, see any foreign matter or achieve a satisfactory wound toilet. A penetrating wound over a vital area should be treated as serious until proven otherwise. Even when a vital organ is not threatened, there is a potential for tetanus and gangrene. There may also be penetration of tendon sheath, joint capsule or bone.

Abrasion

An abrasion is a graze, an injury caused by friction shearing the skin away. It is usually a combination of superficial and partial thickness trauma, but a severe mechanism can produce a much deeper wound. There is usually what Glasgow and Graham (1997) call a 'halo of inflammation' around the overtly damaged skin in superficial injuries. Abrasions are common in patients who have fallen off bicycles.

Minor abrasions can be as painful as a superficial burn. Unfortunately, they are often very dirty, with embedded grit, mud and burned-in discolouration in an area of raw tissue. It is vital to clean an abrasion properly for two reasons. The first is infection. The second is a cosmetic problem. New skin which forms over superfical dirt will preserve it but not hide it, and the patient will have a permanent tattoo. Cleaning may require the use of a local anaesthetic (either infiltrated or applied topically) and a nail or toothbrush. There is sometimes a mutual reluctance to undertake this, but you will do your patient no kindness if you fail to do this job properly.

When is a wound minor?

Chapter 1 discussed the meaning of the word 'minor', in the term minor injury. The term 'minor wound' is a subset of this larger category. The opposite notion, of a 'major' wounds, is not quite so easy to pin down, and it is more important to assess the patient in terms of the history of the entire episode than to focus on the fact that there is a wound. If someone falls 20 feet and lands on his head on concrete, the fact that there is a small gash on the scalp will not be the first concern.

A NP may regard a wound as minor if it presents no complications which oblige a referral of the patient to a doctor. Such complications may include problems with exploration; cleaning or closure of the wound; concern about the size, depth or site of the wound; or mechanism of wounding, such as extreme violence or a human bite. Some complicating factors of wounds will now be discussed.

Factors which complicate wound management

Special types of wound are discussed later in this chapter. A main feature of a traumatic wound, compared with a surgical incision, or even with a pressure sore, is the amount that is unknown, uncontrolled and variable about the cause. For the NP, this means that the priority of management, and the source of most of the problems, is not the closure or the dressing of the wound but the assessment of a range of risk factors which attend the injury. These factors are different from one patient to another. The history and, in particular, the mechanism of injury are the best guides to the possible hazards in any case.

Fractures

Injury to bone can occur with blunt trauma, giving rise to an open or compound fracture. In crush injuries, the wound may be dirty and the fracture comminuted.

Infection

The risk of infection is increased by the presence of dirt, devitalized tissue and haematoma and by a delay in treatment. Puncture wounds and human and animal bites carry risks which will be described below.

Foreign bodies

There are two groups of foreign bodies: those that are **radio-opaque**, (visible on X-ray) and those which are **radiolucent**. Radio-opaque objects include metal, glass, grit and tooth. Wood, a common foreign body in the form of splinters in the hand, is not radio-opaque, although it may be visible on X-ray film if it is covered with a metal-based paint.

Ultrasound may detect foreign bodies which cannot be seen on X-ray films. If there is a strong reason to suspect that a foreign body is present in a wound, refer the patient for investigation.

Damage to an underlying structure

It is important to exclude the possibility that any structure which lies below the skin, in the area which the wound might reach, has been damaged. Over the head, neck and trunk, this may include an injury to a vital organ. In the limbs, the tissues which will be affected are the nerves, blood vessels and the musculoskeletal tissues.

The commonest site of accidental wounding is the hand, and this question is nearly always relevant here. The hand combines power, finesse and mobility in a structure which is not bulky. One of the reasons for this is that much of its muscle power is generated from a distance and transmitted along a network of long, cable-like structures, the tendons, which travel almost to the tips of the fingers. These tendons, and the nerves and blood vessels which accompany them, lie just below the skin, on top of an unyielding surface of bone. They are vulnerable to division by cutting or crush. The hand also has a large number of joints in a relatively small area, and these can be injured by penetrating wounds.

Late presentation

If a wound which requires suture is more than 6 hours old and it has received no treatment, it is assumed that infection has started to develop. Primary closure (see below) may not be appropriate. In fact, a trauma doctor may choose to close the wound if other factors are favourable (such as an absence of dirt and devitalized tissue in the wound), but it is likely that the protocols or guidelines will require referral of such patients to a doctor. Do not close a wound if you are doubtful.

Assessment and Exploration of Wounds

Some considerations have already been discussed, the mechanism of injury, the patient's lifestyle, medical history and medications (with particular interest in antibiotic and elastoplast allergy, anticoagulant, immunosuppressive or corticosteroid medicines, and a history of diabetes). These will inform an assessment of the patient and the wound.

This section will focus on factors specific to the wound.

The Injured Tissue

The assessment of a wound will cover not only the extent of the damage but also the viability and health of the injured tissue. Important factors will include the patient's age, the site of the injury, the patient's health, the quality of the circulation and innervation at the injured area, the frailty of the skin, whether or not the wound will affect a major function such as walking or eating, and the cosmetic significance of the wound. These considerations will influence the management of the injury.

Exploration

A fundamental concept is *never close a wound unless you have seen its base*.

The purpose of wound exploration is to discover the extent of the damage and the threat to the injured tissue. The main categories of problem that will be assessed are damage to underlying structures (see above); the presence of devitalized tissue, which will cause infection; the presence of dirt; and the presence of other foreign materials (commonly, wood, glass and metal).

These risks cannot be assessed if the wound cannot be seen clearly. There must be a good light source (preferably an adjustable spot lamp). Bleeding and pain must be under control.

The initial unpleasantness of bleeding and tearing of skin can make a superficial wound seem worse than it is. The lack of those signs can make a penetrating wound seem trivial. The tendency to underestimate innocuous looking wounds is not confined to patients, and the NP must guard against it. Be extremely curious about every aspect of a wound and answer all the questions before it is closed. It might be expected that an open injury would be easier to assess than a closed one such as a sprain, simply because the access to the damaged tissue is greater. Often, this is not the case.

Penetrating wounds are, by definition, longer than they are wide, and for all that they are open, they are not accessible. Any worrying feature – dirt, foreign body, penetration to a vital area – will lie deep. Penetrating wounds can be assessed indirectly, by probe (do not probe wounds which are near vital organs), and by testing the function of the underlying structures. They can be cleaned by irrigation. They can be X-rayed for foreign bodies. However, except in the cases where surgical exploration is required, they resist a comprehensive inspection and full cleaning. They are prone to many complications and can threaten life and limb.

The difficulty of assessment is not, however, confined to penetrating wounds. Wounds are intrinsically deceptive. Once a wound has stopped bleeding, a clot forms, and the deeper layers of the wound can be covered and held together. Subcutaneous fat is a globular, clustered material and it can be hard to tell if it has been penetrated. Anyone who has experience of wound assessment will remember cleaning an apparently shallow wound which has suddenly popped open to reveal a much deeper injury. This becomes more likely when the wound is a few hours or days old.

Another factor which leads to concealment of the extent of an injury is that the different tissues under the skin have varying degrees of mobility. If a patient closes his fist and punches through a pane of glass, cutting his knuckles and partly dividing his extensor tendon, there is no point in lying the hand flat to explore the wound. The tendon moves over a greater distance than the skin when the hand is opened and closed, and the divided part will no longer be visible in the wound. Find out what position the hand was in when it was injured and explore the cut in that position. It is wise to inspect the wound through the whole range of movement.

A related problem is that tendons which are completely divided by an injury will shrink or be pulled away from the wound by the contraction of muscles and the movement of joints. There is no comfort in the fact that a tendon cannot be seen in a wound if there should be one there. A NP must know the relevant anatomy to assess the wound. Supplement a visual inspection by tests of the function of the local tendons nerves and circulation.

Another difficult feature of wounds is that many of the common complications develop over a period of hours or days. The signs of infection do not usually appear in the first few hours. The loss of sensation which heralds a damaged sensory nerve may deepen over days. A partly divided tendon may fulfil its function, although its action will probably be weak. Later, it may divide completely. Complete division of the central tendon of the extensor mechanism of the finger, at the proximal interphalangeal joint (PIPJ) may be concealed by the fact that the lateral tendons will continue to work as extensors of the PIPJ, perhaps for days; however, the boutonnière deformity (see Ch. 6) will develop eventually. There will be little hope of a good recovery at that stage.

A sterile, round-tipped wound probe can be a helpful aid in wound exploration, for assessing depth in places that cannot be seen and for detecting, by touch, hard foreign bodies. Probes should be used very gently, and only in places where they will do no harm.

The term 'exploration' has been used here to describe a process which is performed in a minor injury clinic. A full exploration of a difficult wound is a surgical procedure, done in theatre conditions with good anaesthesia and instruments, and with the skills and resources to deal with any problems which arise. If your own skills and facilities are not adequate, do not be tempted to go too far. It is easy to stray out of your depth when dealing with wounds.

Other Tests for Complications

Every patient whose wound cannot be seen to the base needs to be sent to a surgeon. The indications for further exploration may include a wound over a vital area, the known presence of a foreign body of fair size, a strong suspicion that a deep structure has been injured or the presence of dangerous contamination.

There are three main methods, in a minor injury clinic, to supplement exploration to exclude complications.

Observation

Observe for external signs of complication. The local signs of wound infection are pain, redness, heat, swelling, offensive discharge and odour, failure to heal and ascending lymphangitis (the 'tracking' red line moving proximally). The lymph nodes in the area may rise (often in the axilla or groin) and systemic signs, pyrexia and malaise, may develop.

Test of Function

Test the function of parts which may be injured. Always assess the nerves and circulation distal to the injury. Test that the patient can feel light touch, that pulses are present and that the colour and temperature of the tissues are normal. In a skin loss injury, assess sensation over the whole injured area to exclude a full thickness wound.

Test tendons carefully. There are two main concerns.

- A problem may be overlooked, for example if a particular function is carried out by more than one muscle and only one of them is damaged. Tendons which move distal joints will also contribute to the movement of every joint that they pass over. Tests can be used which isolate the single tendon that is giving concern.
- A tendon injury can be worsened, for example if there is a piece of glass in a wound and the tendon is mobilized over it, or if a tendon is partly divided and the test completes the job.

A tendon test should be applied against resistance to be conclusive, with power compared with the other side. A patient may retain active movement by using a substitute tendon, or a partly damaged one, but should not have full power. This test has the potential to worsen damage. Do not do it if there are already grounds to think the tendon is cut. Apply and release the resistance gently, and stop at once if there is weakness. Sometimes the pain of the wound prevents the patient from using full power.

Radiography

X-ray can be used to exclude bone injuries where an open fracture is possible and to reveal metal or glass foreign bodies.

Wound Cleaning

Consensus is lacking on certain matters which surround the subject of wound cleaning. Some recommendations, such as those on the role of antiseptics in cleaning, are prone to pendulum swings, which makes confident practice difficult. Topics which are debated include the effectiveness of chemical cleansers in reducing infection and the toxicity of cleansing agents to healthy cells in the wound. In spite of this, the clinicians whose writings are current have a large core of agreement on the advice that they offer for day-to-day treatment of acute wounds.

There are given reasons for cleaning a wound, and a recent, untreated, traumatic wound should always be cleaned thoroughly. However, the fact that the NP sees a wound does not mean that the NP should reflexively clean it. If it is dry, clean and healing, with no signs of infection, leave it. It is also wise to advise patients on such matters. There can be a tendency to overuse powerful disinfectants at home.

Reasons for wound cleaning

Infection

A thorough and effective wound toilet is the key measure which will reduce the risk of infection in the wound. This includes measures such as debriding necrotic or contaminated tissue, evacuating haematoma and getting rid of foreign matter, both small particles of dirt and larger objects. What constitutes an effective wound toilet depends on the nature of the wound and the infection risk factors which apply to the particular injury.

Cosmetic

The discussion on abrasions (above) has already covered the need to remove all dirt embedded in the dermal/epidermal tissue so that it will not form an unwanted tattoo. The cosmetic issue is also linked to the question of infection. An infected wound will not heal, sutured edges will break down, the wound may have to be reopened, and any scarring will be worse than it need have been.

Exploration

A wound cannot be explored if it is covered in dirt, and the discovery of foreign matter of any kind in the wound, which may cause infection, inflammation or injury, is one of the objects of exploration. Cleaning and exploration are reciprocal activities which are discussed separately but carried out together.

Cleaning agents

Water

The effective removal of dirt, as opposed to bacteria, is more a matter of *how much* rather than *what* fluid, and the ordinary tap is the best source of an unlimited supply.

Saline

Normal saline is widely used for cleaning wounds, both for wiping the wound edges and for irrigation of the open area. It will not irritate the damaged tissue but neither does it have any antiseptic effect.

Povidone iodine

Povidone iodine is a combination of substances of which the active agent is iodine, an antiseptic which acts against Gram-positive and Gram-negative bacteria as well as fungi and viruses. The prepartion of povidone iodine which is used as a surgical scrub contains a detergent which is not intended for use in open wounds. Trott (1997) recommends a 1% solution of povidone iodine in saline for wound periphery cleansing. It retains its antibacterial effects with no apparent toxicity problems.

Chlorhexidine

Chlorhexidine is an antibacterial agent which Trott (1997) describes as having strong Gram-positive action but, perhaps, a weaker Gram-negative action than that of povidone iodine. He cites a particular benefit in the use of chlorhexidine as a hand cleaner. It can build up on skin and apparently suppresses bacterial activity over a longer period than other cleansers. He also recommends it as a wound periphery cleanser. He advises against using the detergent-based hand-scrub in the wound itself.

Methods of wound cleaning

Lacerations and cuts

The need for adequate anaesthesia has aleady been discussed above.

Continue cleaning until there is no visible dirt in a wound and the tissue has a pink, fresh look, possibly with a little bleeding.

Cleaning is taken in two stages.

1. The edges of the wound, where tissue is intact, are wiped as vigorously as is required to clean away all visible dirt and blood. The technique is to wipe away from the edge, using a wet gauze swab, so that no contaminants or microbes are carried

into the wound. A patient who is covered in oil or paint may need to use swarfega to clean the skin, avoiding the open wound.
2. Irrigation is considered to be the best way to clean the open wound area because rubbing or scrubbing can damage wound cells, and materials like gauze or cotton wool can leave strands in the wound.

The best way to achieve a reduction in bacteria in a wound is to irrigate under high pressure, regardless of which cleaning material is used. Irrigation is also effective for removing a good deal of visible dirt. If there is serious contamination, other techniques may also be required. High-pressure irrigation is described slightly differently by different clinicians, but the commonest recommendation is to use a 35 ml syringe with a 19 gauge needle and direct fluid from very close range, at full power, into the wound. This is said to create a pressure of 8 psi. A large amount (up to 500 ml) may be required. Splash guard precautions should be taken and there may be a fair amount of mess.

Penetrating injuries are, by their nature, impossible to clean in a satisfactory way, but high-pressure irrigation can be used on the punctures which commonly occur to the sole of the foot or the hand, which do not require surgical exploration.

Abrasions

The particular reasons for the need to clean abrasions thoroughly have already been discussed earlier in this chapter.

A fresh abrasion is very painful. Cleaning may have to be vigorous, often with a brush, and some pieces of dirt may need to be picked out from little sacs of skin with needle or forceps. Dirt may be ingrained like a permanent stain and may not surrender even to scrubbing with a brush. Children are often injured in this manner and the management of a child's distress may be difficult.

Morton and Phillips (1996) recommend the topical application of 2% lidocaine gel to a child's graze, 15 minutes before cleaning, to reduce the pain and give some anaesthesia. Such gel stings on application and is not designated for use on wounds, but it does reduce the discomfort of cleaning in cases where a short scrub with a soft brush will complete the job. Morton and Phillips also recommend, for children, the infiltration of small grazes with an injection of lidocaine. The usefulness of injected local anaesthetic for cleaning abrasions is restricted because larger grazes require amounts which exceed the maximum dose. Extreme care has to be taken in this regard with children. Abrasions which are large, or which are on the face, may require cleaning under a general anaesthetic.

A NP considering treating a child, must think carefully about the possible problems, and refer if there is any doubt.

Debridement

Wound cleaning is part of a continuum which includes surgical techniques to remove contaminants. If these procedures are indicated, the patient requires a medical assessment, not only because of the difficulty which wound cleaning presents but also because that degree of contamination raises other issues, such as wound closure and antibiotic prophylaxis.

Wound Infection

Infection is the main complication of traumatic wounds. The steps that are taken to prevent infection when a new wound is treated may be an important contribution to healing.

A NP may also, depending on local protocols or guidelines, treat established infections which are still local to the area of the wound.

What is a Wound Infection?

The skin, along with other areas of the body, is colonized by **commensal** flora. These are microorganisms which coexist with each other and their host and cause no illness as long as they are checked by their neighbours and stay in their given area. A wound, a break in the skin, allows these microbes to penetrate where they should not be. It also involves the violent invasion, through the barrier of the skin, of some implement from the dirty outer world, shedding its own load of microscopic life forms. The patient then visits a hospital and is exposed to the infection hazards which medical treatment entails.

An organism which multiplies to an extent where it causes harm to its host is called a **pathogen**. The harmful process is an **infection**. The collective term for the organisms which cause most of the wound infections which concern a minor injury clinic is **bacteria**.

Bacteria are subdivided into groups by their shape, their response to laboratory staining and their need of oxygen. Three bacteria are mentioned here. A fourth, which causes tetanus, will be discussed in greater detail below.

Staphylococcus aureus is an aerobic Gram-positive bacterium and it appears, from the frequency with which it is cultured from swabs, to cause most of the traumatic wound infections which are seen in hospital. It is highly resistant to penicillin but sensitive to flucloxacillin and erythromycin. It is a commensal, found in the nares and other sites where there is hair or mucous membranes. It can cause superficial wound infections and abscesses, osteomyelitis and septicaemia. The toxin-producing variety can cause the fatal **toxic shock syndrome**, which is best known in relation to tampon use.

Streptococcus pyogenes is also a Gram-positive aerobic bacterium, and another common offender in traumatic wound infections. It is sensitive to penicillin and erythromycin. It is a commensal in some people and is found in the mucous membranes. It also causes cellulitis and can cause necrotizing fasciitis, septicaemia and toxic shock.

Clostridium welchii is an anaerobic Gram-positive bacterium. It, and other organisms of the same family, cause gas gangrene infection, a dire threat to life and limb. It is a commensal of the human gut and is found in soil. It can form spores and lie dormant in a protective shell, highly resistant to destruction, until conditions are suitable for it to multiply. Anaerobes flourish where oxygen is lacking. Wounds with devitalized tissue are ideal ground for reproduction. The reproducing organism creates gas, hydrogen and nitrogen, and exotoxins' which consume healthy tissue and threaten systemic collapse. *Clostridium welchii* is sensitive to penicillin.

The wounds which are prone to anaerobic infection are those with violent tissue destruction under dirty conditions, such as war injuries and farmyard accidents. As a general rule, these are severe injuries and will not be seen in a minor injury clinic. Among wounds which are likely to be seen in minor injury clinics, dirty penetrating wounds which are difficult to clean at the base are at the greatest risk of anaerobic infection.

A patient who is at a high risk of anaerobic infection may require a combination of prophylactic antibiotics and surgical treatment, with delayed closure of the wound if closure is necessary. (Closure of a dirty wound is a positive encouragement to anaerobic infection.) Refer such patients promptly.

When is a Wound Infected?

A microbiology laboratory will describe a wound as infected if certain levels of bacteria are cultured from a swab. Such levels can often be found in a traumatic wound which has not yet been cleaned and is showing no signs of infection but is more than 6 hours old. (This is why it is preferable not to suture such wounds.)

Laboratory assessment is not of great practical value to the NP. First, a NP will be treating wounds on their clinical appearance, and with the benefit of no more than a few minutes with the patient. Second, a NP will not take swabs unless an infection is already suspected, and initial management of the problem must be decided before a result is received. Third, a positive laboratory finding would not usually lead to treatment of the wound as infected when there are no clinical signs or other risk factors.

The treatment of a wound as infected is based on clinical judgement of two types of factor: indicators for a high risk of infection and clinical signs of infection.

Factors which create a high risk of infection in a wound that does not appear to be infected include:

- wounds which require closure but are not treated for more than 6 hours
- wounds which are very dirty
- wounds which contain devitalized tissue
- penetrating wounds
- bites, animal or human.

A patient with such a wound may be given prophylactic antibiotics (although this may not prevent infection) in addition to the care which the wound itself receives.

The decision to give prophylactic treatment is one that is made in compliance with local protocols or guidelines. The NP may be required to refer any patient with an infection-prone wound to a doctor.

There are a number of clinical signs of infection.

- Pain beyond the expected level (which is usually not great in a healing wound), or worsening instead of settling, suggests infection. Pus collected under a wound causes a throbbing pain. Examine local structures, including tendon, bone and joint for tenderness and other symptoms which suggest a spread of infection.

- Redness is a normal feature of a healing wound, but it should not spread beyond the immediate wound edge. Trott (1997) gives the distance as 5 mm. Spreading redness or redness which tracks proximally, **ascending lymphangitis**, is a sign of infection. Assess the rate of spread and mark its boundaries with a pen so that further assessment can be made.

- Local heat is a sign of inflammation. Assess local structures for spread.

- Swelling can be caused by pus, a localized fluctuant swelling or a general inflammation. If structures such as joints or bursae are swollen, the patient needs orthopaedic review to exclude a joint sepsis. Certain structures, such as the palmar spaces of the hand, can develop abscesses, which need orthopaedic review and drainage.

- A wound which remains moist. Closed wounds should become dry very quickly. Abrasions may exude serous fluid for a few days, but then they should develop a dry fresh granulation. Persistent exudate is a sign of inflammation, and infection is a probable cause. Pus is a sign of infection.

- A wound which does not heal but is not developing any florid signs of infection should be swabbed for culture. This kind of problem is not seen in a minor injury clinic very often. It is a late complication and usually the patient has moved on to the primary care team by then. Obtain a medical opinion. If a wound is not healing you need to know why. A grumbling infection is one, but not the only, possibility. Scarring may be worse if the issue is not settled, and wounds on the lower leg can ulcerate. There may be a foreign body in the wound, a deep infection or an underlying medical complaint. If the patient is a diabetic, has circulation problems or wound healing difficulties for any other reason, there is a risk of gangrene.

- An offensive odour may indicate anaerobic bacteria, a possibility which is greater if the wound is deep, a dirty puncture, one with devitalized tissue, a large haematoma, or an animal bite.

• Raised lymph nodes proximal to the injury indicate an immune response to infection. Assess the axilla or the groin, looking for a difference on the affected side: pea-sized, firm swellings and tenderness.

• Systemic signs of infection may occur, especially feverish shivering. A patient may look pale, tired and unwell, or flushed and sweaty. The patient may complain of malaise, aching joints, tiredness, anorexia or upset stomach. The patient's temperature may be raised and the pulse faster than normal.

Treatment of an Infected Wound

Abscess

A collection of pus, with a painful, fluctuant swelling but no signs of tracking or systemic infection, can be treated by opening the swelling, draining it and letting the open wound heal under the supervision of the practice nurse.

Local treatment is sufficient if there is no cellulitis or other signs of spreading infection.

Spreading infection

A wound should be treated with antibiotics if it shows a spreading redness, a **cellulitis**, an ascending lymphangitis, or it involves bone or joint, shows signs of tissue death, threatens sensitive areas such as the eye (ask for a doctor's opinion of any infection of the face) or is accompanied by malaise.

The infection may require specialist intervention, such as joint aspiration and lavage, wound debridement and, in some cases, life-saving measures to treat septicaemia or toxic shock. Where systemic infection is suspected, blood may be taken to assess the white cell count, which will rise in response to infection, and for culture, to exclude septicaemia.

Treatment is offered on a wide scale, depending on the nature and degree of the problem. When an infection is no longer localized, the patient may require intravenous antibiotics, requiring admittance to hospital.

It is probable that the NP will have a twofold role: to offer definitive treatment where the problem is very localized and to make a referral when a more serious infection is apparent. If a patient is treated without referral, give full advice, so that the patient will return if the infection gets worse or does not improve.

Tetanus

The Joint Committee on Vaccination and Immunisation issues national guidance from the various Departments of Health in the UK in the form of its Green Book: Immunisation against Infectious Disease. The information in this section is largely based on that source.

Tetanus is the disease caused by *Clostridium tetani*, an anaerobic Gram-positive bacillus, which forms spores. *Clostridium tetani* is a commensal of the gut, found in humans and most particularly in grass-eating animals. It passes into the soil, where it can survive as a spore until a suitable host is found. The organism enters through a wound and multiplies in an anaerobic environment, which the injury is more likely to offer if it is a deep puncture, if there is devitalized tissue, haematoma, or if other infection is present. The organism produces an exotoxin which attacks motor nerves. It travels up into the central nervous system and triggers the disease tetanus. The disease may incubate from 4 to 21 days.

There are very few cases of tetanus in the UK because there is a good immunization programme, but this disease cannot be eliminated by reducing its incidence. The spores are still out there, and any patient with a wound who is not properly immunized, is at risk.

The history of the immunization programme indicates that two main groups have received immunizations, everyone who was born after the early 1960s and older people who served in the armed forces from the Second World War onwards. Therefore, older women might be most at risk. There were 145 cases of tetanus in the UK from 1984 until 1995. Women over 65 years are indeed the largest single group of those affected.

There is a national immunization programme for children, which should mean that any person who presents at a minor injury clinic who is under the age of 25 years will be protected. The programme gives children the vaccine in combination with other vaccines, a combined diptheria and tetanus vaccination, in the school years. If a NP is treating a child who has a tetanus-prone wound (see below), and believes that the child should have a booster of adsorbed vaccine, remember that this should be the combined vaccine. If local guidelines do not cover that situation, take advice.

In connection with tetanus vaccine, two terms are used which require explanation. The vaccine is a weak toxin. To increase its effect as an immunogen, it is combined with a preparation which attracts or **adsorbs** it and enhances or **adjuvates** its effect. Aluminium phosphate or hydroxide are the usual agents. The vaccine is called **adsorbed tetanus vaccine** and it is prepared for injection (0.5 ml) by deep subcutaneous or intramuscular route. It causes the host to produce antitoxin and this gives active immunity.

Passive immunity can be provided by giving a dose of **human tetanus immunoglobulin**. This comes in ampoules of 250 IU and is given by intramuscular injection.

A child receives a three-dose initial course of adsorbed vaccine in infancy, followed by two booster doses at 5 and 15 years approximately. This is probably enough to protect for life.

For an adult who has not been immunized, give a dose of vaccine, and arrange for two further doses, each spaced 4 weeks apart, so that a whole course is completed in 2 months approximately. After that, the patient should have a booster dose of vaccine after 10 years, and once more after a further 10 years. This total of five doses is considered sufficient to give lifetime immunity.

Certain wounds are considered to be **tetanus prone** and patients may sometimes require passive immunisation with human tetanus immunoglobulin:

- untreated wounds which are more than 6 hours old
- where devitalized tissue is evident
- punctures
- contamination by soil or manure
- infected wounds.

A thorough wound toilet is vital.

A patient with a tetanus-prone wound and immunizations up to date will not need any further adsorbed vaccine. If the contamination is of very high risk (e.g. manure), the patient may be given a dose of tetanus immunoglobulin. If the patient has had a course of adsorbed vaccine but has not had a booster for more than 10 years, then the NP should give a booster dose of adsorbed vaccine and a dose of immunoglobulin. If there is any doubt that the patient has ever had a course of adsorbed vaccine, give the first injection of the course, and a dose of immunoglobulin, and arrange for the course of adsorbed vaccine to be completed.

The only contraindications which are listed for adsorbed tetanus vaccine are the presence of an acute febrile illness (unless the wound is tetanus prone) and a history of a previous anaphylactic reaction to the vaccine. The vaccine is not live, so there is no contraindication for pregnant women.

The only common adverse reaction is a local, painful, red swelling around the injection site, which may last for a few days.

Wound Treatment

Medical treatment does not repair wounds. The body does that itself. There is, however, scope for intervention to optimize healing, prevent complications and to undo damage nature cannot correct.

If natural processes will see a wound healed, there is no virtue (and perhaps some risk) in any intervention. Understand the process of healing and its problems and ensure that treatments have a clear aim and the likelihood of improving the outcome.

Wound Healing and the Scar

The healing of musculoskeletal injuries has been described in Chapter 5. That process applies to wounds. Healing occurs by the same stages of inflammation, proliferation and maturation. It usually results in an imperfect replacement of the damaged tissue with scar tissue (superficial burns and grazes, where the germinal layer of epithelium is unbroken, can heal without scarring).

The difficulties which a scar can cause in tissues like ligament and muscle have been discussed, and scarring of the skin over a joint can lead to restriction of movement. However, the commonest concern which patients feel about wound scars is their visibility. The term 'cosmetic' has an unfortunate association with ideas of superfical appearance and frivolity. In wound care, it is a vital part of good treatment, connected to notions of self-esteem and confidence, and even mental health. It may have an impact on personal relationships and employment. In cases where the appearance of the wound is not sufficiently considered during treatment, the patient may sue.

The process of wound healing might be summarized as follows. A wound exists from the moment the skin is broken. There is bleeding. The injured skin retracts, closing off small injured vessels at its edges, and other processes (vasoconstriction and the activation of coagulation mechanisms) lead to the development of a clot within a few minutes. The inflammatory phase begins, to combat infection and clear away wound debris by phagocytosis. It lasts for some days. Overlapping with this activity, the base layer of the epithelium starts to propogate the cells of a granulation tissue which covers the wound, usually generating the new cells into the wound from its edges. The processes of establishing new blood vessels, and the development of collagen from fibroblasts, herald the formation of the scar. It will develop, with remodelling, over many months. It will gain in strength, and shrink, and become pale and avascular.

It will not be possible to evaluate the cosmetic effect of the scar fully until this process is complete.

The Aims of Wound Treatment

Wound treatment is intended:

- to repair any damage to deep structures
- to remove foreign material from the wound and minimize the risk of infection
- to promote healing with the minimum of scarring.

The first two of these points are discussed in other sections. The success of the third stage will depend, in part, on the care which has been shown in the first two, especially the second. The condition of the wound, in terms of such factors as the time elapsed since injury, dirt and swelling, skin loss, devitalized tissue, bite injury, will also dictate the approach to the last stage of treatment. There are several options.

Wound Closure

Wound closure is the process of bringing the divided tissues in the wound together, **opposition**, in the anatomical position which the injury has disrupted, from base to surface of the lesion, and stabilizing them in that position until they begin to heal.

Wound closure has functional benefits. It gives the damaged layers of tissue the best chance of resuming their previous relationships and roles. The scar will be minimal, and healing will be quick. The wound will have some external support, and this may allow the patient some use of the injured part while it is healing.

There is a distinction between closure of the layers of tissue, skin, fat and fascia, and repair of vital structures: blood vessels, nerves, tendons. A tidy opposition of the separated edges, with a minimal scar and a minimal loss of function, is the aim of closure. Repair of a specialized tissue, such as a flexor tendon in the hand, is more difficult. Crude opposition of the separated tissues may not restore function.

It is important to reassemble the separated layers from wound base to skin, rejoining each level of tissue, and leaving no gap, no **dead space**, where infection can develop.

Layered closure may sometimes be desirable because the wound tends to gape. A surface closure may not offer sufficient support. The wounds edges may be under great tension, which restricts the blood supply, makes the scar worse and carries the risk of reopening after the sutures are removed. A deep, absorbable suture will reduce tension on the wound edges.

It is likely that local protocols or guidelines will indicate referral to a doctor for a patient whose wound requires layered closure.

Approaches to closure

It is preferable to close a wound, but there are reason why wounds should not be closed because of the risk of complications, which will be worsened by closure or will prevent healing. These include a high risk of infection and an inability to explore the wound fully.

There are also wounds which fall into conflicting categories, where closure may, or must, be achieved, but the risks are too high to perform it at once.

Primary closure (primary intention)

Primary closure is the preferred pathway: the immediate closure at the time of first treatment of a low-risk wound. The wounds which are closed in minor injury clinics are in this category.

Secondary closure (healing by secondary intention)

Healing by secondary intention refers to the method of care for wounds which may not be closed and which will be left to granulate. The main option, in this case, if the final scar is not acceptable, is the grafting of skin to the site.

Small, cosmetically unimportant wounds can be treated by this method in the minor injury clinic, but any which are more difficult will require medical management, possibly by a plastic surgeon.

Delayed primary closure (tertiary closure)

A wound which carries a high infection risk at the time of first treatment may be left open for 4 days, approximately, and then closed. The levels of microorganisms in the tissue will have been reduced by the patient's own defences, and this process may have been assisted by antiseptic wound packs and oral antibiotics. The wound may require 'freshening', debriding the edges partly to restart the healing process.

Delayed primary closure will be managed by a doctor.

Closure with Steristrips

Steristrips are sticky, porous, reinforced paper tapes used in long narrow strips for wound closure. There are other products of this type.

Wardrope and Edhouse (1999) say that 'primary closure by suture is the commonest method of wound closure practised in most A&E departments'. This is not the case in my own place of work, where steristrips are the standard method of closure, and scalp wounds are treated with wound staples. This may be because of the differences in the range of work done in the two settings. It may also be that nurses are more conversant with Steristrips than doctors and use them more widely.

The *advantages* of Steristrips, over sutures, are:

- they are cheaper
- they can be applied very quickly, with minimal preparation and very little equipment
- they are painless to apply, making local anaesthetic unnecessary; this is of great value with children
- there is less traumatic tissue handling
- they can be used on frail skin which would not sustain a suture
- they are non-invasive, leaving no scars and no extra wounds, causing no irritation, and reducing the hazards of infection
- they are not prone to the complications of poor suture technique
- patients can usually remove them themselves at home

The *limits* and *disadvantages* of Steristrips are:

- they can only be used for superficial wounds; they cannot close a dead space
- they have to be kept dry
- they are less robust than sutures on an area like the hand, and patients may be able to perform more of their normal activities with sutures
- Steristrips will not stick in areas where there is hair
- there are problems if they are used on very mobile skin, such as the extensor joints of the fingers: they do not stretch with the skin, they tend not to hold the closure in good position, and they may fall off

Wardrope and Edhouse (1999) make the point that the advocacy of this swift and easy method of wound closure does not imply that cleaning and exploration may be skimped.

Application of Steristrips

Steristrips are supplied in 3 mm × 75 mm width, which is very useful for small, not very tense, superficial wounds. A strip of 6 mm can be used on larger areas. (These are often valuable for pre-tibial lacerations.)

The use of Tincture Benz Co is sometimes advocated for application around the wound edges to increase adhesion. Walton and Matory (1992) say that it dissolves quickly on the skin and becomes ineffective. Steristrips will usually stick, with no other adhesive, if the skin is well cleaned and dried (Fig. 8.1). A problem with adhesion may indicate that there is too much skin tension (in which case a wider strip or suture may be more appropriate) or that haemostasis has not quite been achieved.

It is not usually necessary, with small wounds, to use the full length of the strips, and they are often inconvenient at full length. If strips are used on fingers or toes, they should not pass circumferentially around the digit as they may restrict circulation. If it is intended to put an adhesive dressing on top of the strips then the dressing pad should cover the strips entirely. Otherwise the strips will pull off when the dressing is changed.

The strips are porous, but it is recommended that a space is left between them of approximately 3 mm (i.e. equal to the width of the

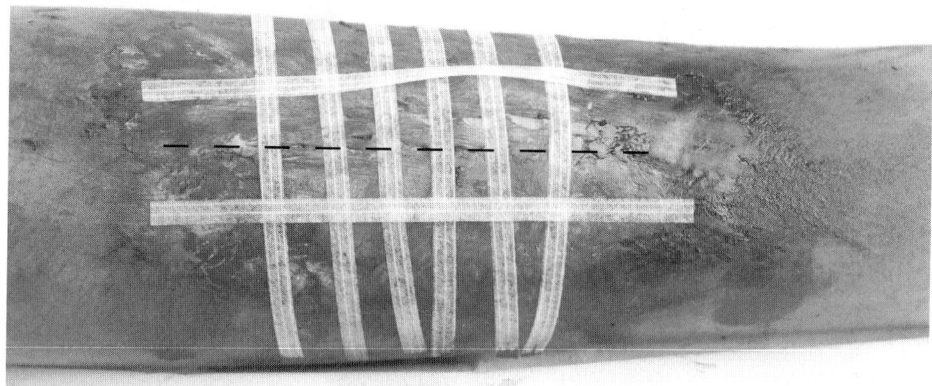

Figure 8.1 The application of Steristrips.

narrow strip). This allows exudate to escape without causing the strips to peel.

Wound closure is usually started at about the middle of the wound. Align the borders, using any irregularity or skin crease to match the sides. Place strips alternately above and below the first strip. This helps to hold the edges in accurate opposition and keeps them in equal tension. The first strip may need to be resited at the end.

Strips may be applied with sterile forceps for an aseptic technique. Place half of the strip on one side of the wound, bring the edges together by pressing the other side into gentle opposition and then passing the strip over. Repeat that over the whole wound.

Place two rows of strips, one on either side of the wound parallel to the wound, across the transverse strips to anchor them.

Closure with an Interrupted Suture

The insertion of an interrupted suture (Fig. 8.2) requires the use of local anaesthetic and sterile instruments.

Local anaesthetic

Lidocaine is the most commonly used infiltrated local anaesthetic. The hazards associated with its use are allergy and toxicity.

Allergic responses are not common, but they can be extreme, including anaphylaxis. Ask the patient for any history of allergy to local anaesthetic. Observe the patient for signs of local reaction, rash, and any signs of swelling or systemic distress.

Toxicity is most likely where the patient receives an overdose of lidocaine or there is accidental injection into a blood vessel. The main toxic effects are to the central nervous system and the heart, causing convulsions and cardiovascular collapse. The patient may appear euphoric, speech may be slurred and the patient may complain of light-headedness, tinnitus and numbness around the mouth. If the clinic is not in a hospital, start resuscitation and transfer the patient as an emergency. If in hospital, commence resuscitation. The priorities are ABC. Give oxygen. Venous access will be needed: for fluids if blood pressure falls and to give diazepam if convulsions develop.

The safe dosage of lidocaine is 3 mg per kg body weight. Lidocaine 1% contains 10 mg per ml, and the maximum dose for an adult is 20 ml. Take care in the calculation of a child's dose.

The addition of epinephrine (adrenaline) to the anaesthetic causes local vasoconstriction. This reduces bleeding in the area, which makes exploration and closure easier. It also slows the absorption of the lidocaine into the circulation, which prolongs its anaesthetic effects.

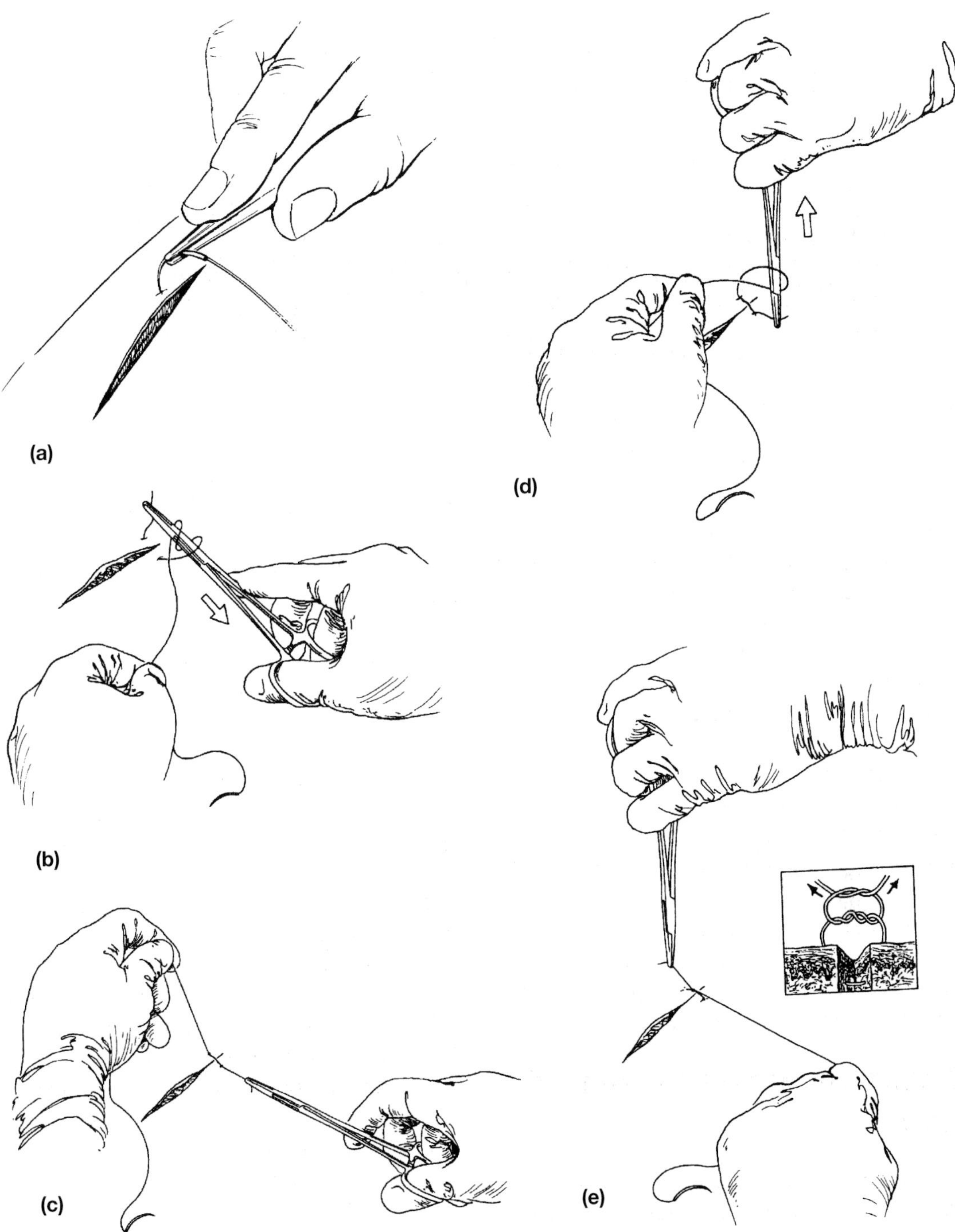

Figure 8.2 **(a) To evert the wound edge, introduce needle at 90° angle to the skin. (b) and (c) pass a double loop round the needle holder. Clamp the free end of the suture and pull it through to the first knot. (d) Pass a single loop in the opposite direction from the first knot, round the top of the needle holder and clamp the free end of the suture. Note in the boxed illustration the final square knot configuration. (e) The position of the suture in a well-everted wound. Note that the knot is to one side of the wound. Align all knots on the same side of the wound. (Reproduced with kind permission of Trott, 1997.)**

The smaller extremities, including the fingers and toes, the nose, the ear and the penis, may suffer ischaemic necrosis from such vasoconstriction, and epinephrine should never be used in these areas.

The types of local anaesthetic which a NP is are allowed to use will be a matter of local policy. Some NPs may be restricted to the use of 1% lidocaine, only for infiltration of the wound edges. Others are permitted to perform digital ring blocks. Lidocaine 1% is not so dense in its anaesthetic effect as a stronger concentration; the patient will feel pressure and tugging on the tissue but will not feel sharpness. The duration of anaesthesia varies, but it is approximately 30 minutes.

Infiltration

Infiltration of lidocaine is shown in Figure 8.3. Draw up the injection, after calculation of the amount to be used and the safe dose for the patient. In practice, the need for a dose that approaches the adult limit would raise the question of whether this wound is minor. Use a fine needle to reduce the discomfort of penetration.

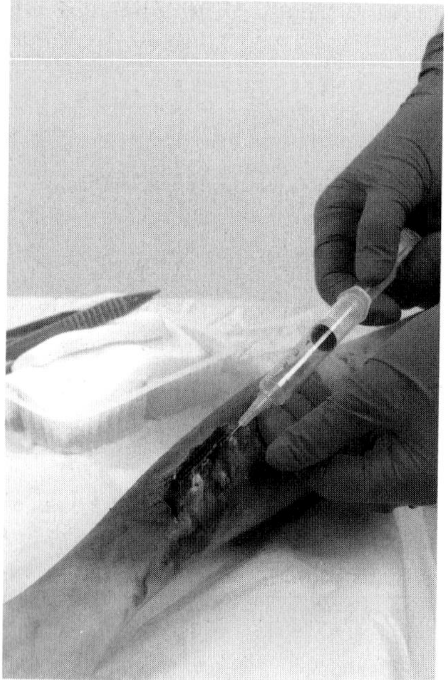

Figure 8.3 Wound edge infiltration with lignocaine.

When infiltrating, remember the risk of intravenous injection. Draw back on the syringe before each compression of the plunger.

There are two common methods of infiltration. Trott (1997) says that injection directly into skin meets with great resistance and injection into deeper fat delays the action of the anaesthetic; consequently the superficial fascia, just below the skin is the proper level for infiltration. Injection can occur through the open wound edges just below the skin. This avoids the discomfort of penetrating the skin but is not advised if the wound is dirty. A sequence of small injections around the whole wound will achieve the purpose. Injection through the skin is started at one end at a little distance from the wound (to ensure numbing of the near corner of the laceration). Pass the needle as far along as it will reach and withdraw it while injecting until lidocaine is infiltrated to the near corner. Without withdrawing the tip; the needle is then passed along the other side of the wound, repeating the process. If the wound is longer than the needle, the remaining part on each side can be anaesthetized fairly comfortably by passing the needle through skin which is already numb.

Digital block anaesthesia

For the treatment of wounds on the fingers and toes, and for some other painful procedures such as incision and drainage of a paronychia or the removal of a splinter from under a nail, it is usually preferable or necessary to achieve local anaesthesia by blockade of the digital nerves. This is achieved by injecting lidocaine *without epinephrine* (adrenaline) into the dorsal finger at its proximal end.

The technique is more invasive than wound edge infiltration and will require training and supervision, in accordance with local policies, to ensure safety and competence.

Potential hazards are:

- intravascular injection of lidocaine
- too much fluid in the small circumference of the finger, threatening compression of the blood vessels and ischaemia.

The targets of the blockade are the four digital nerves which run along the digit close to the bone; there are two on each side, one on the palmar aspect and the other on the dorsum.

There are variations in the recommendations for technique and dosage between various experts, but the use of lidocaine 1% is advocated, and the amount to be injected is set between 2 and 4 ml.

Once the injection has been given, it takes 10 minutes for it to take effect, and the patient's sensitivity to sharpness should be tested before proceeding.

Suture materials

Superficial interrupted suture is the only technique which is required in a minor injury clinic. Interrupted suture is the placing of a series of separately tied sutures in a wound to close it, as opposed to techniques where some form of continuous suture is used.

The fact that the closure is superficial means that a non-absorbable material is used. It will remain visible and accessible, and it must be removed when it has served its purpose. A curved reverse cutting needle is usually considered to be appropriate for closure of skin in traumatic wounds because of its combination of strength, sharpness and smoothness of action. This needle has a triangular cross-section, flattened on its inner curve, with a sharp edge on its outer border.

A synthetic, monofilament, non-absorbent suture, usually nylon (Ethilon) or polypropylene (Prolene), tends to be the material of choice for work on non-cosmetic areas. These sutures are not so easy to handle or tie as the braided materials (silk, cotton and nylon) but they seem to have a lower rate of infection, and silk is thought to leave a larger scar.

The gauge of the suture material is denoted by a numerical configuration, with the lower numbers (e.g. 2/0) denoting the thicker sutures, and the higher numbers (e.g. 6/0) the finer sutures. Thicker material has more strength but is more traumatic. The choice of gauge is largely dictated by the site of the wound on the body. The scalp can be sutured with 2/0, the lower leg with 3/0, the upper limb with 4/0 and the face with 6/0.

Sutures cause additional trauma at a wound site. They make new wounds and lodge foreign material in the tissue. They cause scarring and are infection prone, and their removal is preferable as soon as the wound is able to support itself. Fortunately, the most cosmetically significant area of the body, the face, has an excellent blood supply, high resistance to infection and good healing. Sutures must be removed from the face after 5 days to avoid scarring. In the lower leg, healing is slow, and sutures should be left in place for 2 weeks. Sutures should be left for 2 weeks at sites where the recently closed wound will be exposed to stress and stretching: on the front of the knee, the back of the elbow and the joints on the back of the hand. Wilson et al (1997) recommend that all hand sutures are left in place for longer than usual to allow the patient the freedom to use the hand without concern that the wound will reopen.

Suture instruments

Advice on instrument technique in this section is based on Trott (1997).

For work in the minor injury clinic, three tools are usually adequate: the needle holder, fine-toothed dissecting forceps and suture scissors. Clinics have some form of sterile suture pack, and it is likely that this will also contain curved and straight mosquito type forceps, cleaning materials, gauze swabs and sterile drapes. Clinics also have cleaning fluid, sterile gloves, any splash protection which is needed, local anaesthetic and sutures. A patient trolley is needed in a quiet and clean area with good, adjustable lighting and an adaptable and easily cleaned work surface (often a metal trolley).

Other useful props include an armrest, which can be attached to the trolley, and the working area should be arranged so that the nurse can work comfortably, preferably seated, without stress on the back.

Needle holders

Needle holders are scissor-handled straight instruments, with a locking mechanism and chunky, serrated jaws to hold the suture firmly (Fig. 8.2). Trott (1997) recommends the 4.5 inch size. The needle should be held only at the tip of the jaws, or it may be weakened by the holder's grip. The needle is held at least one third of its length from the suture, where it is strongest, at a right angle to the holder. Trott recommends that, for passing the needle into skin, the holder is not gripped with fingers through its handles but is held cradled in the fingers by its shaft so that the needle can be controlled with fingers which are close to the jaws. The thumb and ring fingers should hold the scissor handles when they are used, leaving the index finger free to control the instrument.

Toothed dissecting forceps

Fine-toothed forceps are a necessary evil as they can damage the tissue which they grip. They are needed to stabilize the skin while it is being sutured. Hold them gently, in the same way as a pencil (i.e. lying on the web of the thumb) rather than enclosed in the hand. Grip the exposed subcutaneous tissue rather than the skin itself, to reduce the trauma.

Suture technique

The principles of suturing are not difficult to grasp, but there are techniques to learn. Competence, dexterity and confidence are only acquired by a programme of training and supervised practice. In addition to skill with the instruments, a NP must understand the difficulties and complications which can arise, the types of wound which require more advanced treatment, and all NPs must know their limits.

Basic technique involves a number of key points.

- Get things right. Do not be afraid to remove and replace a suture.
- The wound edges must be rematched exactly. Any skin crease or peculiarity of the wound might help to do this. The first suture is placed somewhere near the middle of the wound. Is the suture being pulled diagonally by skin tension? Do the subdivided areas of wound, above and below, sit together nicely?
- The suture should not be so tight that the skin is blanched. A loss of circulation at the wound edges will prejudice healing, worsen scarring and encourage infection. The wound edges will swell a little during healing, and a slight space between them is better than making them too tight.
- If the wound edges are slightly everted, or turned outwards, after suture, they will flatten out as the scar shrinks, and the final result should be good from the cosmetic point of view. If the edges are inverted, the scar will tend to form below skin level. Placing the needle into the skin at an angle of 90 degrees and letting the suture describe a square as it passes through the tissue should achieve this result.
- Do not leave the knots over the wound. Site them all on the same side of the wound. This is tidy, which can be important if the sutures are hard to see at removal, avoids irritation of the wound and helps to achieve eversion of the edges.
- The suture should be placed deep enough to close the divided tissue from base to surface so that there is no dead space to act as a refuge for haematoma and infection. The depth of penetration of the needle will depend upon the 'bite' of skin taken. This means that the needle will penetrate more deeply the further from the wound edge that it is placed into the skin. When the needle is brought out through

the skin on the other side of the wound, it should be the same distance from the wound as the opposite needle hole in order to keep the tension equal.

- The right number of sutures should be used. Trott (1997) offers two pieces of advice. First, place just enough sutures to prevent gaps appearing in the wound edges between sutures. Second, as a rule of thumb, the distance between sutures should equal the size of the bite.

A method of tying a suture is illustrated in Figure 8.2.

Closure with Skin Staples

Skin staples have a similar range of application to Steristrips as far as the depth of the wound is concerned. They achieve superficial closure only. They are probably most useful on the scalp, for wounds which are not deep but which cannot be Steristripped because of the hair. They are easiest to place where the bone is fairly superficial and presents a firm base to stabilize the wound.

Hold the wound edges together with one hand and position the gun carefully so that the staple will enter at 90 degrees to the skin and will take an equal bite on either side of the wound. Warn the patient before the staple is placed. Press the gun firmly. A hesitant technique can cause the stapler to jam with a staple caught in the skin but still attached to the gun.

Staples cause pain when they are put in, but it is not extreme and it passes quickly. For small wounds, there is little point in using local anaesthetic, which will probably hurt just as much as the stapling and prolong the whole business.

For a superficial scalp wound, staples can be removed in 5 days.

Staples stand up from the skin, which helps when they are taken out but makes hair combing a matter for care. Hair can be washed gently and the wound should be dried carefully. A hair drier will heat the staple and should be avoided.

Removal involves the use of another gadget, a small, spring-loaded, jawed pincer, which bends the staple and pops it out painlessly. This should also be used firmly or the staple may stick. The patient may need to return to the clinic for removal of the staples as primary care areas may not stock the remover.

Benefits of staples over Steristrips are that they can be used in hair and they can get wet. Disadvantages are that they are painful to put in and they require a return visit for removal. The cosmetic result is not controllable, and they should not be used on the face or hands.

Staples, perhaps surprisingly, given that they are painful to put in, are often successful with children with scalp lacerations, mainly because the procedure ends at the point where the patient is beginning to object. They can be used very swiftly, and the trauma of a prolonged, contested treatment is avoided.

Closure with Skin Glue

Another agent which can be used to close superficial wounds is a medically adapted version of superglue, a sterile preparation of adhesive which polymerizes in the open air within seconds and will seal a wound.

Bleeding must be stopped before the glue is applied, and the edges of the wound must be held firmly closed. The glue should lie on top of and not in the wound, where it would prevent healing.

Glue is applied in a series of spots to the surface of the wound, or in an unbroken line. The glue will become cloudy as it hardens, which usually takes 30 seconds.

It should not be used near the eyes. If glue gets into an eye, flush it with water and leave it to release, which should happen over 2 days. Do not pull at the glued tissue.

Tell the patient that the glued wound will form a scab, which must be kept dry and left alone for 5 days. After that, the glue can be removed by washing.

Glue's advantage is that it is swift and painless. It is limited in use to small superficial wounds, and it is relatively expensive.

Dressings

The economics of the minor injury setting, where patients are treated once and referred to the GP for follow-up, keeps the range of dressings simple. There is no incentive to buy expensive dressings when no long-term benefit, in cost or outcome of treatment, will be seen. The dressing needs of most patients with minor trauma are straightforward, and simple measures will usually do.

The use of a dressing should be an answer to a specific need, and it should be done in the knowledge that it will cause no harm and will bring the patient some benefit.

The common reasons why a patient might require a dressing are:

- to reduce pain caused by exposure to the air (see minor burns, below)
- to keep contaminants out of a wound
- to pad and protect a tender wound
- to protect a wound from disturbance, new trauma and irritation, which may include the patient's own fingers in the case of children
- to soak up exudate
- to keep a topical treatment, such as a magnesium sulphate poultice, or an active dressing, such as kaltostat, in contact with the skin
- to cover a wound and prevent sticking when the patient needs a support bandage over it (this is common practice with pre-tibial lacerations).

Dressing practice in the minor injury clinic is divided into two main areas, the treatment of closed and open wounds.

Closed wounds

The factors which reduce the risk of wound infection have been listed above. There is no evidence that dressing closed wounds reduces the rate of infection. Some closed wounds on sites which are difficult to dress, such as the eyebrow or the scalp, are not covered.

The decision to cover a wound at the time of closure is often taken because the wound is still moist. The decision to continue to cover the wound on subsequent days may be taken for various reasons. Steristrips and wound glue tend to need protection from moisture and rough handling. Sutures are more robust, but an impact can reopen the wound; chafing from clothes and excessive wetting or contamination from everyday substances may slow healing. Patients who are in contact with food which is served to the public, or who provide medical care, should cover their wounds and may be subject to other regulations and restrictions.

Open wounds

Open wounds which are treated with dressings in the minor injury clinic are of three types:

- wounds which will be allowed to heal by secondary intention because there is a complicating factor which prevents closure, such as an unacceptable risk of infection or the presence of swelling
- wounds where skin has been lost, and closure is not possible; bleeding and pain are often the initial problems with these wounds (these will be small injuries, often to fingertips with kitchen choppers; patients with larger, full-thickness skin losses will be referred to hand or plastic surgeons)
- superficial injuries, sometimes over a relatively large area of skin, of the burn, blister and abrasion types; these are tender and have large amounts of serous exudate.

Types of dressing

Wounds which are cut off from the air or are dressed with an overly moist preparation (such as silver sulfadiazine (Flamazine)) become macerated and break down. Wounds which are completely deprived of moisture are slow and less effective in the granulation process.

Closed wounds have a minimal area of open tissue in contact with the air, and it is enough to give them a dry, porous, non-adherent cover (such as Tricotex), which will not bond to the wound and tear off healing tissue when it is removed.

Open wounds which are exuding and, possibly, painful can be covered with one of the vaseline gauze preparations, which maintain a moist environment and are soothing. The vaseline will not stick to the wound while the dressing remains moist, which will usually be for 2 days. Add gauze on top to soak up exudate.

Deep cavities may have to be packed to prevent them from closing over and leaving a dead space and to absorb exudate which gathers below the level of the skin. They should heal from the base outwards. Various absorbent substances are used for packing, and for filling wound craters, including alginate dressings (e.g. Kaltostat) and conforming hydrogel dressings (e.g. Intrasite and Granuflex beads).

Alginate dressing is also for stopping persistent bleeding in skin-loss wounds. It forms a hard shell with the blood and will be difficult to detach from the wound in the next few days (although this can be achieved by soaking the dressing). It will come off as the wound granulates if it is left undisturbed.

Inadine, an iodine impregnated gauze dressing, is one example of an antiseptic, moist wound dressing.

Securing a dressing

There are two basic ways to secure a dressing: with a bandage or with a sticky tape.

Bandages are less secure than sticky tapes because they tend to slacken and slide, and they are difficult to apply to some parts of the body, but they have three advantages:

- avoidance of tape allergy, particularly to elastoplast (always ask the patient about tape allergy when taking the history)
- do not damage frail skin, often an issue with the elderly patient and those who have been on steroids for a long time.
- can combine the holding of a dressing with an element of compression, which may be useful for bleeding or swelling.

The advantages of tapes are:

- they can provide a less bulky, more firmly anchored dressing
- they can be applied in awkward parts of the body
- they can be adapted around joints to leave the patient's range of movement intact.

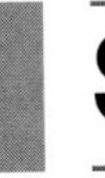

Special Types of Wound

This section will look briefly at some types of wound which are difficult to manage or require special treatment (see also, factors which complicate wound management, above).

Scalp Wounds

A blunt wound to the scalp can cause difficulties on its own, but, in addition, the head injury must be assessed, both in terms of neurological signs and symptoms since the time of injury and the risk of a depressed skull fracture.

A scalp laceration can lose so much blood that the patient can become hypovolaemic. The galea aponeurotica, a layer of connective tissue which joins the frontalis muscle in the forehead, covers the top of the head below the skin. A large tear in this structure can affect the function of the frontalis muscle and also makes it easier for infection to spread to the underlying bone of the skull and even into the intracranial space through the deep circulation. If the galea is torn, layered closure using absorbable sutures may be required, the patient should be referred for assessment by a trauma doctor.

Face Wounds

The medial corner of the eye contains the palpebral ligament and the tear duct, and a wound to the lower eyelid can damage these structures. The levator muscle of the upper eyelid can be divided by a wound. This will cause a drooping, or ptosis, of the lid. Any wounding injury to the surface of the eye should be assessed by a doctor.

Deep wounds over the cheek (below the zygoma and in front of the ear) may penetrate the parotid salivary gland and/or one of the five branches of the facial nerve.

Blunt trauma to the ear, which causes a haematoma, requires referral. The swelling can cause a separation of the soft ear tissue from its cartilage base, which develops into a 'cauliflower ear'. Check the ear canal for internal injury. When a wound to the ear exposes cartilage, there is a risk of infection and tissue death. Treatment may include antibiotic prophylaxis.

Cosmetic implications of face wounds

The cosmetic implications of any wound on the face should always be considered. A lip wound which crosses the lip/skin boundary, called the **vermilion border**, must be realigned so that the line of the lip is smooth, and such injuries should always be referred to a doctor.

Neck and Trunk Wounds

These are dealt with earlier in this chapter.

Hand Wounds

The significance of injuries to the hand and the need to take a good history, including occupation, hobbies and handedness has been discussed in Chapter 6. Musculoskeletal injuries to the hand are also covered in that chapter.

The hand contains many superficial, complicated, easily injured structures. Serious hand injuries can be hard to diagnose, especially at the time of injury. A permanent disability of the hand will bring trouble to *any* patient, and litigation to the NP if the care received was not to standard. The NP must learn the anatomy and function of the hand and the patterns of injury to which it is prone. If there is any doubt about a hand injury, err on the side of caution.

The anatomy and examination of the hand are covered in Chapter 6.

The so-called deep structures of the hand are never very far below the skin. Be suspicious of any wound where you cannot see the base. Watch for divided tendons and nerves. Look for a loss of power, a deformity or a loss of sensation, and relate the findings to knowledge of the local structures.

If there is any chance that there is glass in a wound, request a soft-tissue X-ray. Do not check movement around the injury until this risk is excluded. On occasion, an X-ray film will not reveal a piece of glass if it is lying at an unfavourable angle. If either the patient or the nurse still has concerns after a negative X-ray (usually based on sharp pain on certain movements, or on touching the wound) a trauma doctor's opinion should be sought.

The hand has very little spare skin. A scar over a joint may cause a permanent loss of movement. If a full-thickness skin loss of more than 1 cm × 1 cm occurs, the patient may need a skin graft or a flap repair.

An open crush injury to the tip of a finger may involve tissue loss, with open fracture and/or exposure of bone and a wound to the nail bed. Request an X-ray. These injuries may need reconstruction of the fingertip, with trimming of the bone and cover of the tip with a skin flap, or removal of the nail and suture of its bed. It is not always possible to see if the nail bed is torn, but the possibility must be considered if the nail is torn out at the root or broken. Refer the patient.

Do not suture open crush injuries to the fingertip. They will swell. Steristrips can keep the tissue in loose opposition. Avoid circumferential taping. If the wound is too moist to tape, and loose opposition by suture is needed, the patient will have a ring-block anaesthetic.

A **subungual haematoma** is a collection of blood under the nail caused by a crush injury. It causes painful pressure on the nail bed. The treatment is to trephine (make a hole in) the nail. This can be done by heating the tip of a paper clip in a spirit-lamp flame and touching it to the nail until you feel it give as it passes through. A hole can be bored in the nail with the point of a white, hypodermic needle or a No. 11 scalpel. The hot method is quick except when the nail is very thick. The scalpel makes a bigger hole, which probably improves drainage, but the process is slower and hurts more. Trephining will give no benefit if the blood under the nail has congealed, but this can take quite a few days. There is a chance of a helpful result for up to a week.

Trephining turns a fracture in the underlying bone from closed to open, at least in a technical sense. Different hospitals have different policies, some forbidding trephining if a fracture is present, and others allowing it and giving the patient antibiotics as for an open fracture. The common element is that a fracture should be excluded if it is decided to trephine.

If a nail is loose at a fold, either at the root or the sides, it must be resited to prevent adhesion of the fold tissue.

If a patient brings a piece of **amputated finger**, preserve it for the hand surgeon. Clean it gently with saline, wrap it loosely in sterile swabs, put it in a plastic bag and place the bag in a larger bag of ice. Direct contact between the finger and the ice will damage the skin.

Bites

Bite wounds

A bite wound, from a human or an animal (usually dog or cat), is a complicating factor from the outset. There is a high risk of infection, aerobic and anaerobic, and management is dictated by this hazard. Human bites carry the risk of transmission of blood-borne infection (see above). Exclude injury to bone, joint or other deep structures and the presence of tooth in the wound (tooth is radio-opaque). The wound should be irrigated to reduce contamination (see above). The wound should not be closed. Wounds which cannot be left open for cosmetic or other reasons must be seen by a doctor. Prophylactic antibiotics co-amoxiclav (amoxicillin plus clavulinic acid) are often used if the patient is not allergic to penicillin. This is a matter of local policy, but they are given for deep punctures, when sensitive sites such as hand or face are injured, when the bite is by a human and when the wound has been closed.

Insect bites

An insect bite, often to the leg, can set up an allergic reaction which resembles a cellulitic infection, and sometimes an extremely tender blister will form at the bite.

The patient may complain more of itching than pain if the problem is allergy. Antihistamine (which can be bought at a chemist) is the treatment for allergy. An infection may be accompanied by systemic signs such as raised lymph nodes, pyrexia and malaise. A patient who is not given antibiotics must be told to return if the infection signs get worse. In the case of an infection which is spreading rapidly, the patient may be admitted to hospital for intravenous antibiotics. Ask for a medical opinion if in doubt.

Wasp stings are common in the summer. The patient will have pain at the sting site, with an area of redness and swelling around it. A vinegar pad, if the patient is certain that the attacker was a wasp, eases the discomfort. Once the redness is settling, the patient can be sent home.

Any patient who describes or is seen to be suffering from systemic symptoms after a sting, and especially marked respiratory difficulty and cardiovascular collapse, must be treated for an anaphylactic reaction. The patient will require resuscitation, ABC, with 100% oxygen, intravenous access and intramuscular epinephrine (adrenaline; 0.5 ml of 1 in 1000 solution).

Penetrating wounds to hands and feet

A good deal has already been said about penetrating wounds. Punctures, especially to the sole of the foot, are common in minor injury clinics. These wounds are often inflicted by glass, farm tools, rusty nails or fence spikes and should be assessed in terms of deep structure damage and foreign body (with a soft-tissue X-ray), and should be cleaned with a high-pressure flow of fluid (see above). The tetanus risk is high, and there may be local guidelines or a protocol to issue a prophylactic antibiotic. The hazard of *Pseudomonas* infection, especially if the wound has been inflicted through the sole of a trainer, is leading to a move from the prescribing of flucloxacillin or co-amoxiclav to ciprofloxicin.

Pretibial lacerations

Pretibial lacerations are a very troublesome form of wound. The patient tends to be elderly, with very frail skin which is easily torn at the shin by the slightest knock. Sometimes a paper-thin piece of skin is peeled back in a triangular flap. On other occasions, the wound penetrates through the fat, and a thicker flap is seen. The tissue tends to curl up and retract, and it will often seem that there is a skin loss when there is not. A fresh wound is often very painful to clean.

Open the wound and irrigate any dirt and clotted blood. Moisten the flap with saline and tease it back into shape. Do not put it under any tension, which could tear it, and might reduce its blood supply. Resite the flap with Steristrips. Put a non-adherent dressing over it, with a bandage to secure it. Use no tape on frail skin. Give the patient a support bandage (various types of dressing and support are advocated in different hospitals), advise plenty of rest and elevation and refer the patient to the practice nurse.

The viability of the flap will depend on the circulation which it retains. A proximally based flap, one where the skin is unbroken at its proximal end, will enjoy a direct blood flow and has a better chance of survival.

High-pressure injection wounds

Delayed tissue destruction, caused by high-pressure injection, happens when an industrial device which expels paint or grease through a fine nozzle at high pressure, penetrates skin and discharges into tissue, usually on the hand. The injury may look innocuous at first, but it has the potential to develop into a devastating cocktail of infection, foreign body, chemical injury, necrosis and swelling. The patient may lose the limb if the injury is underestimated. An urgent surgical exploration is needed.

Minor Burns

Triage

There is not a direct relationship between the severity of a fresh minor burn and the triage priority for two reasons.

1. Severe pain is a feature especially of less-serious, fresh burns because the nerve endings in the skin, which can be destroyed by a deeper burn, are intact. Pain is a triage priority. The single measure which brings relief most quickly is cooling of the burn with wet compresses (not ice). Oral paracetamol is valuable, especially for children. Give immediate first aid to patients who present with fresh burns.
2. First aid to a fresh burn, cooling of the injured surface, in the first few minutes may reduce the damage, which continues in the heated tissues after the injury.

The likelihood that a patient with a life-threatening burn will present in a minor injury clinic is not high, but there are some situations where a NP may have to take quick action or exclude serious injury. Always establish the nature of the burning agent at triage.

Chemical burns

In the case of a fresh chemical burn, quick action is needed to return the skin to a neutral pH. Take a history. Get the name of the product. Ask if the patient has brought the container. Ask for any manufacturer's literature on the product and on any antidote. Find out what action the patient has taken, and what effect that has had. Get a colleague to contact the Poisons Information Service while you stay with the patient, to establish the correct initial management of the situation. Assess the risk (especially with a child) that the patient has swallowed the substance. Usually, a recent chemical burn should be irrigated with a lot of water as soon as possible. Do not do this in the unusual case of contact with a water-combustible metal such as sodium or potassium. If the chemical is a dry powder, do not wet it. Brush it off dry. The destructive action of an alkaline agent tends to be more prolonged than that of an acid. Unless there is clear, expert advice, do not put any neutralizing chemical in contact with the substance on the skin. This may trigger further damage or an allergic response, and it may make things worse if the patient is mistaken about the causative agent or if there are other substances mixed with it.

Smoke

A history of exposure to flame in a confined space raises the question of smoke inhalation. The patient may have breathed poisonous or irritant substances. Even when the damage is life threatening there may be no serious signs at once. The patient may progress to collapse caused by swelling in the airway and lungs, hypoxia or poisoning, and the crisis may be irreversible. There is also the danger of a severe pneumonitis caused by irritants in the lungs. A patient who has inhaled dangerous hot gases may have burns and blackening around nose or mouth, singeing of facial hair, a smell on the breath, may be hoarse and sputum may be discoloured. If there is any sign of hypoxia, which may be assessed by physical signs such as cyanosis or a neurological deterioration, or if there is evidence of respiratory difficulty, which may include wheeze, cough or stridor, the patient should be treated as an emergency and resuscitated. ABC is the priority. The airway is in danger and the patient needs oxygen. The most senior anaesthetist available should be called. If the history is the only indication

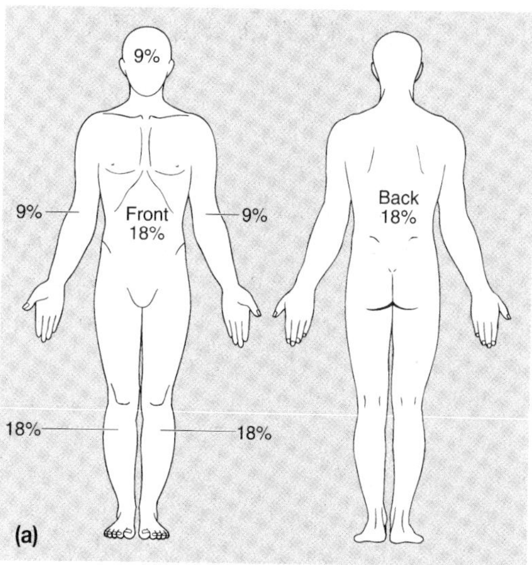

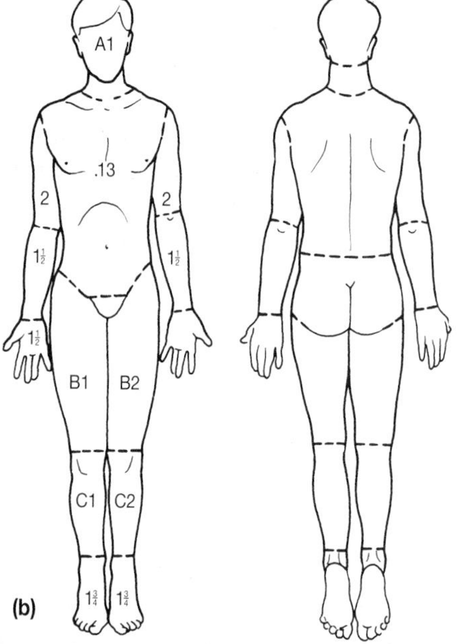

Percentage of body surface at various ages

Percentage of areas affected by growth

	0	1	5	10	15	Adult age
A = $\frac{1}{2}$ head	$9\frac{1}{2}$	$8\frac{1}{2}$	$6\frac{1}{2}$	$5\frac{1}{2}$	$4\frac{1}{2}$	$3\frac{1}{2}$
B = $\frac{1}{2}$ one thigh	$2\frac{3}{4}$	$3\frac{1}{4}$	4	$4\frac{1}{4}$	$4\frac{1}{2}$	$4\frac{3}{4}$
C = $\frac{1}{2}$ one leg	$2\frac{1}{2}$	$2\frac{1}{2}$	$2\frac{3}{4}$	$3\frac{1}{2}$	$3\frac{1}{4}$	$3\frac{1}{2}$

To estimate the total of the body surface area burned, the percentages assigned to the burned section are added. The total is then an estimated of the burn size.

Figure 8.4 Assessing the size and severity of burn injuries. (a) Adult assessment using Wallace's rule of nine; (b) child assessment using the Lund and Browden burn chart. (Reproduced with kind permission from Alexander et al., 2000.)

of risk and the patient seems well, there must still be an immediate medical assessment. A full clinical examination, with chest X-ray and arterial blood gases investigation, will be performed.

Electric shock

A patient who has received a high-voltage electric shock, which is often fatal, is not likely to appear in a minor injury clinic. Patients will present who have suffered shocks from household supplies.

Electricity enters the body through the point of contact, creating a burn, and travels through the least-resistant pathways, which tend to be skin, nerve, muscle and the circulation to an exit point. It then leaves the body, causing a further surface burn. The patient's contact with the power source can be prolonged, and the injury worse, if the voltage is high enough to cause muscle contraction, which will prevent the patient from letting go. There may be injuries at any of the structures involved, and the rhythm of the heart may be disrupted.

Look for burns on the body surface, assess circulation, innervation and movement, check vital signs and perform an electrocardiograph.

Non-accidental injury in children

Glasgow and Graham (1997) cite the probable incidence of 10–15% of burns to children as non-accidental. They estimate that 10% of all physical abuse of children takes the form of burns, and that burns are involved in a smaller number of sexual abuse cases. NPs should be aware with children who have been burned, of other injuries which are consistent with abuse: the small circular mark of cigarette burns, the glove or stocking demarcation line of the burn on a child who has been immersed in hot water, or the mark of a hot contact on a body part, such as the buttocks, which a child would not be likely to injure by accident. More general signs of abuse may include a delay in seeking treatment, an injury which is not compatible with the mechanism described and a history of other attendances. Non-accidental injury is discussed more fully in Chapter 4. If there is any doubt, refer to a pediatrician.

The Commonest types of Minor Burn

These burns provoke most of the minor injury clinic attendances. Scalds and, to an even greater extent, flame and contact burns may also be of the greatest severity.

Scalds (wet heat)

Splashes, spillages and, occasionally, immersion in hot liquids, are the commonest cause of minor burns. Hot water, steam and cooking oil are the main agents. Kitchen and bathroom are the chief sites of injury.

Flames and hot appliances (dry heat)

Dry heat burns is a mixed category of common, non-liquid burns, house fires, objects which produce a flame (gas cookers, cigarettes), appliances which are heated by electric elements (irons, electric cookers, soldering irons) and objects which contain hot water (radiators, hot water bottles, kettles). An object, like a hot water bottle, which is designed to provide heat and which will not cause a burn on a brief contact may inflict a deep burn if the user has a reduced awareness of pain and stays in prolonged contact. This can happen if the user has reduced sensation in the burned area or becomes unconscious because of illness, drink or drugs.

Radiation from the sun

Patients appear every summer with sunburn, or its artificial counterpart the sunbed burn. These burns are painful and sometimes quite large but are rarely serious.

Definition of a Minor Burn

It is easier to define a minor burn in a clear way, than it is to define other types of minor injury. The management of burns is based on reasonably exact calculations of three factors: the size and depth of the surface injury and the part of the body which is injured. There are other indicators of seriousness, such as the risk of inhalation, but burns with such complications are not minor.

Size of the burn

The size of a burn is calculated in percentage of total body area (Fig. 8.4). Erythema, the redness without blister or wound, which is the most superficial burn, is not calculated as part of the percentage.

The 'rule of nines' is a rough guide to estimation of size of a burn. This divides the percentage area of the body into multiples of nine and it is easy enough to learn to carry in the head:

head 9%
each arm 9%
front of trunk 18%
back of trunk 18%
each leg 18%
perineum 1%.

The proportions of a child differ from those of an adult and change dramatically from infancy to adolescence. The Lund–Brouder chart in Figure 8.4 offers a scale of percentages at different stages.

Another useful method of assessing a small burn's percentage size is to calculate that the patient's hand, with the fingers together, will cover about 1% of the body surface. The percentage of burn has to be factored with the other two elements, depth and site, when deciding whether or not a burn is minor, but as a rough guide for an adult patient, burns of less than 5% in area will not require specialist advice or admission. If the burn exceeds 10%, medical guidance is needed.

Depth of the burn

It may not be possible to tell how deep a burn is on first examination, and the patient's pain will be the first priority. However, a history will give the first indication of the depth of the burn. The two factors to be considered are the amount of heat generated by the burning agent and the duration of the contact. The amount of heat may be a question of the boiling point of a particular liquid, such as water or cooking oil, or it may have to do with the voltage of electricity or the strength of a chemical solution.

Burn depth is described as:

1. **Red, unbroken skin (erythema).** It can be very painful, but the burn is superficial and will heal without complication. Milder areas will sometimes disappear on the day after the injury.
2. **Superficial, partial thickness.** There are, or will be, blisters full of serous fluid. When these burst, the underlying skin is pink, tender and exudes for some days. The skin will heal from its own base layer without scarring or contracture of the skin.
3. **Deep partial thickness.** The burn is usually of irregular depth and reaches the base of the dermis. It looks paler than a superficial burn, and sensation may be reduced or absent on its surface. Some hair follicles may be visible in the base tissue.
4. **Full thickness.** This type of burn penetrates through the skin to the level of the superficial fascia. It looks white, the base feels leathery and inelastic. There will be no sensation in the base tissue.

Deep, partial thickness burns and full-thickness burns have lost the capacity to regenerate from the base of the wound. These burns heal very slowly and imperfectly, inwards from the edges, with scarring and contracture.

The patient will carry a permanent reminder of any such burn and may suffer other disadvantages if the injury is large, cosmetically significant or placed over a joint. The management of any deep burn is a matter for a doctor.

SITE OF THE BURN

Three sites, the face, hand and perineum, are vulnerable to complications and special problems if they are burned.

Face

Minor burns to the face, such as erythematous scalds, cannot be dressed and can be very painful at the outset. However, the face heals well and there should be no lasting problem. More serious facial burns, and especially those which are deep, threaten the airway or involve the eyes, require medical referral.

Hands

Even small scars at a joint of the hand can cause contracture and a loss of movement. The sense of touch is most sensitive in the hand, and any damage to the skin may reduce it. Any deep burn should be seen by a doctor. If the hand is restricted by dressings or painful injury, it is prone to stiffness.

Perineum

Burns anywhere in the region of genitals and anus are embarrassing, painful, hard to dress, incompatible with normal movement and prone to infection. There may also be a question of non-accidental injury.

Over joints

In addition to these anatomical sites, close attention should be given to any burn which crosses a joint to assure that the patient will suffer no long-term loss of movement. A burn which is circumferential at any part of the body may act as a tourniquet through swelling around the burn and inelastic, burned tissue; this could cause distal necrosis.

Treatment of Minor Burns

The definition of a burn as minor is meaningless if it ignores other aspects of the situation, such as the inability of an elderly patient to cope at home or a possible non-accidental injury. Assess every situation on its merits.

A minor burn is painful. It may become an open, moist wound, and this may lead to infection.

If the patient presents with a fresh injury, cool it with wet compresses at triage. Take a full history, record the patient's tetanus status, allergies and medical history.

Carry out an initial assessment of the injury, document its site, size and the appearance of the injured skin. A drawing is helpful. Note the presence of erythema, blisters, any broken skin and the apparent depth of the burn. Test awareness of light touch over the injured area.

The priority is to relieve pain. Further assessment of a minor injury can be deferred until the pain has settled.

A NP may give analgesia and will clean and dress the burn. Burns are prone to infection, and dressing technique should be aseptic.

Policies vary from place to place, and person to person, on the treatment of blisters and the dressing of burns. An intact blister which is causing no inconvenience by its position or size, and which is thin walled, is unlikely to cover a deep injury and will not be the site of an infection. It seems reasonable to leave it alone.

In the case of blisters which require treatment, Wardrope and Edhouse (1999) say that deroofing increases bacterial colonization and pain, and they argue for aspiration only, performed under aseptic conditions.

A thick-walled blister should give cause for thought. If the history suggests the possibility of a deep injury, take advice on further management.

Burns to the face and to the perineum may not be suitable for dressing. If the skin is not broken, and the main problem is discomfort from clothes and walking, some perineal burns can be dressed by layering vaseline gauze around the skin creases, moulding and snipping a large wound pad to fit, and holding the dressing loosely in place with an athletic support. This will give comfort but will not help if there is a risk of infection.

A burn to the hand may require a plastic bag dressing. Conventional dressings are difficult to adapt to sizable hand burns and may restrict movement and cause stiffness. Silver sulfadiazine (Flamazine) is often used with a bag. It is soothing, and is active against *Pseudomonas* infections. The silver salt can stain the skin. It also macerates the skin to the extent that it is hard to assess the burn when it is removed. It may be reasonable to use it for the earliest, most painful stage of the burn, and then go on to a vaseline gauze hand dressing when things have settled down. Some health areas favour vaseline gauze or liquid paraffin rather than silver sulfadiazine.

For other areas of the body, standard treatment is a dressing such as vaseline gauze, which puts a moist, soothing layer next to the skin to avoid adherence and encourage healing, combined with an absorbent layer of gauze to soak up exudate and a bandage to secure it.

The burn should be reviewed, either in the clinic, or by the practice nurse, and the patient should be told to attend for redressing if exudate soaks through the bandage.

9 MINOR HEAD INJURIES

CONTENTS

Currie (1993) lists the dilemmas facing the doctor who deals with a head-injured patient. These include which of these patients need a skull X-ray, who should be admitted, have a computerised tomographic (CT) scan, have surgery, be ventilated? The choices facing the NP are much simpler. Should this patient be sent home or does a doctor see the patient? This chapter explores the grounds upon which that choice might be made. Head injuries in children are discussed in Chapter 4.

Anatomy

The brain and spinal cord are, together, the **central nervous system**. The neural tissues of the brain are delicate and damage to them is irreversible.

The **cranial** part of the skull (Fig. 9.1) is a bony box which holds and protects the brain. The bones which contribute to this structure are the **frontal**, **parietal**, **temporal** and **occipital**.

The box is not a sealed container. It has many openings to permit the passage of blood vessels and nerves and a large passage in its occipital floor, the **foramen magnum**, through which the **brainstem** gives way to the spinal cord. It then passes into the vertebral canal of the spine. However, neither these openings nor the joints between the various bones of the cranium provides sufficient leeway to absorb the extra pressure which occurs inside the cranium if there is bleeding caused by injury or if the brain should swell (**cerebral oedema**). The effects of **raised intracranial pressure** are transmitted to the soft brain itself, and its rigid protective environment becomes a liability. Violent impacts or sudden movements of the head can throw the brain against the hard edges and surfaces of the cranial bones, resulting in contusion and damage to the brain.

The brain has other forms of protection. It is covered by three layers of protective fibrous material, the **meninges**. The innermost layer is the **pia mater** (meaning tender mother). This is a fine, richly vascular tissue which clothes the outline of the brain. The middle layer is the **arachnoid** (meaning cobweb), a layer of fine

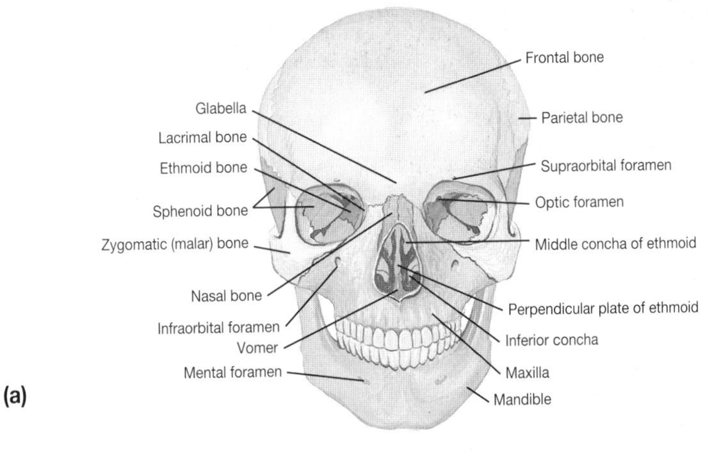

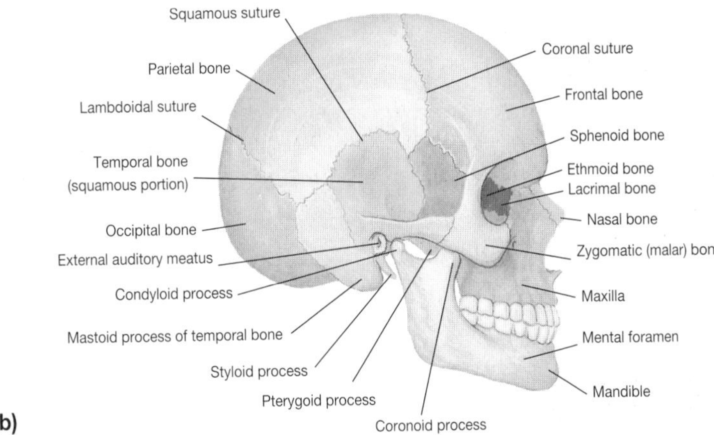

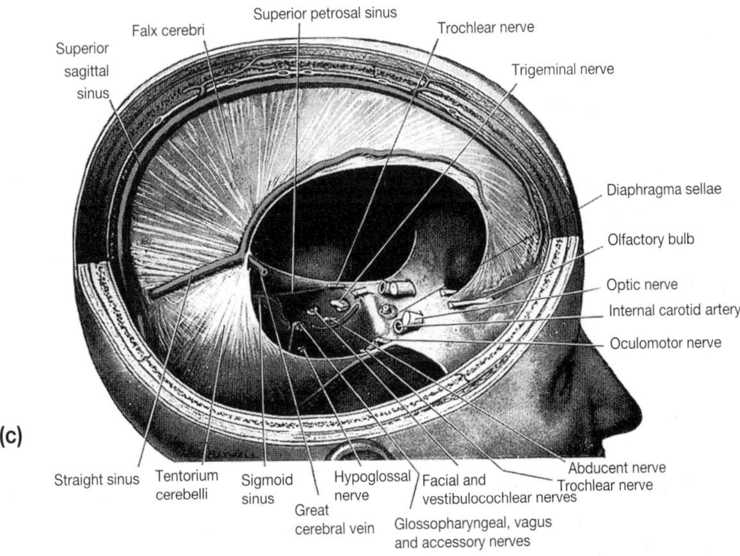

Figure 9.1 **The cranial part of the skull. (a) Anterior view of the skull. (b) View from the right side. (c) The dura mater exposed by removal of part of the right half of the skull and brain. (Adapted with kind permission from (a,b) Thibodeau and Patton (1999) and (c) Williams (1995).)**

Anatomy

tissue which is separated from the pia mater by the **subarachnoid space** and joined to it by web-like attachments, which give the arachnoid its name. The subarachnoid space contains **cerebrospinal fluid** (CSF) and blood vessels. The outer layer is the **dura mater** (meaning hard mother), a tough tissue which covers brain and forms the **dural sheath** around the spinal cord. Bleeding which occurs in the space between the skull and the dura mater (**epidural** haemorrhage) is usually caused by trauma to the temporal bone, causing fracture and bleeding from the meningeal artery. The patient deteriorates very quickly and needs immediate surgery to remove the haematoma. A **subdural** haemorrhage is venous and the patient may not deteriorate so quickly.

The brain floats in, and is protected and nourished by CSF, a liquid formed from, and similar to, plasma. The spinal cord is also surrounded by this liquid. The level of CSF in the brain is delicately regulated to avoid excess pressure.

Our state of consciousness, of awareness in the world, resides in the brain and can be extinguished there. The brain is the centre where all those functions of our inner life that we might call thought and feeling arise. The brain regulates the body, its internal environment and its responses to external changes. It receives the signals from the five senses and translates them into the experiences which we call sight, smell, sound, taste and sensation. It sends out the signals which enable us to act in the world. The vast array of cerebral functions are relegated to specialized zones in the brain. The part of the brain which lies at its base, the brainstem, is of particular concern in the head-injured person who is suffering from the effects of rising intracranial pressure. This area regulates vital functions such as breathing, heartbeat and consciousness itself. Increased pressure on the brain will tend to drive the brainstem into the foramen magnum, the access point to the spinal canal, a fatal process called **coning**.

Assessment of Head Injuries

The assessment of the head-injured patient is, in part, an assessment of external manifestations of the state of health of the central nervous system, the brain and the spinal cord. This can be done by examining the **cranial nerves** and the **deep tendon reflexes**.

Cranial Nerve Assessment

The cranial nerves are a group of 12 nerves, or groups of nerves, which originate in the brain and emerge from there to regulate activity at external sites. A summary of the cranial nerves and their basic assessment is included here, although not all cranial nerves are equally prone to suffer injury as a result of trauma to the head. The tests which would be carried out during a clinical assessment of a patient with a minor head injury are described in the section on examination.

Cranial nerve I: Olfactory

The olfactory nerve is a sensory nerve, for smell. Testing the sense of smell should be done one nostril at a time, with the other one held closed with a finger. The patient should close the eyes and identify different scents. Informal testing may make use of objects such as soap, perfume and fruit. Fracture of the ethmoid bone or trauma to the olfactory nerve may cause **anosmia**, a partial or complete loss of the sense of smell.

Cranial nerve II: optic nerve

The optic nerve is a sensory nerve transmitting visual impulses to the brain. Measurement of visual acuity is described on page 238.

Pupil reactions

Test the reactions of the pupils. The shining of a light on one eye will cause a constriction of both pupils. The constriction on the side affected by direct light is called the **direct light reflex**. The constriction on the other side is called the **consensual light reflex**. Examine the pupils in dim light. Ask the patient to look into the distance to eliminate the **accommodation reflex**, a constriction of the pupils which may occur if the patient looks at something near. Shine a pen torch on the pupils from below and to the sides and observe the direct and consensual responses. If the direct response is absent, but the pupil has a consensual response, the damage is likely to be to the retina or optic nerve (an **afferent** defect, meaning towards the brain). If the pupil is fixed and dilated and lacks the direct response but has the consensual response, the damage may be to the ocular motor nerve or the ciliary ganglion (an **efferent** defect, meaning out of the brain).

Visual Fields

The visual fields should be tested. This can be done by sitting facing the patient, within an arm's length, and comparing the patient's responses to your own. Test each eye in turn, asking the patient to cover the other. Tell the patient to look into your left eye with the right eye and vice-versa. Make sure that the eyebrow and nose do not obstruct vision by asking the patient to tilt the head. Ask the patient to detect finger movements on the periphery of the four fields (named the **upper**, **lower**, **nasal** and **temporal**). Move the finger across the field to detect central defects. There may be defects in one or both eyes, in various patterns. Note the location and disposition of any defects and refer the patient for medical assessment.

A complete examination of the optic nerve includes examination of the fundi with an opthalmoscope.

Cranial nerves III, IV and VI: oculomotor, trochlear and abducent nerves

Cranial nerves III, IV and VI control eye movement and pupil size and are assessed together. The oculomotor nerve supplies the muscles which open the upper eyelids and move the eyeball up, down and towards the nose. It influences, through parasympathetic fibres, the constriction of the pupil and focusing of the lens. Problems with that nerve will lead to impairment of the movements controlled by it, and the eye will move into lateral rotation (**external strabismus**). There may be a drooping eyelid, double vision and difficulty with close focus. The trochlear nerve supplies the muscle which move the eye downwards when adducted. This movement will be reduced by impairment. The abducent nerve supplies the muscle which abducts the eye. Impairment will cause the eye to rotate medially (**internal strabismus**).

The appearance of the patient's eyes is assessed, and their movement is tested. Abnormalities of appearance may include **squint**, or other defects of alignment of the eyes' and **ptosis** (drooping eyelid). Observe the patient's eyes in movement, to the sides and up and down. Is the movement smooth and coordinated? You may observe **nystagmus** on movement. Fuller (1993) defines nystagmus as 'a slow drift in one direction with a fast correction in the opposite direction'. It is seen as an involuntary jerky twitching of the eyeball and it may accompany a fracture of the petrous bone. Ask the patient to follow an object at approximately 60 cm distance horizontally and vertically, moving the eyes but keeping the head still. The patient may report

diplopia, or double vision. Any defect should result in referral for medical assessment.

Cranial nerves V and VII: trigeminal and facial nerves

The trigeminal nerve has a sensory and motor function, and supplies the face (Fig. 9.2).

The sensory function is in three distributions, the **opthalmic** (including the cornea), the **maxillary** and the **mandibular**. The motor nerve supplies the muscles of mastication.

Sensory testing should be to the forehead (opthalmic), cheek (maxillary) and chin (mandibular). The motor nerve can be assessed by resisting opening of the jaw with a hand placed under the chin.

The facial nerve has five main branches which supply the motor function of the face. These can be visualized as five fingers spread against the side of the face, representing, in descending order, the **temporal**, **zygomatic**, **buccal**, **mandibular** and **cervical** branches.

These nerves supply the muscles of facial expression. Taste in the anterior two thirds of the tongue is supplied. The facial nerve also supplies parasympathetic fibres to the lacrimal (tear) and submandibular (salivary) glands.

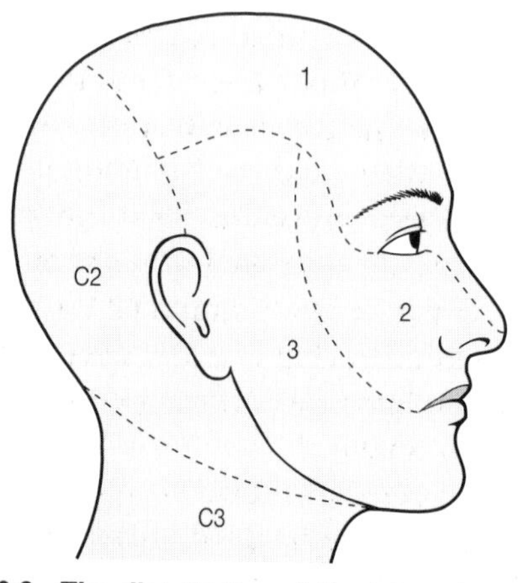

Figure 9.2 The distribution of the trigeminal nerve. (1) Ophthalmic division; (2) maxillary division; (3) mandibular division; C2, second cervical root; C3, third cervical root. (Reproduced with kind permission from Munro and Campbell, 1995.)

To examine the facial muscles, observe the face for symmetry, including actions like blinking and smiling. Ask the patient to look up, screw the eyes tightly shut (try to open them against this resistance), bare the teeth, balloon the cheeks, purse the lips and whistle.

Cranial nerve VIII: vestibulocochlear nerve

Cranial nerve VIII has two major functions, sending sensory information to the brain from the vestibular balance receptors in the inner ear and from hearing receptors in the cochlea. Hearing is assessed by placing a sounding tuning fork on the mastoid process to assess **bone conduction** of sound, and holding it in front of the ear to assess **air conduction**. Vestibular problems will result in vertigo, poor balance, nystagmus and vomiting. The patient's ability to walk toe to heel may be checked for poor balance, with a tendency to fall towards the side of the deficit.

Cranial nerves IX, X and XII: glossopharyngeal' vagus and hypoglossal nerves

The glossopharyngeal nerve provides sensory fibres to the posterior third of the tongue, motor fibres to pharyngeal muscles involved in swallowing and the gag reflex, and parasympathetic motor fibres to the parotid salivary gland. The vagus nerve supplies a large number of efferent parasympathetic motor fibres to heart, lungs and abdominal organs, sensory fibres to the eardrum, outer canal of the ear and the ear itself, and motor fibres to the palate, pharynx and larynx. The hypoglossal nerve supplies motor fibres to the tongue. Look at the uvula, using a tongue depressor, and ask the patient to say 'Ah'. The uvula should rise in the midline. The gag reflex can be tested by touching the tonsil area on each side with an orange stick – the uvula should rise in response. The patient's ability to taste bitter substances may be tested at the posterior third of the tongue. When assessing the larynx, ask the patient to speak, cough and swallow a glass of water. Ask the patient to stick the tongue out.

Cranial nerve XI: accessory nerve

Cranial nerve XI is a combined cranial and cervical spinal nerve which supplies motor fibres to the sterocleidomastoid muscles of the neck and the upper parts of the trapezius.

Make resisted flexion tests of the neck for the sternocleidomastoids by pressing on the forehead, and on the upper trapezius by asking the patient to shrug the shoulders against downwards pressure.

Deep Tendon Reflexes

A reflex is a protective mechanism, an involuntary response to a potentially threatening stimulus. In neurological terms, there is an arc, a linked afferent and efferent response. A specific stimulus to a stretch receptor in a muscle, caused by tapping the tendon with a tendon hammer, will trigger, *on every occasion*, the same motor reaction, a contraction of the muscle. Because the response is predictable and repeated, any deviation from the norm will give a useful indication that something is amiss.

Deep tendon reflexes may be abnormally active, normal, weak or absent. The method of testing five reflexes is shown in Figure 9.3.

What is a Minor Head Injury?

Many patients attend minor injury clinics with injuries to the head or face, which might be called 'head injuries' in the anatomical sense but are more appropriately categorized as lacerations to scalp, or eyebrow or wherever. A common tale is of a clash of heads on the rugby field, where the patient does not know that he is injured until some blood runs down into his eye, or of a workman who stands up below a shelf with a sharp corner and cuts the top of the head. The injured person has an instant of sharp, superficial pain and no other symptom except the bleeding, which brings the patient for treatment. Patients with problems of this kind must be assessed neurologically, and they will be sent home with a sheet of head injury instructions along with advice on the care of staples or sutures.

A NP with experience of treating such injuries knows at once that there is a difference between that kind of event, and the patient who arrives pale and shaken, upset, unable to remember the injury, complaining of a headache and vomiting repeatedly. The patient is brought in by someone who says that the patient has just fallen 10 feet from a ladder and hit the back of the head on a concrete path.

Wrightson and Gronwall (1999) offer a definition of 'mild' head injury for patients when they are first seen which incorporates a minimum degree of severity and an upper limit to the severity of the injury. These are, on the minimum side, that the patient should have suffered 'an injury to the head resulting from physical force' and that neurological function has been disturbed, with symptoms such as confusion, amnesia, altered consciousness, headache or unexplained vomiting. The upper limit of severity in a patient who has just presented is that the **Glasgow Coma Scale (GCS)** (Table 9.1) should not be lower than 13 and that there should be no focal neurological abnormality, such as hemiparesis or cranial nerve damage. Patients with a GCS of 13 may be assessed as having a more severe injury if they do not improve during a period of observation of 4 hours.

Unconsciousness is not mentioned in this definition because it can be hard to find out how long, and how profound an episode has been.

It is clear from the definition, which makes no mention of fracture of the skull, that some evidence of injury to the brain is the element

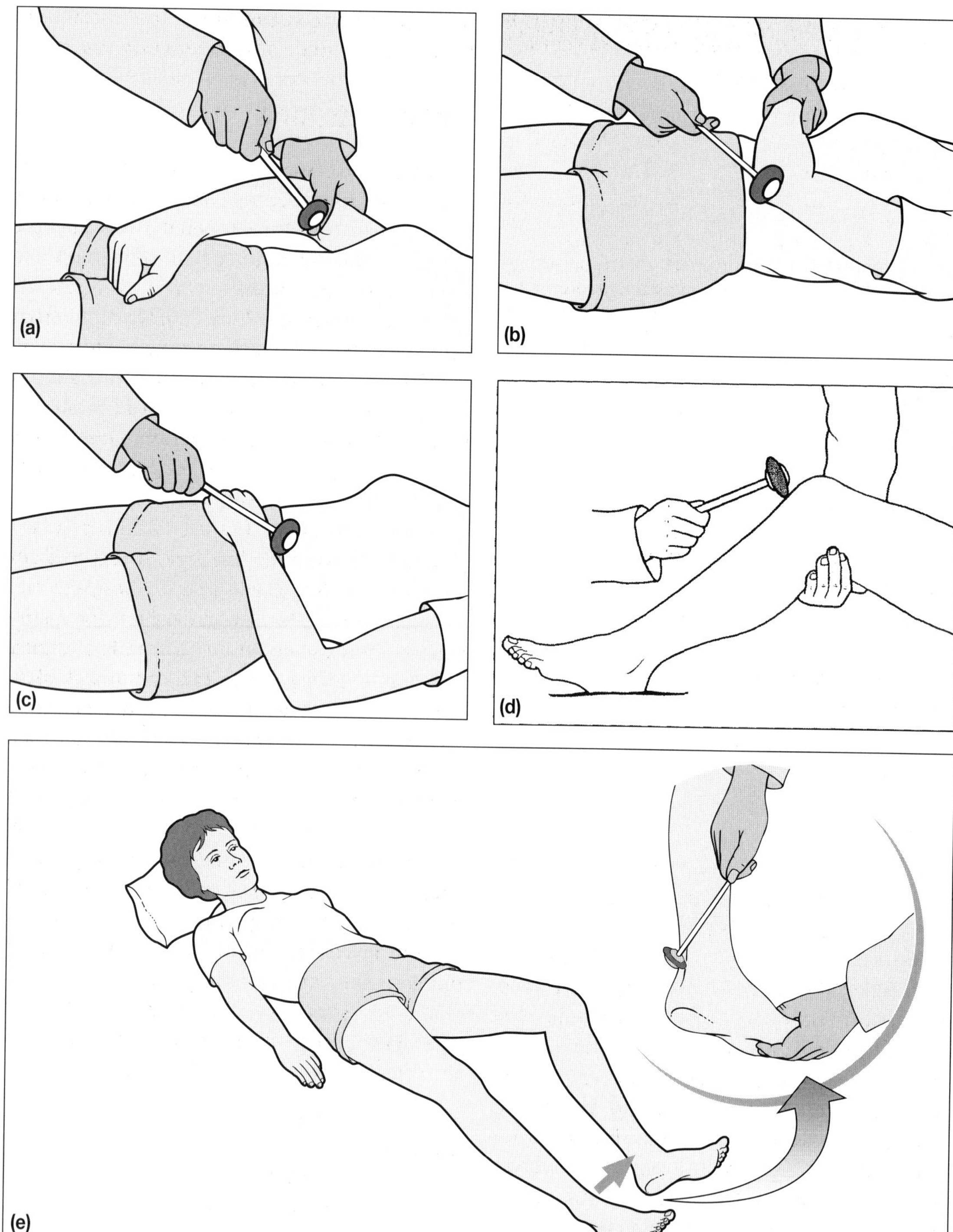

Figure 9.3 **Testing for reflexes. (a) Biceps jerk; (b) triceps jerk; (c) supinator jerk; (d) knee jerk (the legs must not be in contact); (e) ankle jerk. (Reproduced with kind permission from Munro and Campbell, 1995.)**

Testing for reflexes

- Make the patient comfortable.
- Use a tendon hammer to hit the tendon sharply.
- Watch the contraction in the muscle belly.
- Compare with other side.

Table 9.1 Glasgow Coma Scale: the scores are summed to give an overall rating between 3 and 14; minimum score is 3

Category	*Score*
Eye opening	
Spontaneous	4
To speech	3
To pain	2
None	1
Best verbal response	
Orientated	5
Confused	4
Inappropriate	3
Incomprehensible	2
None	1
Best motor response	
Obeying commands	5
Localising	4
Flexing	3
Extending	2
None	1

which is considered to be important, and the NP will be looking for signs of that, and for signs that the patient is getting worse.

The Scottish Intercollegiate Guidelines Network (SIGN) has issued a set of guidelines for the care of head-injured patients. These espouse the principle that the use of reliable *predictors* of brain injury is a preferable way to manage patients, rather than waiting to see which patients will reveal an intracranial bleed by their deteriorating condition. This emphasis is given practical meaning only because CT scanning is increasingly available to A&E departments. CT is very reliable for diagnosis of such injuries, even before the patient deteriorates, while skull X-ray can only give a clearer idea of level of risk.

The two factors which are considered to be of most value in their correlation to a significant brain injury are those patients who have, or have had, impaired consciousness, and those who have, or are suspected to have, a skull fracture.

Investigations

Fracture of the skull is not the same as brain injury, but there are two considerations here. First, a patient who has suffered a skull fracture has been subjected to enough force to produce a brain injury. Second, there is a small incidence of serious, potentially fatal complications from fracture of the skull itself. An open skull fracture is a doorway for infection to enter the brain. An open, depressed skull fracture lodges a piece of bone and, possibly, other foreign matter in the brain and its protective tissues, with the risk of penetrating injury and cerebral abscess.

There is a good deal of discussion about the place of skull X-ray in the management of head-injured patients, partly because a positive finding does not alter the treatment of many patients, and also because a CT scan is of greater value in showing intracranial injury. A skull X-ray is valuable when there is a deep or large scalp wound but no other sign of an intracranial injury. It can be used at a site which has no CT scanner to help a doctor to decide if the patient should be transferred for a scan. The Royal College of Radiologists (1998) has issued guidance on the indications for X-rays of the skull but Currie (1993) emphasizes the need for discretion. The doctor has to judge each case on its merits: 'guidelines are only guidelines'.

The Royal College of Radiologists (1998) lists categories of head injury which offer *low* risk of intracranial injury. The patient has:

- full orientation
- no amnesia
- no loss of consciousness
- no neurological deficits
- no severe scalp laceration
- no haematoma.

They recommend that such patients receive no X-ray or CT scan. They may be discharged with a sheet of head injury advice if they have someone responsible to look after them. An admission for observation may be considered if they have no one at home.

Among the signs which suggest a *higher* risk of intracranial injury are:

- loss of consciousness or altered level of consciousness
- discharge of CSF from nose (rhinorrhoea) or from ear (otorrhoea), or blood from ear
- amnesia
- neurological deficit, including such signs as headache and repeated vomiting
- a second visit to hospital because symptoms are not settling
- a violent mechanism of injury
- a laceration which penetrates to bone or is longer than 5 cm
- a penetrating injury over the skull
- a haematoma to the scalp
- complicating factors, such as alcohol or epilepsy.

These patients will need a doctor's assessment. They may receive a skull X-ray as a first step, or a CT scan may be ordered. In some cases, when the patient has been admitted for observation, imaging may be deferred and only carried out if there is a deterioration in condition. This choice will depend, to some extent, on the facilities which are available.

A NP may need to resuscitate patients who are deteriorating while in the minor injury clinic.

Indications for admission to hospital after a head injury (from SIGN) are:

- Glasgow Coma Scale assessment of less than 15
- post-traumatic amnesia lasting at least 5 minutes
- post-traumatic seizure
- focal neurological deficit
- altered behaviour
- clinical or radiological evidence of skull fracture (which may include nose or ear discharge, full-thickness laceration, boggy haematoma and periorbital bruising) or penetrating injury
- severe headache or vomiting
- medical factors, such as anticoagulant use
- inadequate supervision at home.

Clinical Examination

The History

This section is largely based on the text written by Swann and Yates (1989) for staff in A&E. The taking of a history from a patient who has suffered a head injury is also a form of neurological assessment. The patient's recollection of the injury, and events before and after it, are important measures of condition. This means that the patient may not be a reliable historian and any other accounts, from witnesses to the incident and from people who know the patient, should be used to test the accuracy of the account. A NP may have to rely entirely on witnesses if the patient has no memory of the event. If the NP cannot obtain a history the patient should be referred to the A&E department as most patients are retained until matters are clearer.

The history is also of particular importance in the patient with a head injury because there is very little else to go on. Definitive investigation of every minor head injury is not possible, and a clinical examination may not uncover a developing problem. Patients are pigeon-holed by a series of risk factors in which the history plays a large part, and they are asked to return if it appears that they require promotion to a more urgent category. A full account of the injury is needed (see taking a history, Ch. 3). The timing and sequence of any symptoms are important. A patient who was alert at the time of injury and has had a slow decline in the level of consciousness may have an intracranial bleed, whereas a patient whose responses are sluggish but who is better than at the time of injury may require no more than a period of observation.

Assess the patient using a series of questions.

1. What happened? Direction, speed, duration of force are all important. A direct blow on the head from a hammer may produce a depressed fracture and intracranial damage and infection. It is less likely to cause a neck injury. A patient who is thrown off a horse or a bicycle and lands on the head is prone to neck injury.

2. Was there a fall? The history of a head injury is often the history of a fall, and the NP should always test the patient's notion that it was an injury and not an episode of illness. The elderly are a particular worry in this regard because they may suffer a serious illness such as a myocardial infarction without typical symptoms, and they may present as confused for reasons of long-standing or acute illness as well as trauma. Do not dismiss any symptoms which may relate to a head injury. Patients of this sort are often in the 'hard to assess' category and should be seen by a doctor.

3. Was the patient knocked out? Ask any witnesses what they saw. For how long was the patient unconscious? Ask the witness what is meant by 'unconscious'. Sometimes it is assumed that the patient who fails to get up is unconscious. Ask if the patient moved, spoke, changed colour, vomited, had difficulty breathing, showed signs of a fit? In the end, it may still be unclear whether or not the patient was knocked out.

4. Is there any memory loss caused by the injury? **Retrograde amnesia** refers to forgotten events before the injury and **post-traumatic amnesia (PTA)**, refers to events after the injury until the time of being seen in the clinic. The duration of PTA is a measure of severity of trauma and is correlated to diffuse brain injury. The patient may be able to remember isolated incidents while suffering from amnesia. PTA is measured as the time from the injury until continuous memory returns. It may be possible to establish that PTA has occurred when speaking to the patient, but it may not be clear whether it has ended. Give the patient some simple information which can be asked for later to assess recall. SIGN guidelines provisionally ascribe significance to a PTA of longer than 5 minutes in assessing a patient for admission to hospital.

5. Was the patient using alcohol or drugs? Any use by the patient of alcohol or drugs at the time of the injury will make it difficult to assess the significance of a knockout, drowsiness, disorientation, period of amnesia, headache or vomiting, and it will make the results of examination unreliable. Local protocols or guidelines are likely to require referral for a doctor's assessment, and the patient is likely to be admitted to hospital for observation.

6. Are there any visual problems, especially double vision (diplopia) or blurring of vision since the injury, and are things better or worse? Double vision can be caused by a local injury to the orbit, or pressure of a skull fracture on a cranial nerve. Orbital injury should be signalled by local signs, bruising and swelling. Blurring of the vision in one eye may also have a significant cause. Compression of the optic nerve behind the eyeball by bleeding (retrobulbar haemorrhage) may cause blindness if surgery is not performed quickly. A history of visual disturbance may not herald any major problem, but the patient should be referred for examination by a doctor.

7. Does the patient have a headache? It is very likely, and the progress of the headache in subsequent days is more likely to be important than its presence at the time of injury. A patient will often complain of local pain at the site of the injury. This should be assessed to

exclude a fracture. Other causes of headache include intracranial pathology and neck injury. If the patient is sent home, the NP will advise a return if the headache is not settling.

8. Is there a discharge of fluid from nose or ear, or blood from the ear? This may indicate a base of skull fracture, with leakage of CSF.

9. Does the patient have vertigo? This is dizziness caused by moving the head. This may be related to a fracture of the petrous temporal bone. This bone houses the osseus labyrinth of the inner ear and injury may also cause deafness and tinnitus. There should be other signs that a significant head injury has occurred.

10. Has the patient vomited? Repeated vomiting may be associated with a significant head injury. It is, in any case, a problem in its own right, especially in a child, who may become dehydrated.

11. Does the patient feel any pain or restriction in the neck? Ask if the patient has noticed any weakness or loss of sensation in the limbs or any difficulty walking.

12. Is there any history of allergies? What is the patient's tetanus status if there is a wound, and what are the medical history, medical problems and medications. A patient who is on anticoagulant therapy is at a higher risk of an intracranial bleed and should be referred to A&E for review by a doctor.

Physical Examination

NPs cannot offer an exhaustive examination of a patient with head injury. However, the process of conferring priority on patients with head injury is largely a matter of a careful history, general observation and basic examination at a level which the NP can perform.

1. Record the patient's Glasgow Coma Scale Score (Table 9.1), pulse, blood pressure and respirations. Abnormality caused by the head injury is not likely if the patient seems well, but a baseline will be useful if there is deterioration.

2. Observe the patient coming from the waiting room. Evidence of a focal or general disturbance of movement and coordination will be available from both the gait and the ability to perform simple tasks such as standing up and sitting down.

3. Ask the patient to show the full range of active neck movements (p. 91). Note any restriction and ask if these movements trigger any symptoms such as headache, dizziness, tingling or radiating pain into the arms. Palpate the cervical spine for tenderness.

4. A simple test of arm function is to ask the patient to hold both arms straight out in front with palms up and eyes shut. If an arm is weak, it will drift downwards and into pronation. A more complete assessment of sensation and motor power in the arms is described on page 90.

5. Look carefully at the patient, record any bruising (a fracture of the anterior cranial fossa base may be indicated by two bruised 'panda' eyes; a bruise over the mastoid prominence (Battle's sign) may indicate a fracture of the petrous bone). Record any wounds. Search the scalp carefully. Look for signs of discharge from the ears and nose. Do not put an auroscope into a bleeding ear as it will increase the risk of cranial infection if there is a fracture of the skull.

6. Are the pupils equal and reacting to light? A dilated, non-responsive pupil may be cause by trauma to the eye, fracture of the skull or rising intracranial pressure, Changes in the pupils caused by an increase in intracranial pressure will usually be accompanied by a deterioration in the level of consciousness. The patient with pupil abnormality needs an immediate assessment by a doctor.

7. Check patient's range of eye movements, up and down and to both sides for any difficulty or double vision. A patient with abnormal eye movements or double vision should see a doctor.

8. Visual acuity is tested with a Snellen chart at a distance of 6 metres; it is also valuable to test close vision with a small print chart (see Ch. 10).

9. Hearing can be quickly assessed by closing over one of the patient's ears and testing the other by rubbing two fingers together near it.

10. Assess any loss of the sense of smell.

11. Assess the facial nerves for any asymmetry, loss of sensation and control of facial muscles.

Discharge or Referral

A patient who is not in the higher risk categories listed above and who is examined without revealing any abnormality will usually be sent home.

Patients with minor head injuries receive written advice which lists the ways in which complications may be experienced, advises against driving until the symptoms are settling and against drinking alcohol in case it masks a deterioration in condition.

The most important single provision for the patient's safety is that another adult, someone sensible, who is aware of the situation and has seen the written advice sheet will keep an eye on the patient and obtain help if the patient's condition deteriorates. In a case where the patient has no one to help, a doctor should be consulted for a possible hospital admission.

SIGN criteria for discharge of the patient are:

- adult observation of the patient for at least 24 hours
- the carer will receive verbal and written advice
- the patient should have transport home and be able to obtain prompt medical help if there are problems.

A head injury advice sheet is focused on the first day after the injury. The patient may develop symptoms much later than that and should see a doctor if there are any problems.

Head injury advice includes:

1. Symptoms which should not cause concern unless they become much worse: moderate headache which eases with paracetamol, tiredness, nausea, a loss of appetite and poor concentration.
2. General advice: rest while these symptoms occur; avoid sport, a lot of television and any alcohol.
3. Return to hospital if there is: increasing drowsiness or confusion, vomiting more than once, a headache of increasing severity, disturbed vision, a discharge from nose or ear, a loss of feeling, coordination or power in a limb.

10 THE FACE

CONTENTS

This chapter is devoted to injuries to the face, the eye, and, very briefly, ear, nose and throat (ENT) problems. Wounds to the face are dealt with in Chapter 8. Assessment of the cranial nerves is dealt with in Chapter 9.

The face is capable of sustaining a minor injury, and most injuries to the face are minor. Nevertheless, many of the face injuries presenting at a minor injury clinic are beyond the scope of a NP. The reasons for this are the limits which are placed on the NP's power to request X-ray examination, the delicacy and importance of the structures involved, the cosmetic significance of injuries and the dangerous complications which can occur.

Many injuries, however, require no treatment or straightforward treatment. The NP will also have to assess and correctly refer a great many other problems, and you will need a basic grasp of the anatomy of the face, and the types of injuries which commonly occur.

The Face

The face is the part of the head which lies between the eyebrow and the chin in front, and includes the ears at the sides. It is of unique significance for several reasons:

- it has seven openings, which give access to organs of sense (eyes, ears, nose and mouth); of these, the eyes are the most complex, the most important, the most exposed and the most vulnerable to injury
- the nose and mouth are the external part of the airway; they are used for speech, and the mouth is the upper access to the digestive tract
- the face has a small range of movement compared with, for instance, the limbs, but it has a large supply of nerves and blood vessels, muscles adapted for fine expressive functions, and organs of sense such as the eyes and mouth
- the face gives access to the brain by several pathways, and violent trauma to the face may also cause brain injury or injury to the cervical spine
- certain infections of the face may enter the brain
- many of the signs of brain injury may also be detected in the face
- the face is the part of the body most associated with vital psychological, social and sexual functions.

Faces are intimately associated with the notion of identity. If we think about an absent person, our mental picture is of the face. The face is a repository and a source for many subtle appearances, expressions and emanations, which seem, to other people, to show something which may be called personality, inner being or, for those who use religious language, soul. We reach all manner of relations and accommodations with other people simply by sharing a look with them: attraction, complicity, intimacy, hostility, warning, reassurance, empathy. We communicate emotion, and we conceal our feelings by the ways that we show our faces. In doing this we must have not only a response to the other person's signals but also a sense of how our expressions will be received and understood. An injury which changes our faces, alters or impedes the signals we give, reduces our attractiveness or makes us conspicuous can cause suffering, in ways that have nothing to do with the injury but are related to the **cosmetic** significance of the change. This may also mean that we are less valuable in the world of work or that we become less able to live our normal lives; these are matters which may result in litigation. It is vital, in dealing with injuries to the face, that the importance of this aspect is understood. The word 'cosmetic' sounds frivolous but, in this context, it is not.

Bony Anatomy of the Face

In terms of bone structure, the frontal bone, the parietal, sphenoid and temporal bones at the sides, and the occipital bone at the back enclose the cranial part of the skull, which houses the brain (see Fig. 9.1). Structures such as the orbits, the nasal structures, the zygomas, the maxilla and the mandible are facial.

Many of the joints of the skull are of an immoveable, or only slightly moveable type, and are called **sutures**.

The **orbits** are the bony sockets for the eyes. They also contain muscles to move the eyes, blood vessels and nerves and the lacrimal structures for the production of tears. They are formed by the meeting of several bones of the skull and face, the frontal above, the zygoma on the lateral aspect and the maxilla medially. In the floor of the hollow, the sphenoid, ethmoid, palatine and lacrimal bones contribute to the jigsaw of interlocking bones. There are three major openings in the bony basin: the superior and inferior orbital fissures and the optic canal. These convey nerves and vessels, including cranial nerves, from the brain to the eye and other parts of the face. On the medial side of the socket is the **nasolacrimal duct**, which allows tears to drain from eye into nose.

Between the orbits, the two **nasal bones** meet in the midline of the upper face, forming the bony upper part of the nose called the bridge. Below them, the remaining nasal structures are made of cartilage. The part of the nose which divides the two nostrils is called the **septum. Paranasal sinuses** are air-filled hollows inside adjoining bones of the face; they are lined with mucosal tissue and surround and are linked to the nasal cavity.

The **maxillae** (singular, maxilla) are two bones which meet in the midline of the face above the mouth and form the boundaries of the lower parts of the orbits, the sides of the nose and top half of the mouth. They hold the upper teeth. The maxilla is the main structure in the part of the facial skeleton known as the **middle third** (lying between the frontal bone and the mandible). The maxillary and ethmoid air sinuses lie in this area, and fractures which involve them are treated as **compound**. Backward displacement of the maxilla can compromise the airway.

The **temporal bones** are on the sides of the skull, below the parietal bones and in front of the occipital bones. They correspond, in their frontal parts, to the area called the temple. The temporal bone is subdivided into four regions. The upper part, the **squamous region**, gives rise to the zygoma (see below). The **tympanic region** is the area where the bony structure of the outer canal of the ear is found, the **external auditory meatus**. The **mastoid region** is the site of the **mastoid process**, an attachment point for muscles of the neck. This can be felt as a smooth firm bump behind the ear. The mastoid lies between the middle ear and the brain. It is an area of sinuses which can harbour infection. There is, therefore, a risk, in some cases, that ear infections can pass to the brain through the mastoid. The **petrous region** of the temporal bone forms part of the inside of the cranium and encloses the structures of the middle and inner parts of the ear.

The **zygoma** is the cheekbone. It is one of the bony structures of the middle third of the face. It arises from the **zygomatic processes** of the maxilla and the frontal bone, on the lateral and inferior aspects of the orbit, and passes back along the side of the face towards the ear, as the **zygomatic arch**. It is the distinctive bony ledge which divides the temple from the cheek. It joins the **zygomatic process** of the temporal bone. Here, it forms a roof for the **temporomandibular joint**, the joint between the upper and lower jaws, just in front of the outer canal of the ear. There is a small hollow on the underside of the temporal zygomatic process, called the **mandibular fossa**, which receives the articulating part of the **mandible**, called the **condyle**. The external auditory meatus (see above) lies just below the zygomatic process as it merges with the temporal bone. The zygoma rises from the face and then rejoins it, in an arc something like a single-span bridge. If it suffers a crushing injury, usually from a blow to the side of the face, the span of the bone can be depressed towards the face, a fracture which creates a characteristic asymmetry, a flattening of the outline of the injured cheekbone.

The mandible is the lower jaw bone, the skeletal structure for the lower half of the mouth, the lower teeth and the chin. It comprises two symmetrical L-shaped parts which meet in the midline below the mouth (at the central dip in the chin, called the **mandibular symphisis**). The vertical legs of the bone, called the **rami** (singular, ramus, meaning branch), meet the horizontal parts at the **mandibular angle**, the posterior angle of the chin. The superior part of each ramus is made up of two processes divided by a groove called the **mandibular notch**. The anterior process is called the **coronoid**, and it is the insertion point for the **temporalis** muscle, which arises from the temporal bone and passes under the zygomatic arch to the lower jaw. It closes the mouth. The posterior process of the ramus is the mandibular condyle, which articulates with the mandibular fossa on the inferior surface of the temporal zygomatic process to form the synovial temporomandibular joint. This joint allows movement at the mouth, opening and closing, lateral deviation and protrusion of the mandible (thrusting the lower jaw forward). The mandibular condyles can be felt protruding if the fingertips are placed below the zygoma, just anterior to the entrance to the canals of the ears, and the patient is asked to open his mouth. The condyles become prominent as the mouth opens, and move under the zygoma as it closes.

Fractures of the Face

Any patient who presents with fracture of the face should be referred. Fractures of the face are commonly accompanied by other injuries and often occur in serious incidents such as road traffic accidents or falls from great height. The patients presenting to minor injury clinics are of a different type. There are three common causes of injury:

1. Assault. The face has been punched, kicked or struck with an implement like a baseball bat, a brick, a bottle, a hammer or a metal bar. Issues such as crime (and the injury itself represents a crime), alcohol and drug misuse and domestic violence are often related to the event, and it may be difficult to obtain a clear history.
2. Sports injuries. These include blows to the face with hockey sticks and golf clubs, eye injuries from squash balls and orbit lacerations from clashes of heads at rugby. Patients who fall from bicycles, perhaps because they reflexively squeeze the brakes as they fall, often meet the ground or a wall face first.

3. Elderly people. When elderly people fall, they often fail to put out their hands to break the fall and will take the brunt on their faces. These injuries are often eyebrow and nose lacerations with no fractures. The question of why the fall happened may take more time than the facial injuries.

Facial fractures can obstruct the airway, and any patient is at risk who has suffered an injury which reduces the ability to open and close the mouth or to speak properly, or which produces the sounds of obstructed breathing, stridor or snoring. A fracture of the maxilla which is displaced backwards may endanger the airway and may need prompt reduction. Blood and vomit and broken teeth may be inhaled.

If the airway is threatened, summon emergency help. An anaesthetist will be required, possibly to intubate the patient or perform an emergency cricothyroidotomy.

Make a neurological assessment of a patient with a face injury (Ch. 9), checking both head and neck. Exclude other injuries, especially if the patient is elderly or very young. These are particularly common when the patient has fallen in the street or from a bicycle. Focus, in the patient's history, on why the injury occurred, whether or not the patient was knocked out, whether or not the patient remembers the incident. Has the patient walked since it happened? Find out about past medical history and medications. Anticoagulants are of particular importance if there is a risk of cranial bleeding or bleeding within or behind the eye. Discover if there is a history of falls with an elderly person, or medical conditions which predispose to a fall, of which there are many (the list includes Parkinson's disease, cardiac arrhythmias, arthritis, cataract, transient ischaemic attacks and diabetes). The patient's home circumstances, and whether or not there is someone to provide care, will be important.

A clinical examination of the face should show whether or not a fracture is present. Facial fractures often involve more than one bone, and any separate discussion of the bones should be read with that in mind.

Look for asymmetry or deformity of the face. Look from the front, the sides and from above and behind the patient, looking down. Try to distinguish a genuine bony asymmetry from soft tissue swelling and any imbalance between the sides of the face which is normal for the patient.

Other features which will alert to the presence of a fracture are tenderness, crepitus or gaps in the bone, facial paraesthesia and subcutaneous emphysema (if there is a fracture through an air sinus). There may be a loss of movement of the eye or jaw, a change in the position of the eyes in the orbits or a characteristic pattern of bruising and swelling. Fractures can occur to a number of bones.

The floor of the orbit

A blow on the eye may cause the orbit to give way at its weakest point, the floor. There may be no external bony tenderness. A **blowout fracture** of the floor of the orbit is indicated if the eye is retracted in its socket (**enophthalmos**), if there is loss of upward eye movement or double vision (**diplopia**) on upward movement, a difference in the level of the two pupils, if there is loss of sensation over the area of the infraorbital nerve (on the cheek just below the eye, side of nose, top of lip), a subcutaneous emphysema or a nosebleed on the injured side. There may be herniation of the eye, the fat of the orbit and perhaps the muscles of the eye into the maxillary sinus (the source of any subcutaneous emphysema).

The zygoma

A fracture of the cheekbone, often caused by assault, will cause a depression of the cheek which is plainly visible as an asymmetry.

There may be damage to vital structures within the eye; bleeding behind the eyeball (**retrobulbar haemorrhage**), optic nerve injury and damage to the orbit are common. *Assess visual acuity*. If the eye is protruding (**exophthalmos**), retrobulbar haemorrhage is possible.

Palpate the two sutures at the joints with the frontal bone, on the outer side of the orbit, and with the maxilla below the orbit. Palpate the lower margin of the orbit. Palpate the nasomaxillary and nasofrontal sutures. Assess the temporomandibular joints for disruption. All of these may be involved in the fracture. There may be paraesthesia, as for blowout fracture. A **tripod fracture** of the zygoma and maxilla is usually caused by a punch to the side of the face and is characterized by three fractures. These are found at the zygoma/frontal suture on the rim of the lateral orbit, the zygoma/maxilla suture below the orbit and the arch of the zygoma itself. This fracture disrupts the floor of the orbit.

The maxilla

The maxilla can be fractured by blunt injury, during assault or in sport (although road traffic accidents are the most common cause of fractures). *Assess the airway*. The maxilla may be driven back, obstructing the airway, a very violent injury. Fracture through the maxillary sinus may cause subcutaneous emphysema. Patients should not blow their noses to avoid worsening the emphysema or pushing air into the orbit. A fractured maxilla may drop down, giving the face a lengthened appearance. Maxilla fractures are accompanied by injuries to other parts of the middle third of the face, and this complex of injuries is classified in ascending order of severity as **Le Fort fractures I**, **II** and **III**.

- I The bone containing the top teeth is separated from the face above it.
- II The middle section of the face, including nose and the areas immediately lateral to the nose and the upper teeth, are separated from the face. The face may look elongated, and the front of the face may be mobile.
- III The face is separated in its entirety from the cranium. This is a major injury.

The nose

The nose is often punched, and a sideways impact can easily cause a displacement to the other side, a deformity which most patients will regard as cosmetically serious.

In the initial stage, the priority of management has to do with function. Is there a severe displacement? Are the airways patent? Is there a septal haematoma which should be drained? Is there a severe nosebleed? Are there associated fractures on the face?

Be alert for the presence of cerebrospinal fluid draining from the nose, indicating a fracture of the ethmoid bone. This exposes the cranium to infection. Look also for black eyes and orbital swelling, a flattening of the nose, a very mobile fracture and facial paraesthesia.

If the nose is undisplaced, there is no wound, and its functions are undisturbed, there may be no need, from the point of view of treatment which would follow, to refer the patient for X-ray. Follow local policy on that issue.

If there is a cosmetically significant injury which requires manipulation of the bone or cartilage of the septum, the patient should be referred to the ENT team. There will be a local arrangement for referral. This is usually postponed until the initial swelling is settled, but should be done before manipulation becomes difficult. Hawkesford and Banks (1994) recommend that this should be done in less than 10 days from the time of injury.

Mandible

Assess the airway. The lower jaw may be broken or dislocated at the temporomandibular joints by trauma. There is often more than one fracture, and the point of the impact will not necessarily be the site of the fracture. Check the teeth for injury and the tissues of the mouth for injury and haematoma. There may be paraesthesia of the lower lip. Look for bleeding from the ear. If the jaw is dislocated, there will be deformity and an inability to close the mouth. Is the patient's bite normal? Is the patient swallowing properly? Does speech seem difficult? There may be visible deformity, swelling and bruising, and any fracture may be clearly palpable as a step in the bone.

The Eye

Patients will present to a minor injury clinic with eye problems of every degree of severity and urgency, traumatic and non-traumatic. NPs who deal with eye problems will receive special training to do so and will act within the terms of the protocols or guidelines which they have developed. In many units, patients who present themselves with eye problems are referred to another site. The referral may be to a GP, an A&E department or an eye hospital. This section will give some basic information on first aid to the eye, and on discrimination between problems of different degrees of severity so that an accurate referral can be made. The eye will also need assessing as part of an assessment of the patient after other injuries, such as trauma to the head.

In all dealings with patients with eye problems, the NP must bear in mind that blindness is one of the greatest catastrophes which can befall anyone. No risks should be taken with any eye problem, and a NP should expect patients to be very anxious about anything which affects the eye.

Anatomy of the Eye

Figure 10.1 shows the basic anatomy of the eye. The eyes are protected and lubricated, during reflexive blinking every few seconds, by upper and lower **eyelids**, which are joined at the medial and lateral corners of the eye, at the **canthi**. On the inner surface of the lids are the **tarsal plates**, layers of connective tissue which reinforce the fine skin of the lids. There are many sebaceous glands in the tarsal plates, and these can become blocked and develop cysts which are prominent on the surface of the lids. The upper lid is the larger of the two. The **levator palpebrae superioris** muscle (palpebrae means eyelids) lifts the upper lid to open the eye. The eyelashes have a rich nerve supply at their roots and respond to the slightest stimulus by triggering a reflexive blink. An infection of the sebaceous gland of an eyelash follicle causes a stye.

The **lacrimal gland** produces tears through the **lacrimal duct** to the upper, outer part of the eye. Tears pass across the eyeball surface before draining into the nasal cavity. Tears cleanse the eye and help to suppress infection.

The inner layer of both eyelids is covered by a thin mucous membrane, the **conjunctiva**. At the front, this membrane folds back onto the outer layer of the eyeball, (the **sclera**; see below) and it merges with the epithelial layer of the **cornea**. The conjunctiva lubricates the eye. Irritation of the conjunctiva, often caused by infection or allergy, is called **conjunctivitis**. Foreign bodies often lodge in the conjunctiva of the upper eyelid.

The extrinsic muscles of the eye are shown in Figure 10.2.

The eye is supported in the orbit by pads of fat and held in place at the back by the suspensory ligament. The eyeball is contained separately from the rest of the orbit by a sheet of fibrous tissue.

The eye itself has three layers.

The outermost layer of the eyeball is called the sclera and the cornea. The sclera is the largest part of this layer, covering most of the globe of the eyeball except the front. It is a tough white connective tissue. The colour of this tissue

The Eye

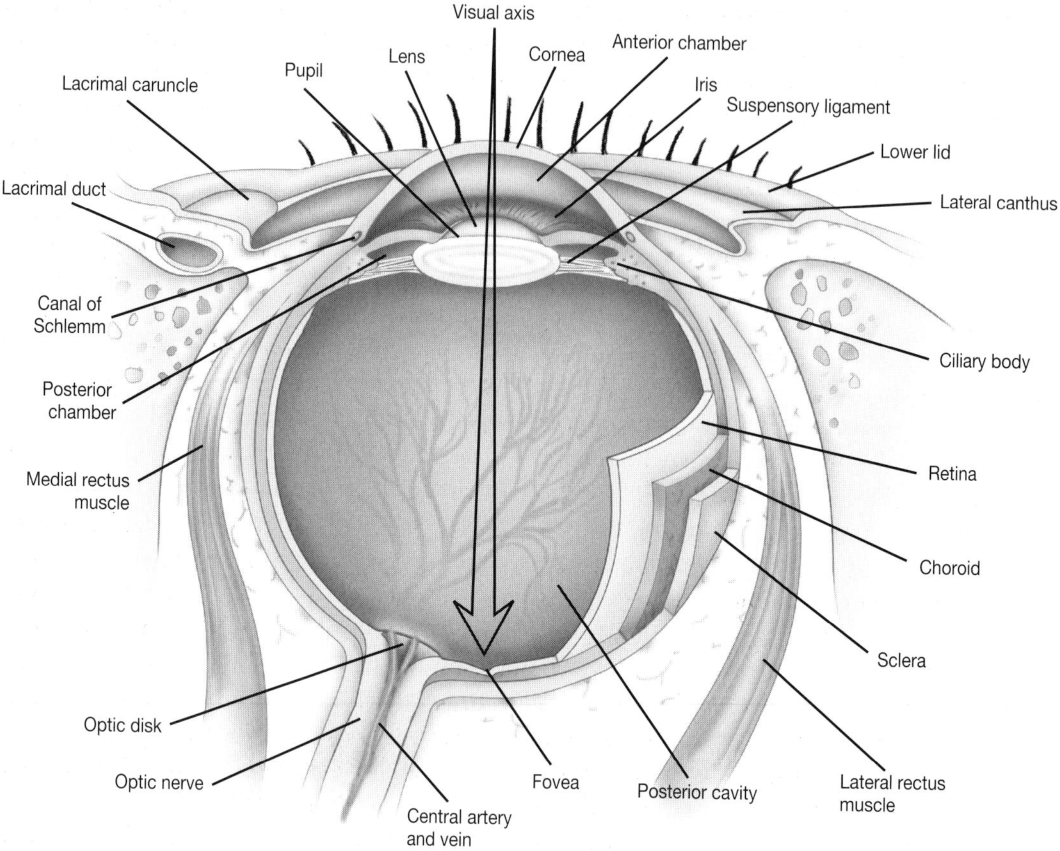

Figure 10.1 Horizontal section through the left eyeball viewed from above. (Reproduced with kind permission from Thibodeau and Patton, 1999.)

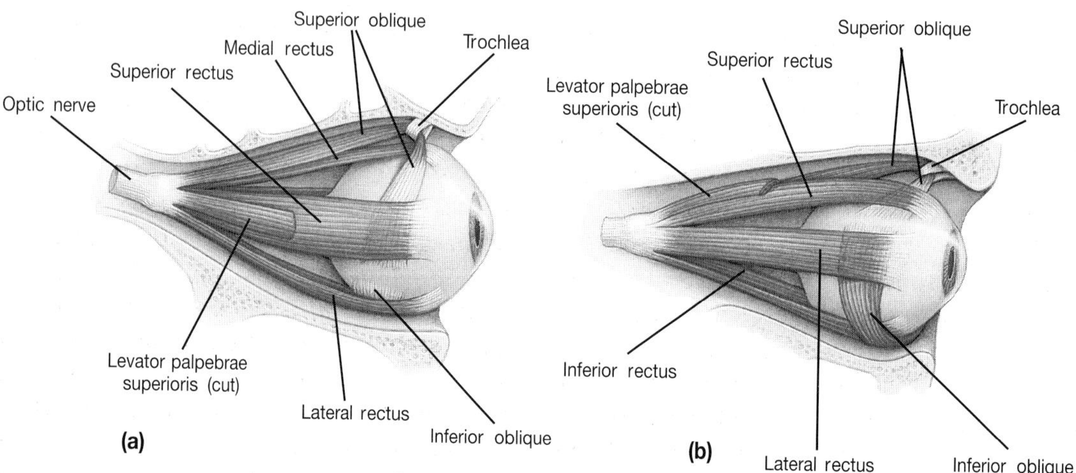

Figure 10.2 The extrinsic muscles of the right eye. (a) Superior view; (b) lateral view. (Reproduced with kind permission from Thibodeau and Patton, 1999.)

gives the eye its white appearance. The tendons of the extrinsic muscles of the eye attach to its posterior area. The **optic nerve** passes through the sclera at the back, and there is a direct connection between the dura mater and the sclera. At the front of the eye, over an area which is one sixth of the globe, the sclera becomes the transparent **cornea** at the corneoscleral junction. The cornea is nerve rich, pain sensitive and moist, but, like the rest of the fibrous layer, avascular. The process of **refraction**, the redirection of light through the front of the eye to the retina at the back, occurs not only at the lens but also through the cornea. Because it is the front surface of the eye, the cornea is exposed to injury. Foreign bodies and wounding objects which pass the defensive blinking reflex, the **corneal reflex**, can cause **corneal abrasions** and damage to deeper structures.

The **uvea** is the middle layer of the eye. From the back of the eye to the front, it is composed of three parts, the **choroid**, the **ciliary body** and the **iris**. The choroid is a membrane which lines the sclera up to the corneoscleral junction. It is pierced by the optic nerve. It has two layers, which correspond to two functions. The outer layer has a brown pigmentation, contributed by melanocytes, which makes it light absorbent. This prevents excessive reflection of light within the eye, which would cause confusion. The inner layer is vascular and supplies the circulation for the other layers of the eyeball. At the front of the choroid is the ciliary body. This is a ring of tissue, mainly muscle, which surrounds the lens of the eye and helps to change its shape so that it can accommodate images from different distances. The **suspensory ligament** is connected to the ciliary body and surrounds the lens, helping to maintain its position. In front of the ciliary body, and continuous with it, is the iris, the part of the eye from which eye colour is derived. The colour of the eye depends directly on the amount of brown pigment in the iris. The iris is placed between the cornea and the lens. It is a membrane laced with two arrangements of smooth muscle fibres, one controlled by the sympathetic and the other by the parasympathetic nervous system. There is a hole in the centre of the iris, the **pupil**. The sympathetic fibres *dilate* the pupil, making it larger to allow more light to reach the lens. The parasympathetic fibres *constrict* the pupil to reduce the flow of light to the lens. This change in pupil size helps the eye to adjust to different lighting conditions. Other factors such as injury to brain, emotional state and the presence in the body of systemic or topical drugs have an effect on the size of the pupils.

The inner, third layer, of the eye is the **retina**. Like the choroid, the retina has an outer pigmented layer, with a similar function to that of the choroid. The inner layer of the retina is transparent. It contains light receptor nerve cells with two basic shapes, **rods** and **cones**. Rods deal with images received in poor light, but indistinctly with poor realisation of colour. Cones give clear, sharp, highly coloured images in good light. The optic nerve passes through the layers of the eye at the back, at a point called the **optic disc**. There are no light receptors at this point, and there is, therefore, a **blind spot** in the eye's field of vision. Lateral to the optic disc is an area called the **macula lutea**, which has a small hollow in its centre, called the **fovea centralis**. This area has a very high density of cone receptors, and vision is sharpest here. Some of the blood supply to the retina is from the choroid, but the largest part is from the **central artery**, a branch of the **ophthalmic artery**, and the **central vein**, which enter and leave the eye through the passage for the optic nerve. The central artery supplies the retina in four branches, and blockage of any branch causes blindness in that area. A separation of the neural layer of the retina from the pigmented layer, usually called a **detached retina**, which may occur spontaneously or as a result of trauma, will impair vision and may cause permanent blindness if it cannot be repaired.

The eye is divided into two **chambers** by the lens and its supporting structures. The front chamber, between lens and cornea, is filled with a watery fluid called **aqueous humour**, a nutrient and cleansing substance which constantly enters and drains from the eye so that a consistent internal pressure of 16 mmHg is maintained. If drainage of aqueous humour becomes blocked, a condition known as **glaucoma**, increasing pressure in the eye destroys the nerves and causes blindness. The rear chamber of the eye is filled with a transparent gel called **vitreous humour**. There is no circulatory change in the vitreous humour. This substance allows the passage of light, maintains the shape of the eyeball and helps to hold the various parts of the eye in place. **Floaters** may be visible defects in the vitreous humour, which literally float in the field of vision as spots or lines. These are a benign degenerative change. However, they may also be symptoms of a retinal detachment or a haemorrhage in the posterior chamber, and a patient should be referred to a doctor if complaining of any sudden change.

Visual Acuity

The most basic measure of the condition of a patient's eye is of its function, which means vision, and this should be assessed in every patient with an eye complaint. Apart from the contribution that this test makes to the clinical picture, eye injuries often lead to court cases, and a formal record of the patient's visual acuity should be documented.

The minor injury NP is not an optician, and there is nothing to gain by making people remove spectacles or lenses before testing them. The purpose of the test is to find any deterioration caused by the injury from the level of correction which the patient normally receives from lenses. Ask patients who are not wearing spectacles if they normally wear glasses or lenses (a point that should emerge during the history). People who attend with fresh injuries to the face or eye often have had to remove these because they have been broken during the incident, the face is swollen or the eye is painful. The eyes are tested one at a time. The eye which is not being tested is covered with an opaque card. Covering the eye with a hand is not adequate because it is hard to be sure that patients are not seeing through a gap in their fingers.

There are visual aids for people who do not speak English, or children who are too young to read, but the standard test is of the ability to name letters on a chart. These are graded in size to reproduce the effect of reading the same size of letter from increasing distances; this avoids the need for an indefinite space to carry out the assessment. As it is, the standard test, the **Snellen**, requires 6 metres (20 feet) from patient to chart (Fig. 10.3). If space is too small for that, a chart with reversed lettering can be hung behind the patient. Reading from that in a mirror from 3 metres (10 feet) effectively doubles the distance to the chart. It is important to test from the correct distance, and there should be a permanent mark at the 6 metre spot. The chart should be evenly lit with, preferably, a spot lamp.

The results of the test are expressed in two numbers. The first one simply tells the

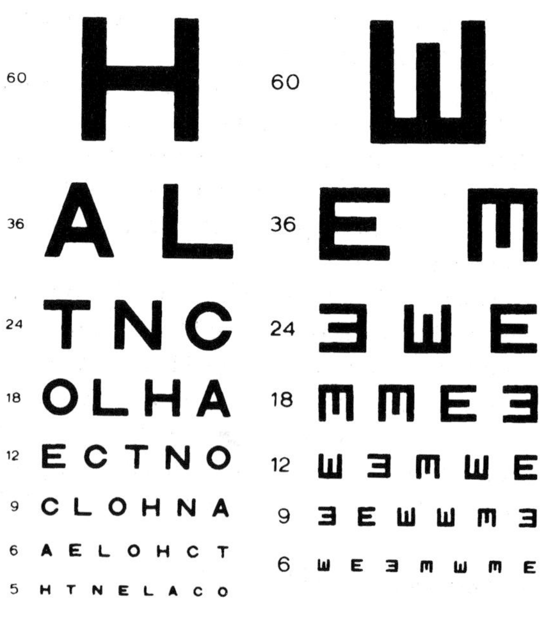

Figure 10.3 The Snellen letter and illiterate E test-types. (Reproduced from Parr J 1989 Introduction to ophthalmology, 3rd edn, Figure 3–14, by permission of Oxford University Press.)

distance to the chart in metres, 6 (when the tests were done in feet, the number was 20). The second number is based on a calculation of how a 'normal' eye, one with no error in refraction, should perform. The top letter on the chart, the largest, should be clear to the normal eye from 60 metres. A patient who can read *only* the top letter from 6 metres will have a test result of 6/60. It follows that the normal eye will achieve a score of 6/6, equivalent to the older non-metric score of 20/20. A separate result is recorded for each eye.

The top line on the chart contains only one letter. The other lines are, in descending order, smaller, with more letters, and meant to be clear from the following distances in metres: 36, 24, 18, 12, 9, 6, 5 and 4.

Patients who cannot read *any* letters from 6 metres are moved closer to the chart. If the patient can read the top letter *only* at 1 metre, this is a visual acuity of 1/60 for that eye.

The patient who cannot see any letters from 1 metre is asked to **count fingers** held up by the examiner. If the patient is able to do that, the result for that eye is charted as **CF**, with the distance in metres. If the patient cannot do that but can detect the movement of a hand waving, record the result as **hand movement** (**HM**). If the patient cannot do that, shine a light into each eye. If the patient sees that, this is marked as having **perception of light** (**PL**); if not, **no perception of light** (**NPL**) is recorded.

Patients who have some kind of refractive defect of their vision will find that reading performance is improved by looking at the chart through a pinhole in a card, and this test may help the assessment of patients who arrive without their spectacles or lenses. An improvement is recorded as 'with pinhole' (with PH).

Examining the eye

Eye medications

Care of minor eye injuries involves the use of three preparations:

- **fluorescein** is a staining substance, yellow-orange in colour, which reveals corneal abrasions when the stained eye is viewed through an ophthalmoscope with a blue filter (or a slit lamp if available); it is available as an impregated paper strip which is moistened and inserted under the lower lid or as eye drops
- **tetracaine** (amethocaine) (tetracaine hydrochloride 0.5% and 1%) is a local anaesthetic eye drop
- **chloramphenicol** ointment or eye drops are used as a broad-spectrum prophylaxis if a corneal abrasion is found or there is an active, superficial eye infection.

Putting in eye drops or ointment

Seat the patient comfortably and explain what you intend to do. Warn the patient if the medication is going to sting.

Eye drops can be put into the eye by asking the patient to look up and gently pulling the lower lid downwards with the tip of the finger. Put two drops into the conjunctival sac, not touching the eye with the dropper. Ask the patient to look down, then gently let the lid return to its normal position.

Place ointment in the same way, then ask the patient to close the eyes for a minute or so.

Eversion of the eyelid

Eversion of the eyelid depends upon the rigidity of the tarsal plate to allow access to the conjunctiva of the upper eyelid, usually to remove a foreign body. A cotton-bud stick is a suitable implement. Lie the stick across the top of the eyelid. Ask the patient to look down. Take the eyelashes between your fingers and pull the lid down and outwards, and then turn it upwards, pressing down gently on the stick at the same time. The lid should fold back along the upper margin of the tarsal plate, and it should stay there as long as the patient is looking down. It will return to normal when the patient looks up and closes the eyes.

To examine the conjunctiva of the lower lid, ask the patient to look up, put your finger on the lid just below the eyelashes and pull the lid downwards.

Irrigation of the eye

Copious irrigation of the surface of the eye with an isotonic solution of normal saline is required for treatment of chemical burns (except burns from lime, a constituent of cement), and it will often remove loose foreign bodies.

The traditional irrigation vessel is the undine, but there is nothing better, for a plentiful irrigation, than an intravenous bag of saline, directed through a giving set. Pull the on/off wheel down close to the external connector of the drip for accurate control of the rate of flow and direction of the stream. You need a receptacle to catch the fluid, and the patient should be wrapped to avoid wetting clothes. The patient lies down on one side with the injured eye below and the head over the basin. Direct the stream downwards from nose to ear, evert both lids one after the other, and ask the patient to look up, down and to both sides while you irrigate.

Eye patches

An eye patch is necessary if local anaesthetic drops have been put in the eye, to protect it from injury while it is desensitized. Eye patches are also helpful to give comfort for a painful eye, for instance after treatment of a corneal abrasion. A double eye patch, with the bottom layer folded double over the eye and a single layer above, held with skin tape keeps the eye closed more effectively.

The closure of one eye deprives the patient of the ability to judge distance accurately, and patients should take care and must not drive.

History

The taking of a history from the patient with an eye injury is the same as for any other injury. The NP should, however, pay particular attention to the patient's ophthalmic history, and whether contact lenses or spectacles are used. The fact that the patient was, or was not, wearing safety goggles may be relevant.

Medical Eye Problems: The Red Eye

Patients often present to a minor injury clinic with a **red eye**. Some of these patients will, in fact, have a trauma problem, such as a foreign body in the eye, and others will mistakenly believe that there must be something in the eye because it is painful. However, the differential diagnosis for the red eye includes a wide range of medical problems, some minor, some urgent and at least one which is an outright emergency. It is unlikely that such problems will be treated in a minor injury clinic, but the NP will need a basic idea of how to discriminate between them so that the level of urgency can be identified and the correct referral made.

1. A red eye with little pain and no disturbance of vision. The redness will tend to be less at the centre of the eye and greater at the conjunctival borders. This will often be a case of conjunctivitis and the NP can refer the patient to the GP.
   - **Bacterial conjunctivitis** is an infection (often *Staphylococcus aureus*) of the conjunctiva of the eye. The vessels of the conjunctiva will be enlarged. There will be a purulent discharge, which makes the eye sticky and difficult to open in the morning. The patient may complain of a 'gritty' feeling (exclude a foreign body) rather than pain. It will probably spread to the other eye. It may be treated with chloramphenicol.
   - **Viral conjunctivitis** is often caused by an adenovirus. The patient may have a history of a recent cold. Both eyes will be gritty, itchy and watery, with widespread redness, deepest at the conjunctiva. Most cases settle in 10 days or so, but some

The Eye

patients develop complications. It is very infectious.

2. A puffy red eye with no disturbance of vision. There may be a viral or allergic conjunctivitis, which the NP should refer to the GP, or a more urgent infection of the orbit.
   - **Allergic conjunctivitis** causes conjunctival redness and swelling, corneal swelling, a clear discharge and itching rather than pain. There may be a history of a contact with a possible allergen, and the patient may have had the same problem in the past. The staple treatment is antihistamine.
   - **Orbital cellulitis** is a bacterial infection of the eyelid and soft tissues of the orbit. It has the potential for dangerous spread in the face and cranial cavity, and the patient may be admitted to hospital for intravenous antibiotics.
3. A very painful eye with photophobia. Is there a foreign body? The treatment of foreign bodies is discussed below. In the case where the eye is painful but no foreign body is found, the patient may need referral to exclude a deep intraocular foreign body or a more severe medical problem.
4. A painful, photophobic, red eye, with impaired vision. The possibilities here include an **acute glaucoma**, which is an emergency, and the patient needs urgent review by an ophthalmologist.
   - **Anterior uveitis**, also called iritis, is an inflammation of the combined choroid, ciliary body and iris. It can cause serious damage to the eye. The patient may have a history of rheumatological problems, or infections such as ophthalmic herpes, and may have had a previous attack of iritis. The redness is not like the redness of conjunctivitis, which tends to be deepest at the conjunctiva. It will surround the inflamed ciliary body on the rim of the iris, an appearance called **ciliary flush** or **ciliary injection**. The vision will deteriorate. The pupil may be small or irregular. Treatment is urgent. Steroids and mydriatics (drops which paralyse the ciliary muscle and thereby dilate the pupil) reduce inflammation and the pain of ciliary spasm.
   - **Corneal ulcer** is an urgent condition, which threatens blindness, although its development may not be sudden. It is caused by infections, and there may have been a predisposing event such as a corneal abrasion or the use of contact lenses. The eye will be very painful. The effect of the ulcer on visual acuity will depend on its site. It can be diagnosed by staining the eye with fluorescein and viewing it through an ophthalmoscope with a blue filter. Refer to an ophthalmologist urgently if the history suggests the possibility.
   - **Acute angle closure glaucoma** is most likely to attack a person who is over 50 years of age and one who is long-sighted. The flow of aqueous humour from the rear part of the anterior chamber to the drainage channels at the front is prevented by the lens lying too close to the iris. This causes the iris to push forward and block the drainage channels of the humour, causes a rise in intraocular pressure. There is a sudden onset of pain in the eye and temporal headache, corneal oedema, a 'muddy iris', with redness of the eye and ciliary injection, vomiting, impaired vision and haloes around lights. The pupil is fixed and semi-dilated. This condition may cause blindness, and emergency relief of the pressure is required. Medications which may be used include acetazolamide, a systemic drug which reduces the secretion of aqueous humour, and pilocarpine drops, which contract the ciliary muscle and constrict the pupil, removing the obstruction to the drainage of humour.

It can be summarized from the above that conditions with pain and visual impairment, signs of spreading infection and any systemic malaise should be treated with greater caution. Some red eye presentations are a threat to the patient's sight, and all patients with a red eye should be assessed by a doctor, more or less urgently.

The Injured Eye

The following discussion is a general one on the subject of eye trauma. It is targeted at the likely range of presentations at a minor injury clinic, of which, as is usually the case, the less serious are the more common. However, it is not a guideline. There is likely to be a particularly large variation in the scope which NPs are allowed with eye problems from place to place, and the NP will be guided by local policies, protocols and guidelines (see also Ch. 8). There are four main types of eye injury:

- chemical burns
- corneal abrasion
- blunt trauma
- foreign body: subtarsal, corneal, intraocular (penetrating injury).

Chemical burn

Splash burns to the eye with chemical substances constitute an emergency until proven otherwise. Alkaline burns are particularly destructive, and lime may linger in the eye as trapped particles in the further reaches of the conjunctiva even after a thorough irrigation. The basic elements of initial treatment are local anaesthetic, irrigation, examination and removal of particles. Evert the lid, and then lift the everted lid away from the eye (this is called **double eversion**, and it exposes the upper fold of the conjunctiva) to search for lodged particles. The patient requires urgent referral to an ophthalmic surgeon.

Corneal abrasion

A corneal abrasion is a superficial wound to the surface of the cornea, removing a part of the epithelium. It is often inflicted by foreign bodies, the leaves of plants, fingernails or claws, branches and contact lenses.

The eye is very painful and local anaesthetic is usually required before examination. Stain the eye with fluorescein and view the injury with a blue-filtered ophthalmoscope. A corneal abrasion will appear to be green. Remove any foreign body.

The patient should be given antibiotic drops or ointment, which will protect against infection and lubricate the eye. Patients may also benefit from other medications if pain is severe; for example, **cycloplegic** eyedrops, paralyse the ciliary muscle (and are used to dilate the pupil for examination of the fundus) and can help to control painful ciliary spasm. An eyepad may be helpful while the eye is healing, a process which should only take a couple of days.

If the pain does not settle, the patient should return. There is, in addition to the possibility of infection, the risk of corneal ulceration.

A **flash burn** is similar in its effect and is diagnosed and treated in the same way as a corneal abrasion. Flash burns are radiation injuries to the cornea caused by exposure of the naked eye to a sun lamp or welder's flash. The symptoms develop some hours after the injury. The pain can be severe.

Blunt trauma

Blunt trauma is an injury to the eye and its surrounding tissues, usually inflicted by a fist or an object like a squash ball. (A small ball is more likely to injure the eye itself than a large one, which will be deflected by the orbit.) The patient may have a black eye, and the eye may be closed and difficult to examine.

A first priority is function of the eye. A full test of visual acuity may not be possible, but the NP should try to find out if the patient can see. If the eye is open, and there is a defect in visual acuity, the patient must be referred to the ophthalmologist.

Check the eyeball for damage. There may be a corneal abrasion. Is there **hyphaema** (visible blood in the anterior chamber of the eye)? The lens may be dislocated or the iris or pupil injured. (Beware of changes in the pupils. Assess the patient as having a potential head injury.) There may be haemorrhage in the posterior chamber, and detachment of the retina.

Facial fractures are discussed above (p. 233, for blowout fracture). Palpate the orbit and the zygoma for signs of fracture.

Clearly, there is great potential for significant damage with injuries of this type, and the patient will require referral at least to an A&E doctor for full examination.

Foreign bodies in the eye

Subtarsal foreign body

Typically, the patient presents with a watery, painful eye and a history of something, supposed to be grit, blowing into the eye outdoors in windy conditions. The discomfort may be localized to an area under the upper lid. If the cornea has been scratched by the grit, the discomfort may be less well localized.

Lie the patient down with the head back, and ask the patient to look down. Evert the upper lid (see above) and look for the foreign body. It can usually be lifted off with a cotton bud. The eye should be stained with fluorescein and examined under a blue filter for corneal abrasion. If this is found, a topical antibiotic is prescribed (often chloromycetin) in accordance with local practice.

Corneal foreign body

A foreign body lying on the corneal surface may be slightly embedded. The injury may have been of a higher velocity injury than a subtarsal injury, or the patient may embed the object by rubbing the eye. It may involve something flying from a hammer and chisel or a metal grinder, and it is often a sharp piece of metal. The object is usually visible on the eye surface and can be made more prominent by side-lighting the eye.

Beware of a serious intraocular injury caused by a deep penetrating foreign body, which may cause blindness.

Anaesthetise the eye with tetracaine (amethocaine) drops. Tell the patient to gaze at a fixed point. Hold the eyelids with one hand. A very superficial object can be lifted off the cornea with a cotton bud. An embedded object should be lifted out with the point of a sterile hypodermic needle. Use the needle point obliquely to avoid penetration of the eye if the patient moves. If it is deeply embedded, or a rust ring remains when it has been lifted out, refer the patient to the ophthalmology service.

Use antibiotic prophylaxis, as for a corneal abrasion, and protect the anaesthetized eye with a pad. If the foreign body was large, the eye may require a pad for a couple of days to allow healing.

Intraocular foreign body and penetrating injury

A history of a high-velocity foreign body is always, potentially, the history of a deep penetration injury into the eye. If the object is buried deep in the eye, there may be very little to see on the surface, no more than a tiny, inconspicuous entrance wound. In all of these cases, the patient will, at the very least, require X-ray examination to exclude an intraocular foreign body (IOFB). The patient may become blind if that diagnosis is missed.

A larger than normal object embedded in the cornea may penetrate to a much greater depth than its external appearance suggests. If the history suggests a large object, or if it resists removal, take care and refer the patient. Do not subject the eyeball to any pressure. If there is a projecting, penetrating object, leave it alone and make sure that the patient does the same. Make an urgent transfer of the patient to an ophthalmic surgeon.

Ear, Nose and Throat

In the minor injury clinic there are three common ENT presentations: bony injuries to the nose, nosebleed (**epistaxis**) and foreign body. Patients will attend with a nosebleed or a recent history of repeated nosebleeds. Parents will bring children who have inserted foreign bodies into the nose or the ear, or both. Adults who have ignored the injunction to stick nothing smaller than the elbow into the ear will present with cotton wool buds lodged in the outer canal. Patients will also present declaring that they have a fish or chicken bone stuck in the throat.

Nosebleed

A nosebleed feels, and looks, alarming. On occasion, there can be sufficient blood loss to make transfusion necessary. It may also be a persistent or a recurring phenomenon, either because a vessel in the nose is tending to bleed, in which case cauterization may be the only effective treatment, or because there is an underlying medical cause, such as hypertension or a blood coagulation disorder. This would need treatment before the bleeding will stop. The patient may also, in addition to bleeding from the nose, bleed into the back of the throat and swallow blood, which is later vomited.

Nosebleed which follows face or head injury may indicate a leakage of cerebrospinal fluid or a blowout fracture of the orbit. If a nosebleed follows a blow to the nose, consider the possibility of a fracture. With small children, check whether there is a foreign body in the nose.

Common causes for a nosebleed are nose picking or an infection of the upper respiratory tract, with sneezing and blowing of the nose. Bleeding, especially in children and young adults, is usually in **Kiesselbach's area**, in the anterior part of the nasal septum. In older patients, the source of the bleeding can be much further back in the nose and much less accessible.

Take a history which includes any relevant medical facts, including a history of hypertension and anticoagulent medicines such as warfarin, and the frequency and duration of bleeding episodes. Check the patient's blood pressure.

This may have to be postponed until after first aid. It is usually possible to stop a nosebleed by:

- seating the patient, leaning forward to discourage bleeding down the throat.
- getting the patient to apply firm pressure, at the bleeding nostril, with the tip of a finger to the side of the nose at the top of the soft part; this has to be maintained for 10 minutes without interruption.
- telling the patient to breathe through the mouth and spit any blood in the mouth out, rather than swallow it.

If the bleeding stops, observe the patient for a further half hour. Tell the patient not to blow the nose or otherwise dislodge the forming clot. Check the throat for back flow of blood. There are various methods, and you will have access to your own, for packing a nose to stop bleeding, including gauze packs, special tampon devices and inflatable pressure devices. A bleeding point which is very high up can be blocked with a foley catheter. This is passed up the nose to the back of the throat, its balloon inflated and the catheter pulled forward until it lodges in the posterior nasal area. There will be local protocols or guidelines for the referral and treatment of patients.

Foreign Bodies in the Nose, Ear and Throat

Children often put things into nose and ears, and a presentation with a foreign body in one orifice should lead the NP to check the other three. An undeclared foreign body may lie in the nose for weeks until the patient develops tell-tale symptoms, a purulent, runny nose, bad breath and alteration in the sound of the voice caused by nasal obstruction. Small beads, sweet corn, beans, pebbles and leaves are among the possibilities.

Removal of a foreign body from a child's nose or ear is a touchy business. Cooperation is difficult to obtain for work on such a delicate area. Any mishandling may make the situation worse. It can be difficult to get a child to blow the nose to dislodge the object. Children will tend to inhale, with the possibility of achieving the reverse of the desired result. There is also a small risk that a nasal foreign body will travel into the airway. Refer such patients to a doctor, in line with local policy.

Removal of a cotton wool ball from an adult's ear can usually be achieved by using crocodile forceps. Be careful to avoid pushing the ball further into the ear.

The patient who feels that there is a fish or chicken bone stuck in the throat will require examination by a doctor. Perforation of the oesophagus by a foreign body is a serious risk, and the sensation of a foreign body may indicate a stricture or other medical problem.

Teeth that have been Avulsed

In descending order, the best options for a patient who has suffered a traumatic avulsion of an adult tooth and has the tooth are:

- it can be cleaned with saline
- preserve the tooth by replanting it in the socket and biting down lightly on it
- tuck it between the gum and cheek, so that it is bathed in saliva
- put it in milk.

The patient needs a dentist at once.

References

Adams J, Yates D 1995 Foreword. ABC of emergency radiology (authors Nicholson & Driscoll) BMJ Publishing Group, London, p viii

Alexander M, Fawcett J, Runciman P 2000 Nursing practice – the adult-hospital and home, 2nd edn. Churchill Livingstone, Edinburgh

Apley A G, Solomon L 1997 Physical examination in orthopaedics. Butterworth–Heinemann, Oxford

Beattie T F, Hendry G M, Duguid K P 1997 Pediatric Emergencies. Mosby–Wolfe, London

Burn L 2000 Back and neck pain the facts. Oxford University Press, Oxford

Chartered Society of Physiotherapy 1998 Guidelines for the management of soft tissue injury with protection, rest, ice, compression and elevation during the first 72 hours. Association of Chartered Physiotherapists in Sports Medicine, London

Clinical Standards Advisory Group Committee 1994 Back pain. HMSO, London

Corrigan B, Maitland G D 1998 Vertebral musculoskeletal disorders. Butterworth–Heinemann, Oxford

Crown J 1989 Report of the advisory group on nurse prescribing DoH, London

Currie D G 1993 The management of head injuries. Oxford University Press, Oxford

Cyriax J H, Cyriax P J 1993 Cyriax's illustrated manual of orthopaedic medicine, 2nd edition. Butterworth–Heinemann, Oxford

Dandy D J, Edwards D J 1998 Essential orthopaedics and trauma, 3rd edn. Churchill Livingstone, Edinburgh

Dean C, Pegington J 1996 Core anatomy for students, vol 1. WB Saunders, London

DHSS 1986 Neighbourhood nursing – a focus for care. HMSO, London (The Cumberlege Report)

DoH 1996 Immunisation against infectious disease. The Stationery Office, London

DoH 1997 Guidelines on post-exposure prophylaxis for health care workers occupationally exposed to HIV. DoH, London

DoH review of prescribing, supply and adminstration of medicines 1998 A report on the supply and administration of medicines (Crown report). DoH, London

DoH review of prescibing supply and administration of medicines 1999 Final report (Crown report). DoH, London

Ellis H 1983 Clinical anatomy 7th edn. Blackwell, Oxford

Fuller G 1993 Neurological examination made easy. Churchill Livingstone, Edinburgh Glasgow J F T, Graham H K 1997 Management of injuries in children. BMJ Publishing Group, London

Glasgow JFT, Graham HK 1997 Management of injuries in children BMJ, London

Hawkesford J, Banks J G 1994 Maxillofacial and dental emergencies. Oxford University Press, Oxford

Hogg C 1997 Emergency health services for children and young people. Action for Sick Children, London

Hollinshead W H 1982 Anatomy for surgeons, 3rd edn. Harper Row, Philadelphia, PA

Manchester Triage Group 1997 Emergency triage. BMJ Publishing Group, London

Marieb E 1995 Human anatomy and physiology, 3rd edition. Benjamin–Cummings Publishing Co Inc, California

McRae R 1994 Practical fracture treatment, 3rd edition, Churchill Livingstone, Edinburgh

Meadows J T S 1999 Orthopedic differential diagnosis in physical therapy. McGraw Hill, New York

Morton R J, Phillips B M 1996 Accidents and emergencies in children 2nd edition. Oxford University Press, Oxford

Munro J, Campbell C R W 1995 MacLeod's clinical examination, 9th edn Churchill Livingstone, Edinburgh

Parr J 1989 Introduction to ophthalmology, 3rd edn. Oxford University Press, Oxford

Raby N, Berman L, de Lacey G 1995 Accident and emergency radiology. Saunders, London

Rogers A W 1992 Textbook of anatomy. Churchill Livingstone, Edinburgh

Royal College of General Practitioners 1996 Clinical guidelines for the management of acute low back pain. Royal College of General Practitioners, London

Royal College of Radiologists 1998 Making the best use of a department of clinical radiology. Royal College of Radiologists, London

Rutishauser S 1994 Physiology and anatomy: a basis for nursing and health care. Churchill Livingstone, Edinburgh

Scottish Intercollegiate Guidelines Network 2000 Early management of patients with a head injury. SIGN, Edinburgh

Spitzer W O, Skovron M L, Salmi L R 1995 The Quebec Task Force on whiplash associated disorders. Spine 20–8S, 1S–73S

Stiell I G, Greenburgh G A, McKnight R D et al 1993 Decision rules for the use of radiography in ankle injuries. Journal of the American Medical Association 269: 1127–1131 (the 'Ottawa ankle rules')

Swann I J, Yates D W 1989 Management of minor head injuries. Chapman and Hall, London

Thibodeau G A, Patton K T 1999 Anthony's textbook of anatomy & physiology, 16th edn. Mosby, London

Trott A T 1997 Wounds and lacerations emergency care and closure, second edition. Mosby, St Louis

Walsh M 1999 Clinical nursing and related sciences, 5th edition. Baillière Tindall, London

Walton R L, Matory W E 1992 Wound care. In: CE Saunders, MTHo. Current emergency diagnosis and treatment, 4th edition. Appleton & Lange, Connecticut

Wardrope J, Edhouse J A 1999 The management of wounds and burns, second edition. Oxford University Press, Oxford

Wardrope J, English B 1998 Musculoskeletal problems in emergency medicine. Oxford University Press, Oxford

Waugh A, Grant A 2001 Ross and Wilson anatomy and physiology in health and illness, 9th edn. Churchill Livingstone, Edinburgh

Williams P L 1995 Gray's anatomy, 38th edn. Churchill Livingstone, Edinburgh

Wilson G R, Nee P A, Watson J S 1997 Emergency management of hand injuries. Oxford University Press, Oxford

Wrightson P, Gronwall D 1999 Mild head injury. Oxford University Press, Oxford

Bibliography

The main works which have not been directly referred to in the text, but which have contibuted to it, are listed below

Agur A M R 1991 Grant's atlas of anatomy, ninth edition. Williams and Wilkins, Baltimore

American Society for Surgery of the Hand 1990 The hand, examination and diagnosis, third edition. Churchill Livingstone, Edinburgh

American Society for Surgery of the Hand 1990 The hand, primary care of common problems, second edition. Churchill Livinstone, Edinburgh

Anderson M K, Hall S J 1995 Sports injury management. Williams and Wilkins, Baltimore

Apley A G, Solomon L 1993 Apley's system of orthopaedics and fractures, seventh edition. Butterworth–Heinemann, Oxford

Buttaravoli P, Stair T 2000 Minor emergencies: splinters to fractures. Mosby, St Louis

Cooke M, Jones E, Kelly C 1998 Minor injuries unit handbook. Butterworth–Heinemann, Oxford

Cyriax J 1982 Textbook of orthopaedic medicine, vol 1, 8th edn. Baillière Tindall, London

Cyriax J 1984 Textbook of orthopaedic medicine, vol 2, 11th edn, Baillière Tindall, London

Fitzgerald M J T 1992 Neeuroanatomy basic and clinical, second edition. Balliere Tindall, London

Gross J, Fetto J, Rosen E 1996 Musculoskeletal examination. Blackwell Science, Massachusetts

Guly H R 1996 History taking, examination, and record keeping in emergency medicine. Oxford University Press, Oxford

Hislop H J, Montgomery J 1995 Daniels and Worthingham's muscle testing, 6th edn. WB Saunders Company, Philadelphia

Kendall F P, McCreary E K, Provance P G 1993 Muscles testing and function, 4th edn. Williams and Wilkins, Baltimore

Khaw P T, Elkington A R 1994 ABC of eyes, 2nd edn. BMJ Publishing Group, London

Kisner C, Colby L A 1996 Therapeutic exercise, foundations and techniques, 3rd edn. F. A. Davis Company, Philadelphia

Loudon J, Bell S, Johnston J 1998 The clinical orthopedic assessment guide. Human Kinetics, Champaign Illinois

Macnicol M F 1995 The probleem knee. Butterworth–Heinemann, Oxford

Martin D S, Collins E D 1998 Manual of acute hand injuries. Mosby, St Louis

McRae R 1990 Clinical orthopaedic examination, 3rd edn. Churchill Livingstone, Edinburgh

Nicholson D A, Driscoll P A 1995 ABC of emergency radiology. BMJ Publishing Group, London

Palastanga N, Field D, Soames R 1998 Anatomy & human movement structure & function. Butterworth–Heinemann, Oxford

Peterson L, Renstrom P 1986 Sports injuries their prevention and treatment. Martin Dunitz, London

Petty N J, Moore A P 1998 Neuromusculoskeletal examination and assessment. Churchill Livingstone, Edinburgh

Tubiana R, Thomine J-M, Mackin E 1996 Examination of the hand and wrist. Martin Dunitz, London

Index

Note: References to figures are indicated by 'f' and references to tables are indicated by 't' when they fall on a page not covered by the text reference.

T